Atlas of
INFECTIOUS DISEASES

Volume I

AIDS

Atlas of
INFECTIOUS DISEASES

Volume I
AIDS

Editor-in-Chief
Gerald L. Mandell, MD

Chief, Division of Infectious Diseases
University of Virginia Health Sciences Center
Charlottesville, Virginia

Editor
Donna Mildvan, MD

Division of Infectious Diseases
Beth Israel Medical Center
New York, New York

DEVELOPED BY CURRENT MEDICINE INC.

PHILADELPHIA

CURRENT MEDICINE
20 NORTH THIRD STREET
PHILADELPHIA, PA 19106

Library of Congress Cataloging-in-Publication Data

AIDS/volume editor, Donna Mildvan.
      p.   cm.–(Atlas of infectious diseases; v. 1)
  Includes bibliographical references and index.
  ISBN 1-878132-50-4 (hardcover)
  1. AIDS (Disease)–Atlases. I. Mildvan, Donna. II. Series.
  [DNLM: 1. Acquired Immunodeficiency Syndrome–diagnosis–atlases.
2. Diagnosis, Differential–atlases. WD 308 A28733 1994]
RC607.A26A34413 1994
616.97'92–dc20
DNLM/DLC
for Library of Congress

94-28724
CIP

Development Editor:	Lee Tevebaugh
Art Director:	Paul Fennessy
Designer:	Patrick Whelan
Illustration Director:	Larry Ward
Illustrators:	Larry Ward, Ann Saydlowski, Lisa Weischedel
Production Manager:	David Myers
Typesetting Director:	Colleen Ward

Printed in Hong Kong by Paramount Printing Group Limited.

10 9 8 7 6 5 4 3 2 1

PREFACE

The diagnosis and management of patients with infectious diseases are based in large part on visual clues. Skin and mucous membrane lesions, eye findings, imaging studies, gram stains, culture plates, insect vectors, and preparations of blood, urine, pus, cerebrospinal fluid, and biopsy specimens are studied to establish the proper diagnosis and to choose the most effective therapy. *The Atlas of Infectious Diseases* will be a modern, complete collection of these images. Current Medicine, with its capability of superb color reproduction and its state-of-the-art computer imaging facilities, is the ideal publisher for the atlas. Infectious diseases physicians, scientists, microbiologists, and pathologists frequently teach other health-care professionals, and this comprehensive atlas with available slide atlas is an effective teaching tool.

Dr. Donna Mildvan planned, organized, and edited this superb volume on AIDS. She assembled a team that is expert in various aspects of this amazingly complex disease. We are continually reminded that manifestations of disease in patients with HIV infection may be unique or atypical, and this volume is a vivid indication of this phenomenon.

Gerald L. Mandell, MD

Chief, Division of Infectious Diseases
University of Virginia Health Sciences Center
Charlottesville, Virginia

CONTRIBUTORS

Edward J. Bottone, PhD
Director of Consultative Microbiology
Division of Infectious Diseases
The Mount Sinai Hospital
Professor of Medicine, Microbiology, and Pathology
Mount Sinai School of Medicine
New York, New York

Mary Ann Chiasson, PhD
Assistant Commissioner
Disease Intervention Research
The New York City Department of Health
New York, New York

David A. Cooper, DSc, MD
HIV Medicine Unit
St. Vincent's Hospital
National Centre in HIV Epidemiology and
Clinical Research
Syndney, Australia
University of New South Wales
Kensington, Australia

Janet L. Davis, MD
Assistant Professor
Bascom Palmer Eye Institute
University of Miami School of Medicine
Miami, Florida

Gregory J. Dore, MBBS, BSc
HIV Medicine Unit
St. Vincent's Hospital
Sydney, Australia

D. Peter Drotman, MD
Assistant Director for Public Health
Division of HIV/AIDS
National Center for Infectious Diseases
Centers for Disease Control and Prevention
Atlanta, Georgia

W. Christopher Ehmann, MD
Assistant Professor
Department of Medicine
Division of Hematology
The Pennsylvania State University College of Medicine
Hershey, Pennsylvania

M. Elaine Eyster, MD
Distinguished Professor
Department of Medicine
Division of Hematology
The Pennsylvania State University College of Medicine
Hershey, Pennsylvania

Judith Feinberg, MD
Assistant Professor of Medicine
Division of Infectious Diseases
The Johns Hopkins School of Medicine
Baltimore, Maryland

Margaret A. Fischl, MD
Professor of Medicine
Director, Comprehensive AIDS Program
University of Miami School of Medicine
Miami, Florida

Alvin E. Friedman-Kien, MD
Professor of Dermatology and Microbiology
New York University Medical Center
New York, New York

Christopher D. Gocke, MD
Department of Pathology
The Pennsylvania State University College of Medicine
Hershey, Pennsylvania

Deborah Greenspan, BDS, DSc, ScD(hc)
Clinical Professor of Oral Medicine
Department of Stomatology
Clinical Director, Oral AIDS Center
School of Dentistry
University of California San Francisco
San Francisco, California

John S. Greenspan, BSc, BDS, PhD, FRCPath, ScD(hc)
Professor of Oral Biology and Oral Pathology
Chair, Department of Stomatology
Director, Oral AIDS Center
School of Dentistry
Professor of Pathology
Director, AIDS Clinical Research Center
School of Medicine
University of California San Francisco
San Francisco, California

Carl Grunfeld, MD, PhD
Department of Medicine
University of California San Francisco
Metabolism and Infectious Diseases Sections
Medical Service
Department of Veterans Affairs Medical Center
San Francisco, California

Peter Jensen, MD
Department of Medicine
University of California San Francisco
Metabolism and Infectious Diseases Sections
Medical Service
Department of Veterans Affairs Medical Center
San Francisco, California

Harold A. Kessler, MD, FACP
Professor of Medicine and Immunology/Microbiology
Associate Director, Section of Infectious Disease
Rush Presbyterian-St. Luke's Medical Center
Chicago, Illinois

Susan E. Krown, MD
Member and Attending Physician
Memorial Sloan-Kettering Cancer Center
New York, New York

G. Diego Miralles, MD
Division of Infectious Disease and International Health
Duke University Medical Center
Durham, North Carolina

Susan Morgello, MD
Department of Pathology
The Mount Sinai Medical Center
New York, New York

Alan G. Palestine, MD
Clinical Associate Professor of Ophthalmology
Georgetown University
Washington, DC

Josephine Paredes, MD
Memorial Sloan-Kettering Cancer Center
New York, New York

Mark J. Rosen, MD
Division of Pulmonary and Critical Care Medicine
Beth Israel Medical Center
New York, New York

Michael S. Saag, MD
Associate Professor of Medicine
Director, AIDS Outpatient Clinic
Associate Director for Clinical Care and Therapeutics,
* AIDS Center*
The University of Alabama at Birmingham
Birmingham, Alabama

David M. Simpson, MD
Department of Neurology
Director, Neuro-AIDS Research Center and Clinical
* Neurophysiology Laboratories*
The Mount Sinai Medical Center
New York, New York

Michele Tagliati, MD
Department of Neurology
The Mount Sinai Medical Center
New York, New York

Hedy Teppler, MD
Assistant Professor of Medicine
Division of Infectious Diseases
Jefferson Medical College
Philadelphia, Pennsylvania

Sten H. Vermund, MD, PhD
Chief, Vaccine Trials and Epidemiology Branch
Clinical Research Program
Division of AIDS
National Institute of Allergy and Infectious Diseases
National Institutes of Health
Bethesda, Maryland

Christine A. Wanke, MD
Assistant Professor of Medicine
Division of Infectious Diseases
Harvard Medical School
New England Deaconess Hospital
Boston, Massachusetts

Kent J. Weinhold, PhD
Department of Surgery
Duke University Medical Center
Durham, North Carolina

Thomas C. Wright, MD
Assistant Professor of Pathology
Department of OB and GYN
College of Physicians and Surgeons of Columbia University
New York, New York

Ram Yogev, MD
Professor of Pediatrics
Northwestern University Medical School
Director, Section of Pediatric and Maternal HIV Infection
The Children's Memorial Hospital
Chicago, Illinois

CONTENTS

CHAPTER 1

Epidemiology, Natural History, and Prevention

Sten H. Vermund
D. Peter Drotman

EPIDEMIOLOGY OF THE WORLD PANDEMIC

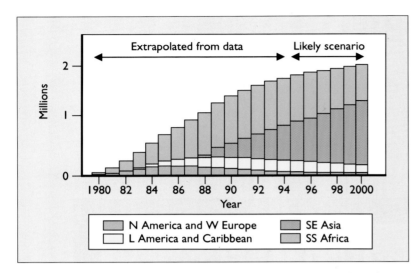

FIGURE 1-1 Annual HIV infection rates have been projected to the year 2000 by the World Health Organization based on conservative assumptions from HIV and AIDS reports and estimates. The epidemics in North America and Europe have stabilized, with the number of new infections and the number of deaths from AIDS coming into equilibrium. The epidemic in Latin America substantially exceeds that in North America. The epidemic in Asia began in the late 1980s but has been growing at least as rapidly as did the African epidemic 5 to 10 years earlier. New Asian cases may exceed 1 million/year by 2000. The African epidemic is of almost unimaginable magnitude; the projected decline in incident HIV cases in the late 1990s is a consequence of a saturation with HIV infection of at-risk persons rather than due to prevention successes; ie, the number of *new* HIV infections will be limited by a decreasing pool of susceptible persons. (World Health Organization: *The HIV/AIDS Pandemic: 1993 Overview.* Geneva: WHO; 1993, and Dr. James Chin, personal communication, 1994.)

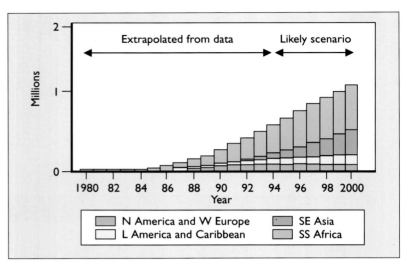

FIGURE 1-2 Annual AIDS case rates projected to the year 2000 by the World Health Organization based on conservative assumptions from HIV and AIDS reports and estimates. The number of AIDS patients worldwide will rise inexorably on all continents, reflecting the incident HIV infections from earlier years. The delay in time from the incident HIV infections to AIDS averages a decade for this long-latency virus. Few data are available to suggest that the time from HIV infection to AIDS differs in various parts of the world. (World Health Organization: *The HIV/AIDS Pandemic: 1993 Overview.* Geneva: WHO; 1993, and Dr. James Chin, personal communication, 1994.)

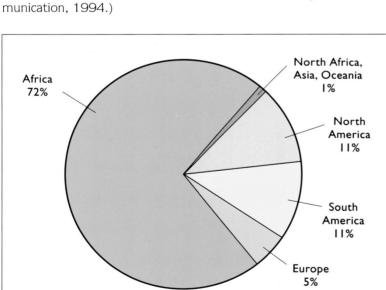

FIGURE 1-3 Global distribution of HIV-infected adults. As of 1991, 84% of global HIV infection cases were found in developing nations, whereas only 16% were in North America and Europe. The proportion of cases in the industrialized world will further decline over time, given the magnitude of the growing epidemic in Asia, Africa, and South America. (World Health Organization: *The HIV/AIDS Pandemic: 1993 Overview.* Geneva: WHO; 1993.)

AIDS incidence rates per 100 person-years by sex and age in Rakai District, Uganda

Age, *yrs*	Men (±95% CI)	Women (±95% CI)
13–16	0	0
17–19	0	8.0 (±3.8)
20–24	4.9 (±2.8)	6.4 (±2.8)
25–29	9.8 (±4.9)	1.4 (±1.4)
30+	2.2 (±1.0)	1.0 (0.7)
All ages	2.6 (±0.7)	2.7 (0.7)

FIGURE 1-4 The rural Rakai District in Uganda has been studied for rates of HIV seroincidence (expressed per 100 person-years of observation). These data illustrate the intense HIV transmission occurring in adolescents and young adults near the time they become sexually active. Because somewhat older men have sexual relations with younger women, the risk for young women begins earlier than for young men. (Wawer MJ, *et al.*: HIV incidence in rural Rakai District, Uganda. *BMJ* 1994, in press; with permission. Wawer MJ, *et al.*: Dynamics of spread of HIV-1 infection in a rural district of Uganda. *BMJ* 1991, 303:1303–1306.)

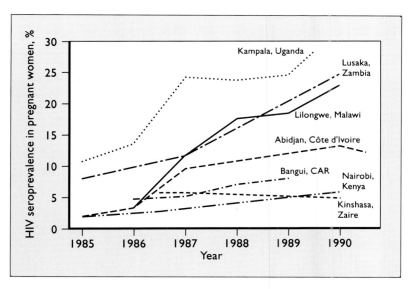

FIGURE 1-5 Recent survey data on women delivering infants in various parts of Africa suggest more than 30% of this general population is now infected with HIV in certain regions. The implications for the future health of these women, the probable HIV status of their sexual partners, the risk for HIV infection to their newborn infants, and the risk of orphaning surviving children are all exceedingly worrisome. (*Adapted from* Mann J, *et al.*, eds: *AIDS in the World*. Cambridge: Harvard University Press; 1992; with permission.)

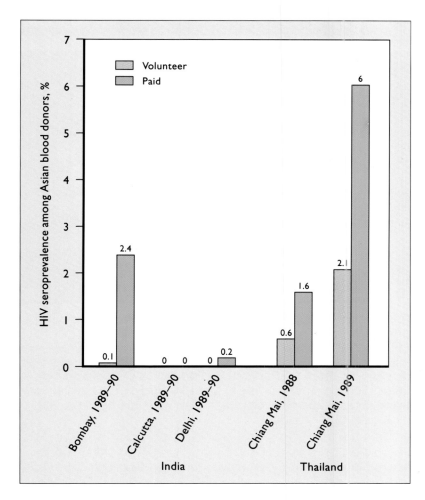

FIGURE 1-6 The rising incidence of HIV infection in Asia. Although the Asian AIDS epidemic started later than that seen elsewhere in the world, even as early as 1989 and 1990, data from blood donors in cities such as Bombay, India, and Chiang Mai, Thailand, suggested HIV-1 seroprevalence rates rivaling the highest general population rates seen in highest risk neighborhoods in the US, *ie*, over 2%. The current situation is even more dramatic, with very high seroincidence rates among persons at highest risk (*eg*, sex workers and injection drug users) as well as in persons reflecting the general population (*eg*, Thai soldiers). (*Adapted from* Mann J, *et al.*, eds: *AIDS in the World*. Cambridge: Harvard University Press; 1992; with permission. *Also see* Nelson KE, *et al.*: Risk factors for HIV infection among young adult men in northern Thailand. *JAMA* 1993, 270:955–960.)

EPIDEMIOLOGY OF THE EPIDEMIC IN THE UNITED STATES

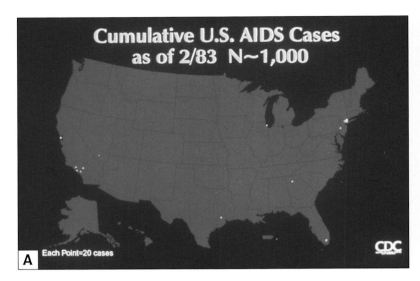
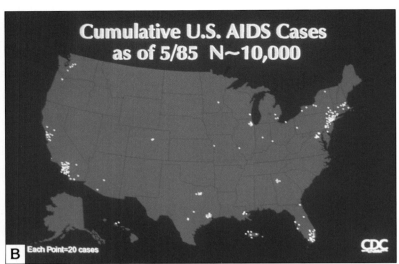
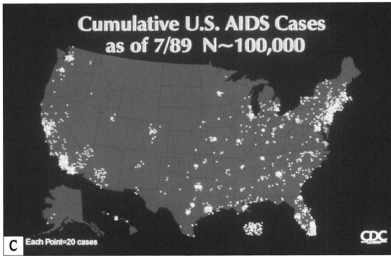

FIGURE 1-7 The expansion of AIDS in the United States, 1983 to present. Each map illustrates the approximate distribution of reported AIDS cases. Each dot represents 20 cases. (Centers for Disease Control and Prevention: US cases reported through December 1992. In *HIV/AIDS Surveillance Reports*. 1993, [Feb]:1–23.) **A**, The first 1000 AIDS cases, February 1983. Urban areas with cases included New York, San Francisco, Los Angeles, Philadelphia, Miami, Atlanta, Chicago, and Houston.

B, The first 10,000 AIDS cases, May 1985. Urban areas with cases now include over 30 metropolitan areas. **C**, The first 100,000 AIDS cases, July 1989. Urban areas with cases are now too numerous to count easily, and many smaller towns are now represented. **D**, The first 330,000 AIDS cases, August 1993. The magnitude of the epidemic is noted in the density of white dots, which now coalesce in many urban areas to reveal thousands of local cases.

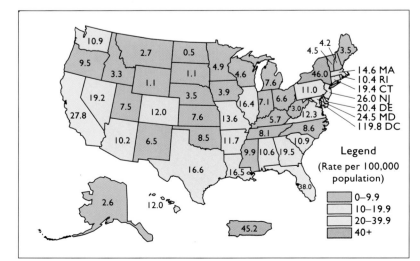

FIGURE 1-8 The states and territories in the United States with the highest AIDS rates in 1992. They included the District of Columbia, New York, and Puerto Rico, with over 40 cases/100,000 population reported. States with 20–40 cases/100,000 included Florida, California, New Jersey, Maryland, and Delaware, whereas Connecticut, Georgia, and Nevada nearly reach this case threefold.

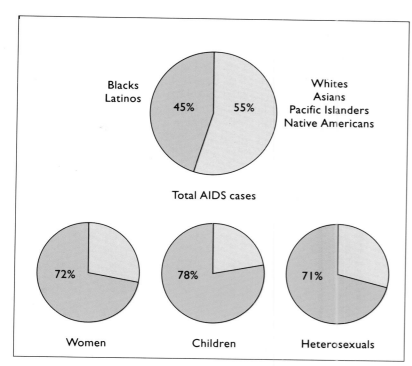

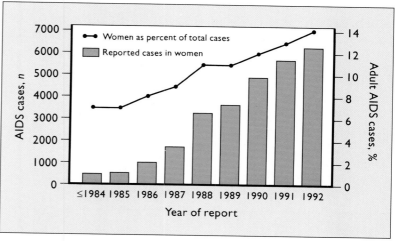

FIGURE 1-10 Women with AIDS. As the number of women with AIDS rises in the United States, so does the proportion of women in the total number of AIDS cases. Although under 8% of the reported cases prior to 1985 were women, over 14% of reported cases since 1992 have been among women.

FIGURE 1-9 Minority composition of AIDS cases. Through 1992, 45% of all AIDS cases reported to the CDC were among persons of African-American and Hispanic/Latino background, more than double what would be expected from their proportion in the US population. These minority groups represent about three quarters of the women and children reported with AIDS. Since 1992, 52% of all new AIDS reports have been among these minority racial and ethnic groups.

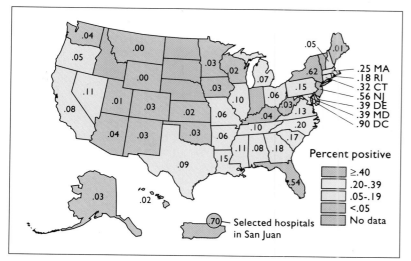

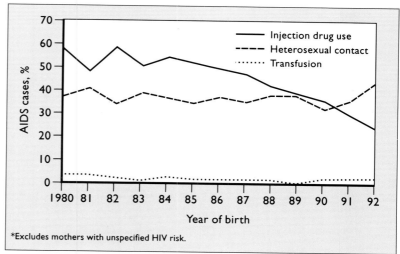

FIGURE 1-11 HIV seroprevalence rates among child-bearing women in the United States, as estimated from newborn infant surveillance statistics. Seroprevalence rates exceeding 4/1000 women were noted in 1991 in the District of Columbia, New York, New Jersey, Florida, and Puerto Rico. Cases from injection drug use and cases among women are closely associated, because over 70% of HIV infections are attributable to injection drug use by the woman or her sexual partner.

FIGURE 1-12 Maternal risk factors and pediatric AIDS. Since 1991, mothers of babies with perinatally acquired AIDS are more likely to have acquired their infections from heterosexual exposure than from injection drug use, reflecting the substantial increase in heterosexually acquired infection in recent years. Transfusion-related AIDS cases are still reported from HIV infections occurring prior to 1985, but new HIV infections from transfusion have been reduced to near-zero since the start of blood and blood-product HIV screening in 1985.

AIDS cases reported in children (< 13 yrs of age) in the United States

Transmission category	Year of report			
	1982–1991		1992	
	Cases, n	Cases, %	Cases, n	Cases, %
Perinatally acquired	3665	86	697	90
Transfusion associated	306	7	19	2
Hemophilia	188	4	21	3
Other/under investigation	90	2	34	4
Total	4249	100	771	100

FIGURE 1-13 Causes of AIDS in pediatric patients. Currently, over 90% of pediatric (< 13 years of age) AIDS cases reported in the United States are attributed to transplacental or intrapartum perinatal transmission. Transfusion-related AIDS cases are still reported from HIV infections occurring prior to 1985, but new HIV infections from transfusion have been reduced to near-zero since the advent of blood and blood-product HIV screening in 1985.

Adolescent sexual behavior

	Men*	Women†
Age of first heterosexual intercourse	50% by age 16	32% by age 16
	86% by age 19	75% by age 19
Mean number of lifetime sex partners	5.1	3.3
Condom use at last sexual intercourse	57%	32%

*National survey of adolescent men 15–19 year olds, 1988.
†National survey of family growth 15–19 year olds, 1988.

FIGURE 1-14 A majority of adolescents aged 15–19 years report high-risk sexual behaviors, including failure to use condoms, early onset of sexual activity, and multiple sexual partners. As the epidemic expands, adolescents who have acquired HIV are being recognized with increasing frequency, particularly in areas of highest background HIV seroprevalence. (*National Survey of Adolescent Men, 15–19 Year Olds, 1988*, and the *National Survey of Family Growth, 15–19 Year Olds, 1988*. Washington, DC: National Center for Health Statistics, Centers for Disease Control and Prevention; 1989.)

HIV-1 seroprevalence among adolescents ≤ 19 years of age

Clinical setting	Clinics, n	Patients tested, n	HIV-1 seroprevalence	
			Median, %	Range, %
STD clinics	111	99,667	0.30	0.00–4.05
Women's health clinics	146	91,614	0.08	0.00–1.61
Correctional facilities	29	13,054	0.22	0.00–4.23
Adolescent clinics	19	9844	0.16	0.00–1.04
Homeless youth	5	4185	1.20	0.00–4.43

FIGURE 1-15 HIV-1 seroprevalence was tested among adolescents < 20 years of age from 210 clinical sites from 1988–1992. Homeless youth from five sites had a median 1.2% seroprevalence with a range from 0 to 4.4%. Sexually transmitted disease (STD) clinic and correctional facility youth also had rates over 4% at some sites. Three rates strongly suggest the need for preventive programs targeting adolescents at risk. (Centers for Disease Control and Prevention: National HIV Serosurveillance Summary: Results through 1992. 1992, 3:1–38.)

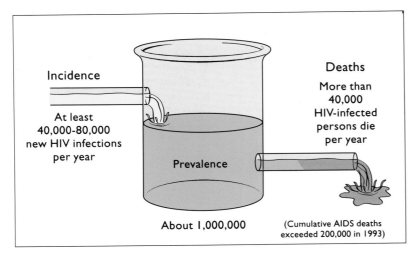

Incidence

At least 40,000–80,000 new HIV infections per year

Prevalence

Deaths

More than 40,000 HIV-infected persons die per year

About 1,000,000

(Cumulative AIDS deaths exceeded 200,000 in 1993)

FIGURE 1-16 The US AIDS epidemic has been fairly stable for several years since the number of HIV-related deaths has approximated the number of new HIV infections (> 40,000/year). Thus, the prevalence of HIV is about stable at somewhat below 1 million infected Americans. (Centers for Disease Control: HIV prevalence estimates and AIDS case projections for the United States: Report based upon a workshop. *MMWR* 1990, 39[RR-16]:1–31. For a nontechnical review of these estimates, *see* Vermund SH: Changing estimates of HIV-1 seroprevalence in the United States. *J NIH Res* 1991, 3[Jul]:77–81.)

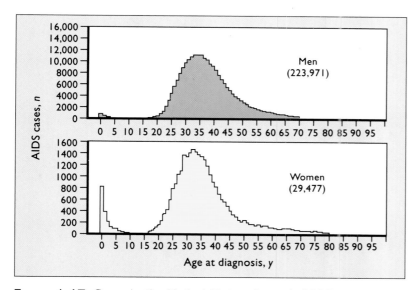

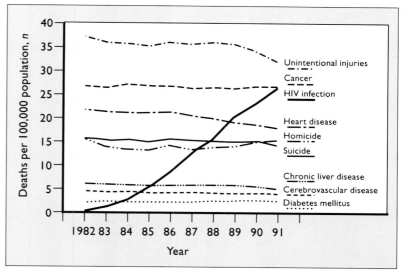

FIGURE 1-17 Cases in the United States through 1992 reported by age and gender demonstrate that AIDS is primarily a disease of young and middle-aged adults. (For an update on death rates among young Americans, *see* Selik RM, *et al.*: HIV infection as leading cause of death among young adults in US cities and states. *JAMA* 1993, 263:2991–2994.)

FIGURE 1-18 As of 1991, AIDS rivals cancer as the second leading cause of death among Americans aged 25–44 years. In 1994, AIDS is likely to become the leading cause of death in this age group in the US. By 1992, AIDS was already the leading cause of death among men. (*From* Vermund SH: Rising HIV-mortality in young Americans. *JAMA* 1993, 269:3034–3035; with permission.)

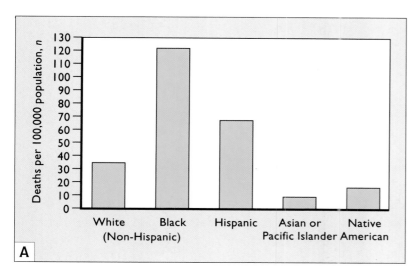

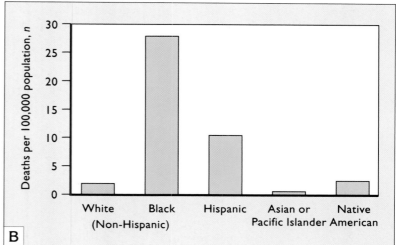

FIGURE 1-19 **A** and **B**, Death rate attributable to HIV infection among US men (*panel 19A*) and women (*panel 19B*) aged 15–44 years in 1991. The impact of the epidemic on men and women of minority ethnic and racial origin is notable, particularly among US-

born African-Americans and Hispanic/Latino men, especially of Puerto Rican background. (National Center for Health Statistics: Advance report of final monthly statistics, 1991. *Mon Vital Stat Rep (Suppl)* 1993, 42[2].)

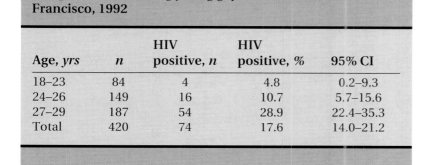

HIV prevalence among young gay and bisexual men in San Francisco, 1992

Age, yrs	n	HIV positive, n	HIV positive, %	95% CI
18–23	84	4	4.8	0.2–9.3
24–26	149	16	10.7	5.7–15.6
27–29	187	54	28.9	22.4–35.3
Total	420	74	17.6	14.0–21.2

FIGURE 1-20 In a population-based survey in the areas of San Francisco where many gay and bisexual men live, high HIV prevalence was noted among young men. In the first 420 men studied, about 5% of 18–23 year olds, 11% of 24–26 year olds, and 29% of 27–29 year olds tested HIV seropositive. This suggests continued high transmission among young gay men sampled from this general urban population. Seroincidence rates may be close to half those noted in the 1979–1984 period in this part of San Francisco, perhaps reflecting a partial impact of safer sex messages. (*From* Osmond DH, *et al.*: Human immunodeficiency virus infection in homosexual/bisexual men, ages 18-29: The San Francisco Young Men's Health Study. *J Acquir Immune Defic Syndr* 1994, in press.)

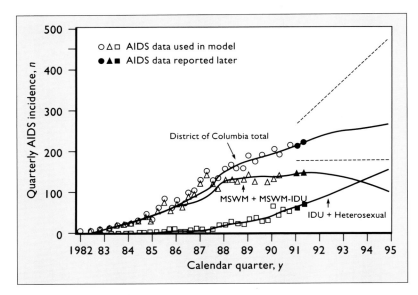

FIGURE 1-21 A projection of the AIDS epidemic in Washington, DC, suggests that by the mid-1990s, more drug users and heterosexuals will develop AIDS than gay men. This pattern is typical of one being seen in many urban areas in the United States, in that HIV prevention messages have had impact among communities of gay and bisexual men, whereas drug users and inner-city heterosexuals continue to have increasing risk for HIV. Also worth noting in Washington, DC, is that about half the gay men developing AIDS are from African-American backgrounds, suggesting that the epidemic, even among gay men, is hitting minority communities especially hard. (*From* Rosenberg PS, *et al.*: Population-based monitoring of an urban HIV/AIDS epidemic: Magnitude and trends in the District of Columbia. *JAMA* 1992, 268:495–503; with permission.)

1993 AIDS SURVEILLANCE CASE DEFINITION

A. 1993 Expanded CDC surveillance case definition for AIDS	**B. 1993 Expanded CDC surveillance case definition for AIDS**
Category A	**Category B**
One or more of the following conditions in an adolescent or adult ($\geq$ 13 years of age):	Symptomatic conditions in an HIV-infected adolescent or adult that are not included in clinical category C and
Asymptomatic HIV infection	Are attributed to HIV infection or a defect in cell-mediated immunity, or
Persistent generalized lymphadenopathy	Have a clinical course or require management complicated by HIV infection
Acute (primary) HIV infection with accompanying illness or history of acute HIV infection	Bacilliary angiomatosis
	Oropharyngeal candidiasis (thrush)
	Vulvovaginal candidiasis (persistent, frequent, and poorly responsive)
	Cervical dysplasia; cervical carcinoma *in situ*
	Consitutional symptoms lasting > 1 month
	Hairy leukoplakia, oral
	Herpes zoster (shingles) in 2 episodes or > 1 dermatome
	Idiopathic thrombocytopenic purpura
	Listeriosis
	Pelvic inflammatory disease
	Peripheral neuropathy

FIGURE 1-22 A, B, and **C**, 1993 CDC surveillance case definition for AIDS comprises three categories, A–C, of increasing severity. **D**, In 1993, the case definition was revised to add three new clinical conditions to the 1987 definition: pulmonary tuberculosis, recurrent pneumonias, and invasive cervical cancer. All persons with a single CD4+ T-cell count < 200 cells/mm³ or a CD4+ T-cell proportion of total lymphocytes < 14% are now included in the AIDS case definition. (*From* Centers for Disease Control and Prevention: 1993 revised classification system for HIV infection and expanded surveillance case definition for AIDS among adolescents and adults. *MMWR* 1992, 41[RR-17]:1–19.) *(continued)*

C. 1993 Expanded CDC surveillance case definition for AIDS

Category C

AIDS indicator conditions
Candidiasis of bronchi, trachea, or lungs
Esophageal candidiasis
Cervical cancer, invasive
Coccidioidomycosis, disseminated or extrapulmonary
Cryptococcosis, extrapulmonary
Cryptosporidiosis, chronic intestinal
Cytomegalovirus disease (other than liver, spleen, nodes)
Cytomegalovirus retinitis (with loss of vision)
HIV-related encephalopathy
Herpes simplex: chronic ulcer, bronchitis, pneumonitis, or
  esophagitis
Histoplasmosis, disseminated or extrapulmonary
Isosporiasis, chronic intestinal

Kaposi's sarcoma
Burkitt's lymphoma
Immunoblastic lymphoma
Primary brain lymphoma
Mycobacterium avium complex or *M. kansasii* infection, dissem-
  inated or extrapulmonary
M. tuberculosis, any site
Mycobacterium species, disseminated or extrapulmonary
Pneumocystis carinii pneumonia
Recurrent pneumonia
Progressive multifocal leukoencephalopathy
Salmonella septicemia, recurrent
Brain toxoplasmosis
Wasting syndrome due to HIV

FIGURE 1-22 *(continued)*

D. Conditions included in the 1993 AIDS surveillance case definition for adolescents or adults with documented HIV infection*

< 200 CD4$^+$ T-lymphocyte cells/μL (or < 14% CD4$^+$ T-lymphocyte cells of total lymphocytes)
Pulmonary tuberculosis
Recurrent pneumonia
Invasive cervical cancer

*In addition to all conditions in the 1987 case definition.

1993 Revised classification system for HIV infection and expanded AIDS surveillance case definition for adults and adolescents ≥ 13 years of age*

	Clinical categories		
CD4$^+$ T-cell categories	**(A)** Asymptomatic, acute (primary) HIV, or PGL	**(B)** Symptomatic, not (A) or (C) conditions	**(C)** AIDS-indicator conditions
(1) ≥ 500/μL	A1	B1	C1
(2) 200–499/μL	A2	B2	C2
(3) < 200/μL AIDS-indicator T-cell count	A3	B3	C3

*HIV-infected persons classified in A3, B3, or any C cell meet the 1993 AIDS surveillance case definition.

FIGURE 1-23 The 1993 revised AIDS surveillance case definition is a component of the overall HIV infection classification system. This classification system categorizes persons aged 13 and older on the basis of their clinical manifestations and their CD4% or CD4$^+$ T-lymphocyte counts. (*From* Centers for Disease Control and Prevention: 1993 revised classification system for HIV infection and expanded surveillance case definition for AIDS among adolescents and adults. *MMWR* 1992, 41[RR-17]:1–19.) (PGL—persistant generalized lymphadenopathy.)

COFACTORS FOR TRANSMISSION AND MARKERS OF CLINICAL PROGRESSION

Adolescent risk factors for HIV infection

Multiple sexual partners
Drug use, including cocaine
Resident of community with high incidence of HIV
Coexistent sexually transmitted diseases

FIGURE 1-24 Adolescents may be at especially high risk for HIV. Specific behaviors or risk factors include multiple sexual partners, drug use, high-risk activities in an area with prevalent HIV, and sexually transmitted diseases as cofactors for HIV transmission or acquisition. In addition, adolescent condom usage rates are low. Ectopia are common in the immature cervix, possibly increasing the exposure of friable tissue more easily infected by HIV and other sexually transmitted diseases. (Bowler S, *et al.*: HIV and AIDS among adolescents in the United States: Increasing risk in the 1990s. *J Adolesc* 1992, 15:345–371.)

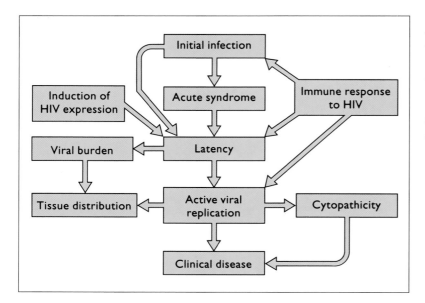

FIGURE 1-25 A model of HIV pathogenesis highlights the interaction of the HIV with host immune response, showing that many tissues are seeded with HIV, not merely circulating CD4+ T cells. Increased viral replication may be the consequence of immune activation or the nature of the viral type, or it may interact with host genetic factors influencing HLA–viral interactions, for example. (*From* Fauci AS: Multifactorial nature of human immunodeficiency virus disease: Implications for therapy. *Science* 1993, 262:1011–1018; with permission.)

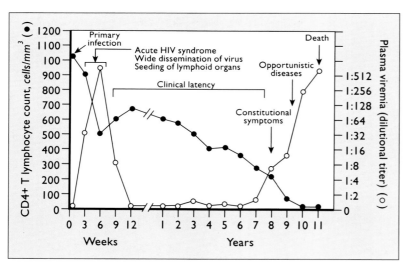

FIGURE 1-26 Typical course of HIV infection. Primary infection is a devastating immunologic event which typically results in the loss of 30% of circulating CD4+ T-cell volume (*solid circles*). As the host immune response is mounted, viremia (*open circles*) drops and some immunologic recovery is typical. However, many cells have been seeded by HIV, and typically, 60 CD4+ T cells/mm^3 are lost per year. AIDS may typically manifest about a decade after infection, though there is wide variation. As the immune system deteriorates, more or less unbridled viral replication may ensue. (*From* Pantaleo G, *et al.*: New concepts in the immunopathogenesis of human immunodeficiency virus infection. *N Engl J Med* 1993, 328:327–335; with permission.)

Cumulative incidence of *P. carinii* pneumonia among HIV-seropositive men, according to CD4⁺ cell count at base line*

Baseline count, n	Subjects, n	Patients with PCP, n	Cumulative patients with PCP, %[†]			
			6 mos	12 mos	24 mos	36 mos
≤ 200	77	19	8.4	18.4	25.3	33.3
201–350	217	47	0.5	4.0	15.0	22.9
351–500	389	39	0.0	1.4	5.7	9.0
501–700	483	43	0.0	0.4	3.2	8.3
≥ 700	499	20	0.0	0.0	1.3	3.8

*Participants receiving prophylactic medication were excluded from the analysis. PCP denotes *P. carinii* pneumonia.
[†]According to Kaplan-Maier estimates. $P < 0.001$ by the log-rank test for global differences.

FIGURE 1-27 The major cause of morbidity and mortality from HIV disease in industrialized countries has been *Pneumocystis carinii* pneumonia (PCP). A threshold of risk is noted at about 200 CD4⁺ T lymphocytes/mm³, which suggests that PCP prophylaxis be instituted when patients reach this count. In addition, regular CD4⁺ T-cell monitoring is advisable for persons who near this therapeutic threshold. (*From* Phair JP, *et al.*: The risk of *Pneumocystis carinii* pneumonia among men infected with human immunodeficiency virus type 1. *N Engl J Med* 1990, 322:161–165; with permission. *Also see* Centers for Disease Control [PHS Task Force]: Guidelines for prophylaxis against *Pneumocystis carinii* pneumonia for persons infected with human immunodeficiency virus. *MMWR* 1989, 38[S-5]:1–9; and Hirschel B, *et al.*: A controlled study of inhaled pentamidine for primary prevention of *Pneumocystis carinii* pneumonia. *N Engl J Med* 1991, 324:1079–1083.)

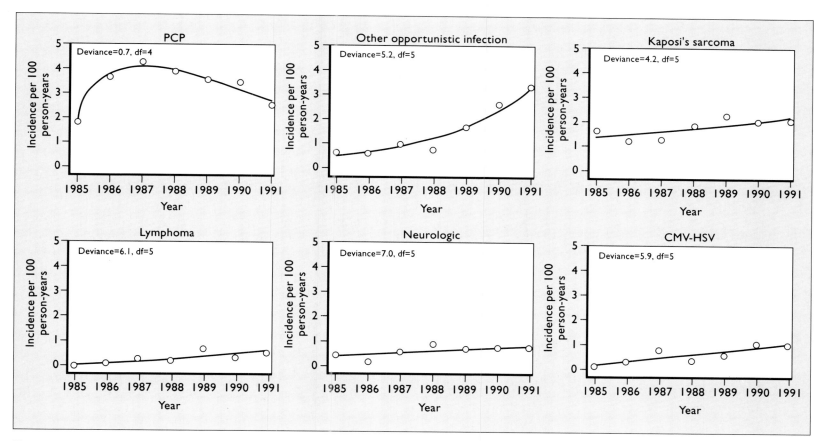

FIGURE 1-28 The Multicenter AIDS Cohort Study has followed about 5000 gay and bisexual men since 1984. Because most seropositive men acquired their disease prior to 1986, it would be expected that all AIDS-related conditions would increase in frequency over time. Although this is true for most opportunistic infections and malignancies, a dramatic downward trend in incidence has been seen for *P. carinii* pneumonia. This result can be attributed to the use of prophylactic antiviral and PCP prophylaxis. (*From* Muñoz A, *et al.*: Trends and explanatory factors for the incidence of initial AIDS-defining outcomes in the Multicenter AIDS Cohort Study: 1984-1991. *Am J Epidemiol* 1993, 137:423–438; with permission.)

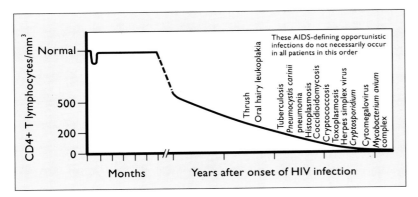

FIGURE 1-29 The appearance of opportunistic infections in relation to CD4+ T-cell count. Several opportunistic infections characteristically appear earlier in the course of HIV-related immune suppression, including oral candidiasis, oral hairy leukoplakia, and pulmonary tuberculosis. Conditions that occur typically when the CD4+ T cell count has fallen below 200/mm³ include *P. carinii* pneumonia and various fungal and parasitic conditions. Conditions seen most often in the profoundly immunosuppressed (CD4+ T-cell counts < 50/mm³) include cytomegalovirus and *Mycobacterium avium* complex. Opportunistic malignancies might be expected to become more common as persons live longer in immunosuppressed conditions, including non-Hodgkin's lymphomas, cervical and anal cancer, and other tumors that may grow in the absence of an intact immunologic surveillance system. Kaposi's sarcoma can appear when a patient is profoundly immunosuppressed but also can be seen much earlier in the course of HIV disease, even when CD4+ T-cell counts are > 500/mm³.

Association of SIL (PAP smear) with HPV, stratified by HIV immune status

| | Patients with SIL, *n*(%)* | | |
	HIV+ CD4 < 20%	HIV+ CD4 > 20%	HIV–
HPV–	1/16 (6%)	0/29 (0%)	8/113(7%)
HPV+	12/21 (57%)	8/19 (42%)	6/26 (23%)
Or (95% CI)†	20 (2.2–180)	43.6(2.3–820)‡	3.9 (1.2–13)
P value	< 0.01	< 0.001	0.025

*224 with CD4+ cell measurements within 6 mos.
†Odds ratios (95% CI) for the association between SIL and HPV.
‡0.5 added to each cell.

FIGURE 1-30 The association of human papillomavirus (HPV) and cervical squamous intraepithelial lesions (SIL) stratified by HIV immune status. When HIV-related immunosuppression is present, a synergism is evident, increasing the magnitude of the HPV–SIL association. This result suggests that women who live longer in an immunosuppressed state may be at higher risk of cervical cancer and should be the target of Papanicolaou smear screening efforts. (*From* Klein RD, *et al.*: Squamous intraepithelial lesions and genital human papillomavirus infection in women with HIV infection. *J Infect Dis* 1994, in press. *See also* Vermund SH, *et al.*: High risk of human papillomavirus infection and cervical squamous intraepithelial lesions among women with symptomatic human immunodeficiency virus infection. *Am J Obstet Gynecol* 1991, 165:392–400.)

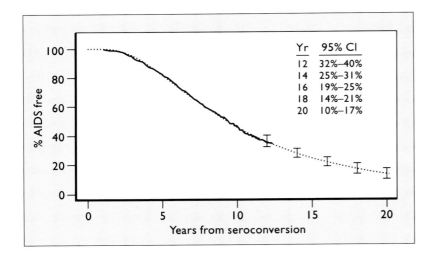

FIGURE 1-31 A median time from HIV infection to development of AIDS of 7–11 years has been estimated by various cohorts. In the Multicenter AIDS Cohort Study, a 9-year median has been noted among more than 400 seroconverters. Using a log-normal model, a projected 10% to 17% of men with HIV will remain AIDS-free 20 years after seroconversion. AIDS is rare in the first 3 years after seroconversion. (Kirby AJ, *et al.*: Long term survivors with HIV-1 infection: Incubation period and longitudinal patterns of CD4+ lymphocytes. Submitted.)

PREVENTION OF HIV INFECTION

PREVENTION OF HIV INFECTION

A. Interventions for HIV prevention

Sexual transmission

Reduce sexually transmitted diseases
Create and/or improve barriers
Treat HIV-infected persons with antiviral medication
Improve behavioral interventions

B. Interventions for HIV prevention

Perinatal transmission

Identify HIV-positive pregnant women and offer prenatal care
  and antiviral therapy
Provide noninvasive prenatal and intrapartum care to reduce
  blood exposures
Provide sexually transmitted disease diagnosis and treatment
Minimize time of delivery after membrane rupture
Do cesarean section, when indicated

C. Interventions for HIV prevention

Parenteral transmission

Medical exposure
  Provide clean blood supply
  Prevent nosocomial and iatrogenic spread
Injection drug use
  Expand drug prevention and treatment programs
  Provide needle exchange programs, including "clean works"
    education
  Minimize sexual transmission

FIGURE 1-32 HIV prevention strategies. It is widely accepted that more could be done with existing prevention modalities to control HIV. In addition, many important research projects can be performed to assess whether novel control strategies are efficacious. **A.** Regarding sexual transmission, it is not known to what extent different sexually transmitted disease control strategies might work to prevent HIV transmission. Although male condoms are important to prevent HIV, many female-controlled methods remain untested, such as available virucides, female condoms, or cervical caps and diaphragms. Treating HIV-infected persons with antiviral medications may reduce their infectiousness, but the duration or magnitude of any protective effect is not known. Finally, practical and effective behavioral interventions remain elusive. (For virucide and microbicide review, *see* Elias CJ, Heise L: *The Development of Microbicides: A New Method of HIV Prevention for Women.* New York: The Population Council, 1993, Programs Division Working Paper no. 6.) **B.** Perinatal transmission. In the wake of 1994 results suggesting that zidovudine given antepartum, intrapartum, and to the newborn infant prevents 67% of perinatal HIV transmission, a number of challenges remain in efforts to block perinatal transmission. These efforts include the effective identification of HIV-infected women to offer state-of-the-art prenatal care, including antiviral therapy when indicated and intrapartum and postpartum care designed to avoid potentially infectious blood contaminations to the infant. Sexually transmitted diseases can be screened and treated in pregnancy. Several studies suggest that prolonged rupture of membranes increases risk of perinatal transmission. Cesarean section might be protective for infants born to HIV-infected mothers, and studies should assess the costs and benefits to enable women and their health-care providers to make informed decisions. (*See* Important therapeutic information on the benefit of zidovudine for the prevention of the transmission of HIV from mother to infant. *NIAID Clin Alert* 1994, [Feb 20].) **C.** Parenteral transmission can result from a contaminated blood supply where HIV testing is not readily available, such as in developing countries. Occupational or iatrogenic exposures must be minimized for health-care workers by using universal precautions for all patients with unknown or HIV-seropositive status. Providing treatment to all drug users who wish to take advantage is a goal to which we should strive. Until treatment is available to all and for those who do not avail themselves of treatment opportunities, needle exchange and education to clean the needle injection equipment might be expected to slow the epidemic of HIV among injecting drug users. Many drug users are exposed through high-risk sexual activities. (For needle exchange discussion, *see* Kaplan EH: Needle exchange or needless exchange? *Infect Agents Dis* 1992, 1:92–98.)

PREVENTIVE HIV VACCINES

Challenges in AIDS vaccine development

State of protective immunity against HIV is unknown
Genetic variation of HIV
HIV latency
Cell-to-cell transmission of HIV
Lack of ideal animal model for HIV and AIDS

FIGURE 1-33 Challenge in AIDS vaccine development. To blunt the burgeoning worldwide HIV pandemic, vaccines are needed due to their theoretical ease of administration and low cost. However, HIV infection differs from the vaccine-preventable diseases in several ways. We do not know what correlates with immune protection and therefore do not have a clear surrogate result in early trials, which can reliably guide us in choosing products for large-scale testing. HIV is highly variable genetically. HIV is a latent virus, which can continue replication in lymph nodes and other parts of the reticuloendothelial system even when it seems quiescent, from peripheral blood measurements. Cell-to-cell transmission of HIV may occur, suggesting that a humoral immune blockade may not be adequate to protect from infection. Also, the animal models for HIV are useful but are not ideal. For example, chimps can be infected with HIV, but do not experience disease analogous to AIDS in humans. Macaques can be infected with SIV and they can get simian AIDS from SIV. However, SIV is different in several ways from HIV. New models and chimeric viruses are being studied.

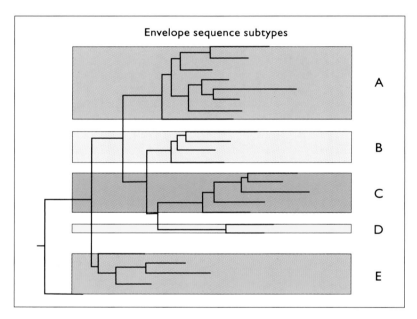

Envelope sequence subtypes

A
B
C
D
E

FIGURE 1-34 There are five or more different genetic groups of HIV-1, termed *clades*, and envelope genetic sequences can differ by up to 40% across viruses in different clades. Most HIV vaccinologists anticipate needing vaccines engineered toward one clade or as cocktails to induce an immunogenic response to multiple viral strains. (*Adapted from* Myers G, Korber B: The future of HIV. *In* Morse SS, ed. *Evolutionary Biology of Viruses.* New York: Raven Press, 1994; with permission.)

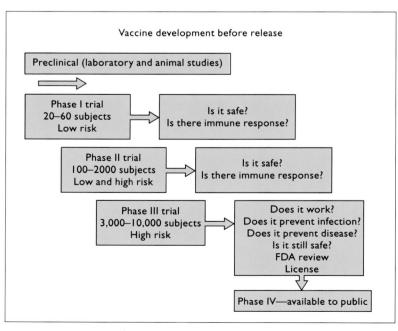

Vaccine development before release

Preclinical (laboratory and animal studies)

| Phase I trial 20–60 subjects Low risk | → | Is it safe? Is there immune response? |

| Phase II trial 100–2000 subjects Low and high risk | → | Is it safe? Is there immune response? |

| Phase III trial 3,000–10,000 subjects High risk | → | Does it work? Does it prevent infection? Does it prevent disease? Is it still safe? FDA review License |

Phase IV—available to public

FIGURE 1-35 Over a dozen HIV vaccine candidates are in human trials at present. Only two candidates are in phase II trials in early 1994; both are recombinant subunit gp120 products. No products are in large-scale phase III efficacy trials in 1994, though such trials could begin in the mid-1990s.

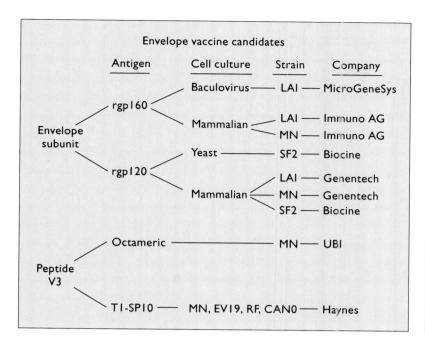

Envelope vaccine candidates

Antigen		Cell culture	Strain	Company
Envelope subunit	rgp160	Baculovirus	LAI	MicroGeneSys
		Mammalian	LAI	Immuno AG
			MN	Immuno AG
	rgp120	Yeast	SF2	Biocine
		Mammalian	LAI	Genentech
			MN	Genentech
			SF2	Biocine
Peptide V3	Octameric		MN	UBI
	T1-SP10	MN, EV19, RF, CAN0		Haynes

FIGURE 1-36 Among the first-generation HIV vaccine products are the envelope subunit products. These are manufactured by several companies, using different parts of the envelope, different cell culture systems, and different viral strains. Products that are based on peptides are also in phase I trials. If immunogenic and safe, these peptide products might be cheaper for worldwide use than most other conceivable vaccines. (*From* Dr. Patricia Fast, personal communication.)

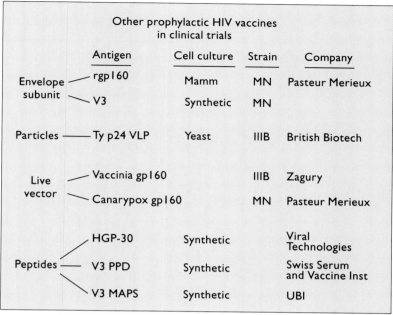

Other prophylactic HIV vaccines in clinical trials

	Antigen	Cell culture	Strain	Company
Envelope subunit	rgp160	Mamm	MN	Pasteur Merieux
	V3	Synthetic	MN	
Particles	Ty p24 VLP	Yeast	IIIB	British Biotech
Live vector	Vaccinia gp160		IIIB	Zagury
	Canarypox gp160		MN	Pasteur Merieux
Peptides	HGP-30	Synthetic		Viral Technologies
	V3 PPD	Synthetic		Swiss Serum and Vaccine Inst
	V3 MAPS	Synthetic		UBI

FIGURE 1-37 Along with recombinant subunits and peptides, other products now in human vaccine trials include viruslike, genetically engineered particles and live virus vector primes with subunit or peptide boosts. A theoretical advantage of these approaches might be the production of cytotoxic T lymphocytes against HIV-infected cells, complementing the humoral immune responses. Many of these products are grown in a variety of culture systems from various viral strains, resulting in different conformational epitopes being presented by different vaccine products. In phase I and II trials, over 1400 patients have been studied through early 1994. Side effects of HIV vaccines have been mild and typical of other licensed vaccines. There are no data to suggest that immunologic enhancement is likely, but this will be the topic of intense scrutiny in all large-scale trials. (*From* Dr. Patricia Fast, personal communication.)

What do trials require?

Virology and vaccines
  Circulating virus genetically characterized
  Vaccine candidate appropriate to circulating virus
  Vaccine candidate demonstrated safe and immunogenic
Infrastructure
  Transportation and communications adequate
  Trained and experienced local collaborators
  Laboratory and clinical facilities adequate
Population
  Population at high risk of seroconversion despite other interventions
  Seroincidence rate documented
  High-risk population willing to cooperate with the needs of the protocol
Political and ethical
  National and community political support for study
  Protocol in conformity with national legal and ethical codes
  Realistic community expectations

FIGURE 1-38 Four key elements are needed for large-scale efficacy trials to be indicated and successful: a promising vaccine given the circulating virus; an adequate research infrastructure; a study population at-risk, which is willing to participate in the multiyear trial; and the resolution of key social, ethical, and political concerns. A vaccine product must have a clear biological rationale for its effect, with preclinical and early human data to back up its claim. The criteria for selection of a candidate for an efficacy trial are the subject of intense debate.

Prophylactic HIV vaccines

Range of effects on natural infection
Seronegative/no viremia
Seroconversion/no detectable viremia
Seroconversion/transient viremia
Seroconversion/low-level viremia
Seroconversion/normal-level viremia
Seroconversion/high-level viremia

FIGURE 1-39 Possible effects of an HIV vaccine. If a patient were to remain seronegative without viremia, despite exposure, this would suggest that the vaccine had induced a *sterilizing immunity*. If a patient were to seroconvert, but there were no viremia or immunologic deterioration, this might imply an *abortive infection*. If a patient had a transient viremia but with an arrested course of immune deterioration, this might result in a *"cleared"* virus, analogous to the effect of many other viral vaccines. If a low-level viremia persisted, then perhaps the HIV disease course would be *modulated* and the patient might be both clinically stable and minimally infectious. Seroconversion with a normal viral replication implies an *ineffective* vaccine, whereas the sixth scenario would suggest *immunologic enhancement*. (Vermund SH, *et al.*: Prevention of HIV/AIDS with vaccines. *Curr Opin Infect Dis* 1994, 7:82–94.)

HEALTH-CARE WORKERS

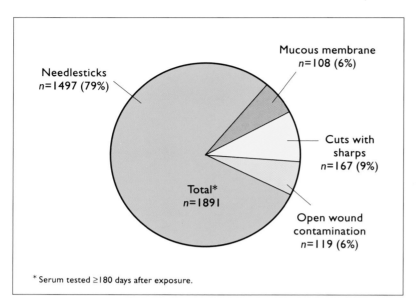

FIGURE 1-40 From 1983 to 1993, occupational exposures to HIV were reported to the CDC from 1891 health-care workers. Fully 79% of these exposures were due to needlesticks, 9% were from cuts with sharp objects, 6% from open wound contaminations, and 6% from HIV-infected fluids contacting the mucous membranes of the health-care worker. (Tokars JI, *et al.*: Survival of HIV infection and zidovudine use among health care workers with occupational exposure to HIV-infected blood. *Ann Intern Med* 1993, 118:913–919.)

Location of exposure for exposed health-care workers*

Location of exposure	Patients, *n(%)*†
Hospital room/ward	1236 (65)
Intensive care	209 (11)
Clinical laboratory	110 (6)
Emergency room	104 (5)
Operating room	97 (5)
Procedure room	70 (4)
Morgue/autopsy	28 (2)
Other/unknown	37 (2)

*Serum tested ≥ 180 days after exposure.
†*n*=1891.

FIGURE 1-41 Of 1891 occupational HIV exposures in the health-care setting, nearly two thirds occurred in hospital rooms or wards, followed by intensive care (11%), clinical laboratories (6%), emergency room (5%), and operating room (5%). (Tokars JI, *et al.*: Survival of HIV infection and zidovudine use among health care workers with occupational exposure to HIV-infected blood. *Ann Intern Med* 1993, 118:913–919.)

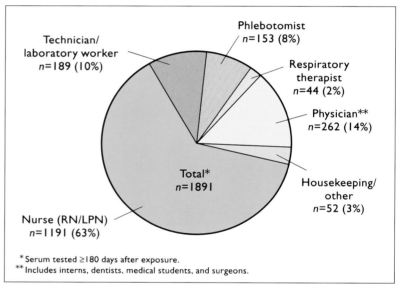

*Serum tested ≥180 days after exposure.
**Includes interns, dentists, medical students, and surgeons.

FIGURE 1-42 The occupations involved in 1891 reported HIV exposures within the health-care setting show nursing personnel (63%) at highest risk. True exposure rates are not known because these data reflect only those reports received at CDC, and the denominator of total procedures and total health-care workers is not known. Nonetheless, this suggests the need for special precautions and training targeting nursing personnel.

HIV seroconversion rate among enrolled health-care workers*

Exposure type	Positive cases, *n*	Patients enrolled, *n*	Seroconversion rate per 100 (upper 95% CI)
Percutaneous	4	1243	0.32 (0.73)
Mucous membrane/non-intact skin	0	161	0.00 (1.83)

*Serum tested at baseline and ≥ 180 days after exposure.

FIGURE 1-43 Of 1404 health-care workers with HIV tests at least 6 months after exposure, only four had seroconverted, all of whom had percutaneous needlestick exposure. The 0.3% seroconversion rate underscores the need for training and precautions in needle manipulation.

Description of enrolled health-care workers who seroconverted after exposure

Needle size	Severity of injury	Retroviral illness	Time until positive HIV antibody tests[†]	Postexposure zidovudine
Large bore	Deep	14 days	184 days	No
21- and 25-Gauge*	Moderate	4 weeks	121 days	No
21-Gauge	Deep	4 weeks	121 days	No
21-Gauge	Deep	38 days	121 days	Yes

*Two needlestick injuries 10 days apart.
[†]EIA and Western Blot.

FIGURE 1-44 All four health-care workers who were documented to have seroconverted had moderate to severe needlestick injuries. One person seroconverted despite zidovudine prophylaxis, suggesting that such therapy does not provide absolute protection. At least 6 months of follow-up testing is advisable as 4–6 months passed before all four persons had seroconverted.

Conclusions: HIV exposures and HCWs

Risk of HIV infection after percutaneous exposure of HIV-infected blood is approximately 0.3%

Risk after mucous membrane or nonintact skin exposure is lower than 0.3%, but is not well quantified

Side effects of zidovudine after short-term exposure is 74% (relatively minor) and after long-term exposures is unknown

Failures indicate that if zidovudine is protective, any protection provided is not absolute

If zidovudine is used, possible risks and benefits must be carefully considered

FIGURE 1-45 Without controlled clinical trials of postexposure zidovudine prophylaxis, no definitive recommendations can be made regarding its use in exposed health-care workers. It is assumed that risk of seroconversion is low, as per the results of surveillance to date, but certain factors are likely to increase this risk, including deep, severe injury; viremic, immunosuppressed patient; large inoculum, as with a large-bore needle; and highly infectious viral strain.

Universal precautions

Barrier precautions as appropriate
Handwashing
Injury control
Environmental control

FIGURE 1-46 Universal precautions are now the standard of medicine and nursing for all patients, not merely those for whom these precautions had applied in the past. To protect oneself from HIV, a health-care worker must consider all patients as potentially HIV-infected. These precautions will also help protect patients from a far less likely event, *ie*, inadvertent HIV transmission from an infected health-care worker to a patient. (*From* the Centers for Disease Control and Prevention: Guidelines for prevention of transmission of human immunodeficiency virus and hepatitis B virus to health-care and public-safety workers. *MMWR* 1989, 38:1–36; and Centers for Disease Control and Prevention: Recommendations for preventing transmission of human immunodeficiency virus and hepatitis B virus to patients during exposure-prone invasive procedures. *MMWR* 1991, 40[RR-8]:1–9.)

Wear gloves for phlebotomy

When health-care worker has cuts, scratches, or other breaks in skin

When health-care worker judges that hand contamination with blood may occur

For finger and heel sticks on infants and children

When receiving training in phlebotomy

FIGURE 1-47 Gloves should be used at all times when procedures risk blood contamination. Thus, gloves should be worn during phlebotomy. It is feasible for a health-care worker to practice phlebotomy using gloves with equivalent skill to that without gloves.

Exudative lesions and weeping dermatitis

No direct patient care and handling patient-care equipment until condition resolves

FIGURE 1-48 Given the theoretical increased risk for transmission or acquisition of HIV through epithelial mucosa whose integrity has been violated, health-care workers who have dermatitis or any exudative dermatologic process must not practice any patient care or patient equipment tasks until the lesions are fully resolved.

Injury prevention

Needles should not be recapped by hand, purposely bent or broken by hand, removed from disposable syringes, or otherwise manipulated by hand

After use, disposable syringes and needles, scalpel blades, and other sharps should be placed in puncture-resistant containers, located as close as practical to the use area

Large-bore reusable needles should be transported to reprocessing area in a puncture-resistant container

FIGURE 1-49 Standards of current practice include minimal manipulation of needles after use, thereby assuring lower risk of needle-stick related to needle discarding.

Precautions for invasive procedures

Routinely use appropriate barrier precautions to prevent skin and mucous-membrane contact with blood and other body fluids requiring universal precautions

Wear gloves and surgical masks for all procedures

Wear protective eyewear and face shields during procedures likely to generate droplets of blood, other body fluids requiring universal precautions, or bone chips

Wear gowns or aprons during procedures likely to generate splashes of blood or other body fluids requiring universal precautions

FIGURE 1-50 Precautions for invasive procedures are designed to minimize risk of direct contact with a patient's blood and body fluids using barrier clothing such as gloves, eyewear, gowns, aprons, and face shields.

SELECTED BIBLIOGRAPHY

Centers for Disease Control and Prevention: US cases reported through December 1992. *HIV/AIDS Surveillance Report.* 1993, (Feb):1–23.

World Health Organization: *The HIV/AIDS Pandemic: 1993 Overview.* Geneva, WHO, 1993.

Tokars JI, et al.: Survival with HIV infection and zidovudine use among health care workers with occupational exposure to HIV-infected blood. *Ann Intern Med* 1993, 118:913–919.

Centers for Disease Control and Prevention: National HIV serosurveillance summary: Results through 1992. 1993, 3:1–38.

Centers for Disease Control and Prevention: 1993 revised classification system for HIV infection and expanded surveillance case definition for AIDS among adolescents and adults. *MMWR* 1992, 41(RR-17):1–19.

CHAPTER 2

Human Immunodeficiency Virus

Michael S. Saag

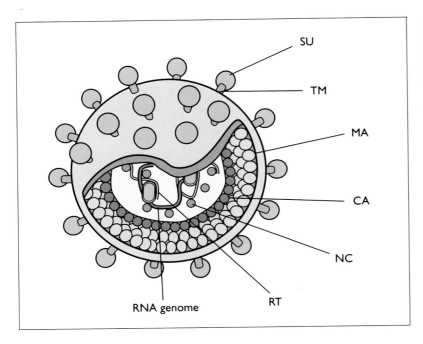

SU

TM

MA

CA

NC

RNA genome

RT

FIGURE 2-1 Structure of HIV. AIDS is caused by a retrovirus known as the human immunodeficiency virus type 1 (HIV-1). In certain regions of the world, primarily west Africa, AIDS may be caused by a related virus, HIV-2, which differs from HIV-1 in some of its genetic products (Vpx) and its lower pathogenicity. The virus consists of an outer lipid bilayer coat studded with surface (SU,gp120) and transmembrane (TM,gp41) glycoprotein complexes. Just beneath the lipid bilayer are matrix proteins (MA) and beneath that, the virion, consisting of internal capsular (CA) and nuclear capsid (NC) proteins, which surround the single-stranded RNA genome. The unique feature of retroviruses is the presence of reverse transcriptase (RT), an enzyme that is capable of transcribing RNA into DNA. (*Courtesy of* Eric Hunter, PhD.)

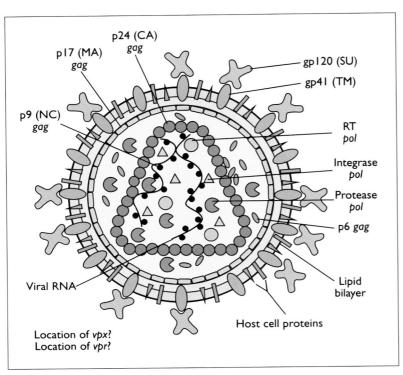

p24 (CA) *gag*

p17 (MA) *gag*

p9 (NC) *gag*

gp120 (SU)

gp41 (TM)

RT *pol*

Integrase *pol*

Protease *pol*

p6 *gag*

Viral RNA

Lipid bilayer

Host cell proteins

Location of *vpx?*
Location of *vpr?*

FIGURE 2-2 HIV virion. A more detailed view of the HIV virion shows its components and their genetic source. In addition to the matrix (MA), internal capsular (CA), and nuclear capsid (NC) proteins, which are produced by the *gag* region, the virion contains gene products of the *pol* region, including the enzymes reverse transcriptase (RT), integrase, and protease. As the virion buds from the membrane of an infected cell, it picks up host cellular proteins on its coat, which may be important in the lack of antigenic response against the virus. Certain gene products, such as Vpr in the case of HIV-1 and Vpr and Vpx in the case of HIV-2, are of uncertain function and location within the virion. (*Adapted from* Hahn BH: Viral genes and their products. *In* Broder S, Merigan TC, Bolognesi D (eds): *Textbook of AIDS Medicine.* Baltimore: Williams & Wilkins; 1994:21–44; with permission.)

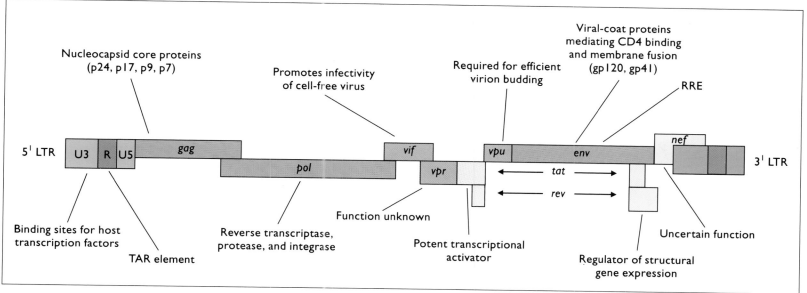

FIGURE 2-3 HIV genome map. This genetic map of the HIV-1 viral genome depicts the structural and regulatory genes in their relative positions as well as their products and functions. The 9-kb RNA virus is flanked by a long terminal repeat (LTR) section on both the 5' and 3' ends of the virus, which serves as a promoter and binding site for host and viral transactivating factors. The TAR element exists within the R region of the LTR and serves as a binding point for the *tat* gene product (a potent transcriptional activator). The *gag* region encodes the nucleocapsid core and matrix proteins. The *pol* gene codes the reverse transcriptase, protease, and integrase enzymes. The envelope region (*env*) is responsible for the viral-coat glycoproteins, gp120 and gp41, which mediate CD4 binding and membrane fusion. The remaining genes (*vif, vpr, vpu, rev,* and *nef*) are regulatory genes whose products play critical roles in controlling viral expression, trafficking of viral gene products within the infected cell, and viral infectivity. The *rev*-responsive element (RRE) is the binding site for the *rev* gene product, which is important for the transport of unspliced and singly spliced RNA messages from the nucleus. (*Courtesy of* Beatrice Hahn, MD.)

HIV-1 AND RELATED RETROVIRUSES

Primate lentiviruses*

Virus	Host	Natural	Pathogenic	Origin
HIV-1	Humans	No	Yes	—
HIV-2	Humans	No	Yes	—
SIV$_{agm}$	African green monkeys	Yes	No	Africa
SIV$_{mac}$	Macaques	No	Yes	Asia
SIV$_{sm}$	Sooty mangabeys	Yes	No	Africa
SIV$_{mnd}$	Mandrills	Yes	No	Africa
SIV$_{cpz}$	Chimpanzees	Yes?	No?	Africa
SIV$_{syk}$	Sykes monkeys	Yes	No	Africa

*Only those species from which viral sequence data are available are included.

FIGURE 2-4 Primate lentiviruses. HIV is a human lentivirus, which exists in the family of primate lentiviruses. Although similar in structure, human and primate lentiviruses have important genetic and functional differences. This table presents a summary of lentiviruses from which viral sequence data are currently known. The simian immunodeficiency viruses (SIV) occur naturally in African green monkeys (SIV$_{agm}$), sooty mangabeys (SIV$_{sm}$), mandrills (SIV$_{mnd}$), chimpanzees (SIV$_{cpz}$), and Sykes' monkeys (SIV$_{syk}$). The virus isolated from macaques (SIV$_{mac}$) is not found among macaques captured in the wild but is isolated only from those animals infected in captivity. SIV$_{mac}$ shares common features with HIV-1 and HIV-2 in that the virus is pathogenic in macaques, whereas other SIV occurring within their native species are generally not pathogenic. (*From* Hahn BH: Viral genes and their products. *In* Broder S, Merigan TC, Bolognesi D (eds): *Textbook of AIDS Medicine.* Baltimore: Williams & Wilkins; 1994:21–44; with permission. Markovitz DM: Infection with the human immunodeficiency virus type 2. *Ann Intern Med* 1993, 118:211–218.)

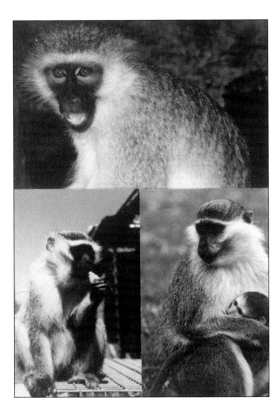

FIGURE 2-5 African green monkeys. Studies of the African green monkeys and their related simian virus (SIV$_{agm}$) yield important information in our understanding of HIV-1 and HIV-2. Shown here are three major species of African green monkeys indigenous to Africa. (*Courtesy of* Jon Allan, PhD.)

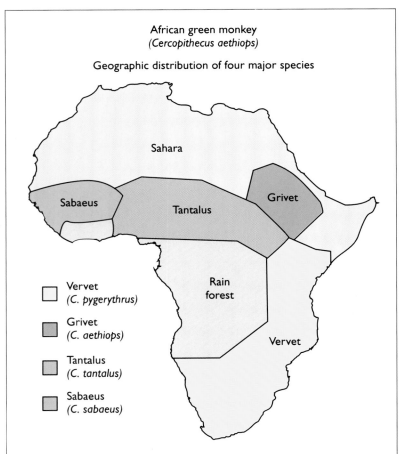

African green monkey
(*Cercopithecus aethiops*)

Geographic distribution of four major species

Vervet (*C. pygerythrus*)
Grivet (*C. aethiops*)
Tantalus (*C. tantalus*)
Sabaeus (*C. sabaeus*)

FIGURE 2-6 Geographic domains of African green monkeys. This map of Africa indicates the native locations of different species of the African green monkey. Within each species, a unique family of SIV$_{agm}$ has been shown to exist. (*Courtesy of* Beatrice Hahn, MD.)

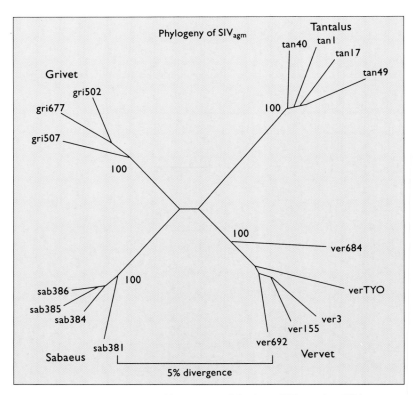

Phylogeny of SIV$_{agm}$

FIGURE 2-7 Phylogenic differences of SIV$_{agm}$. When the SIV$_{agm}$ from different species of African green monkeys are genetically mapped, the phylogenic tree demonstrates unique clustering of SIV$_{agm}$ based on the species of African green monkey from which the virus was obtained. This particular phylogenic tree demonstrates genetic distances within a region of over 382 amino acid residues in the *env* gene. (*From* Hahn BH: Viral genes and their products. *In* Broder S, Merigan TC, Bolognesi D (eds): *Textbook of AIDS Medicine.* Baltimore: Williams & Wilkins; 1994:21–44; with permission.)

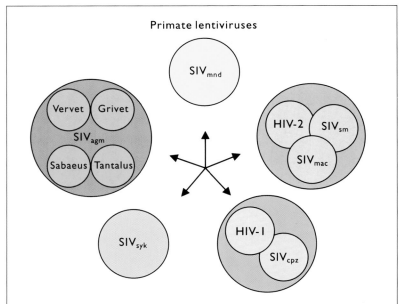

Primate lentiviruses

FIGURE 2-8 Subgroups of SIV. When viewed in the context of the primate lentiviruses, SIV$_{agm}$ has several subspecies, based on the species of African green monkey from which the viruses were obtained. Other SIV, such as SIV$_{mnd}$ and SIV$_{syk}$, form their own subspecies of lentiviruses. Interestingly, SIV$_{mac}$ and SIV$_{sm}$ are more closely linked to HIV-2, whereas SIV$_{cpz}$ (obtained from chimpanzees) is more closely related to HIV-1. (*From* Hahn BH: Viral genes and their products. *In* Broder S, Merigan TC, Bolognesi D (eds): *Textbook of AIDS Medicine.* Baltimore: Williams & Wilkins; 1994:21–44; with permission.)

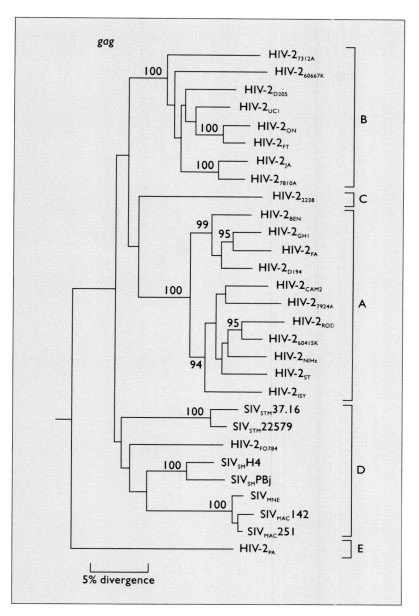

FIGURE 2-9 Phylogenic subgroups of HIV-2. This phylogenic tree demonstrates the multiple subgroups within the HIV-2 viral family. Horizontal branch lengths represent the relative genetic distances between each group (*ie*, the further the branch occurs from the left-hand margin, the greater is the confidence that the grouping is a separate family) and are drawn to scale; vertical branches are for clarity only. The numbers noted on the nodes (vertical branches) represent the percentage of bootstrap samples (*ie*, a statistical description of the strength of the distribution as shown), which support the clustering. Only values > 80% are shown. Five roughly equidistant genetic lineages are identified, noted as subgroups A to E. Viruses within subgroup D are more related to SIV$_{mac}$ and SIV$_{sm}$, whereas viruses from subgroups A and B are more related to themselves (*ie*, HIV-2) than to SIV. (Gao F, Yue L, Robertson DL, *et al.*: Genetic diversity of HIV 2: Evidence for distinct sequence subtypes with differences in virus biology. *J Virol* 1994, in press.)

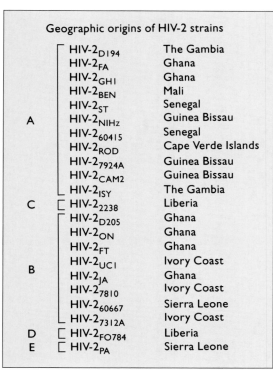

FIGURE 2-10 Geographic origins of HIV-2 strains. HIV-2 predominantly comes from western Africa. Within each subgroup of HIV-2, there are several countries from which different viral strains have originated, however, there is no correlation between the geographic origin of an HIV-2 isolate and its phylogenic clustering. Moreover, identification of intersubtype recombinant variants requires the simultaneous spread of divergent viral strains in the same population. Each strain has a different ability to be cultured *in vitro* and varying expression of clinical disease. (*Illustration courtesy of* Beatrice Hahn, MD. Boeri E, Giri A, Lillo G, *et al.*: *In vivo* genetic variability of the human immunodeficiency virus type 2 V3 region. *J Virol* 1992, 66:4546–4550. Gao F, Yue L, White AT, *et al.*: Human infection by genetically diverse SIV$_{sm}$-related HIV-2 in west Africa. *Nature* 1992, 358:495–499. Gao F, Yue L, Robertson DL, *et al.*: Genetic diversity of HIV 2: Evidence for distinct sequence subtypes with differences in virus biology. *J Virol* 1994, in press.)

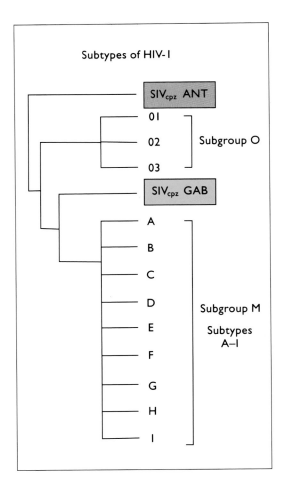

Subtypes of HIV-1

SIV_cpz ANT

01
02 Subgroup O
03

SIV_cpz GAB

A
B
C
D   Subgroup M
E   Subtypes A–I
F
G
H
I

FIGURE 2-11 Subtypes of HIV-1. A phylogenic tree indicates the relative genetic distances between different subtypes of HIV-1. Each subtype has been isolated from patients in specific geographic locations, underscoring the relative spread of a given viral genotype within each "mini-epidemic" of the global pandemic. Note the relatively new addition of subgroup O, which is equidistant from other known HIV-1 isolates (subgroup M, ie, subtypes A–I) and SIV_cpz (Myers G, Korber B, Smith R, et al. (eds): *Human Retroviruses and AIDS 1993*. Los Alamos, CA, Los Alamos National Laboratory, 1993.)

Geographic distribution of HIV-1 subtypes

Central and West Africa
United States, Europe, South America, Africa, Asia
South Africa, India, Zambia, Djibouti
Central Africa
Thailand, Central African Republic, India
Brazil, Romania, Zaire
Africa
Africa
Africa

FIGURE 2-12 Geographic distribution of HIV-1 subtypes. Geographic associations of the HIV-1 subtypes are shown with the region of the world from which the subtype was initially isolated. As opposed to HIV-2 strains, most HIV-1 isolates are readily isolated in tissue culture and most appear virulent in humans. Although some strains may be less pathogenic than others, the relative pathogenicity of a given strain does not correlate with a specific subtype or apparent geographic origin. (*Courtesy of Beatrice Hahn, MD.*)

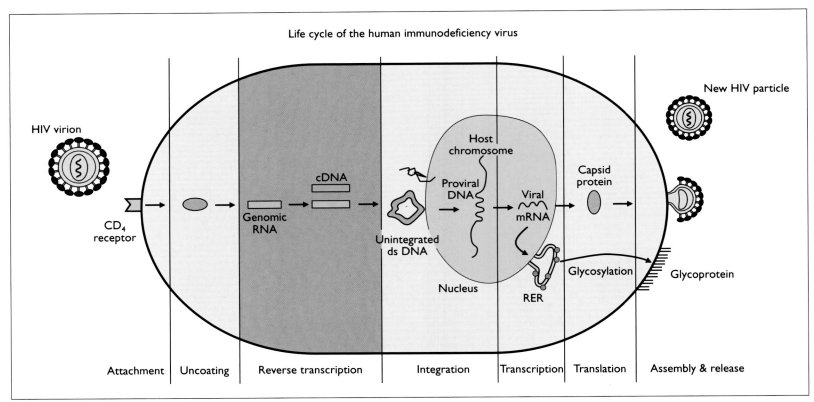

FIGURE 2-13 Lifecycle of HIV-1 (not drawn to scale). The HIV-1 virus binds to the CD4 receptor complex on the surface of CD4+ cells. The virion then enters the cell, uncoats, and undergoes the process of reverse transcription (*red area*) in which viral RNA is transcribed into complementary DNA. This is the portion of the lifecycle at which all currently available antiretroviral agents are designed to intercede. After reverse transcription, the DNA becomes double-stranded and migrates to the cell nucleus, where it is integrated into the host genomic DNA as a provirus. The virus can then be transcribed back into mRNA and genomic RNA, and the resultant proteins and genomic RNA are assembled near the surface of the cell and packaged into a new virion, which buds from the cell membrane. (Flier JS, Underhill LH, Crumpacker CS: Molecular targets of antiviral therapy. *N Engl J Med* 1985, 321:163–172.)

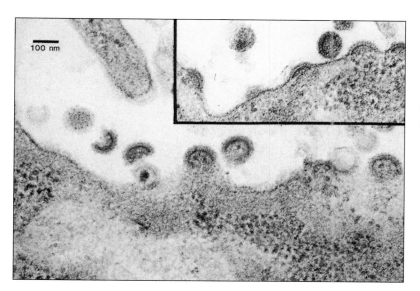

FIGURE 2-14 Viral budding. In this electron micrograph, the virus can be seen budding forth from the surface of a cell. Note how the outer membrane of the virus is composed of the lipid bilayer membrane of the host cell studded with integrated protein products (envelope proteins) of the virus. (*From* Barre-Sinnoussi F, Chermann JC, Rey F, *et al.*: Isolation of a T-lymphotropic retrovirus from a patient at risk for acquired immune deficiency syndrome (AIDS). *Science* 1983, 220:868–871; with permission.)

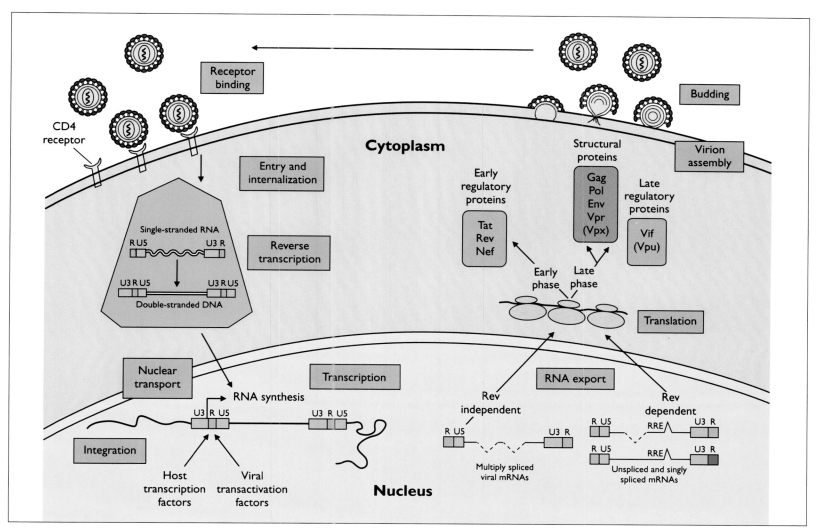

FIGURE 2-15 Viral replication. Once HIV enters a cell, undergoes reverse transcription, and is integrated into the nucleus (integration), several host transcriptional and viral activational factors stimulate viral replication (transcription). Regulatory proteins, such as Tat, Rev, and Nef, are generally produced early and, in the case of Tat, stimulate the virus to replicate. REV-dependent mRNA usually results in unspliced or singly spliced RNA products via the "chaperone" effect of Rev, which escorts the unspliced message from the nucleus to the cytoplasm. Once in the cytoplasm, the long messages are translated into structural proteins, such as Gag, Pol, and Env, usually as a later event in the replication cycle (translation, late regulatory proteins). The production of these proteins is augmented by the help of late regulatory proteins such as Vif. Once the proteins and genomic RNA have been produced, they aggregate near the cell surface, where an immature virion buds on the cell membrane. After release of the immature virion from the cell, the activity of the protease gene results in development of a mature virion. (*Figure adapted from* Hahn BH: Viral genes and their products. *In* Broder S, Merigan TC, Bolognesi D (eds): *Textbook of AIDS Medicine.* Baltimore: Williams & Wilkins; 1994:21–44; with permission. Cullen BR: Mechanism of action of regulatory proteins encoded by complex retroviruses. *Microbiol Rev* 1992, 56:375–394.)

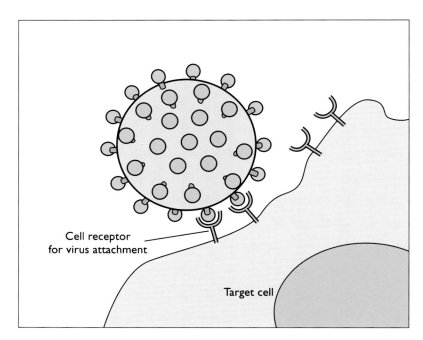

FIGURE 2-16 HIV binding via CD4 receptor (not drawn to scale). The HIV virus binds to the cell surface of a CD4+ lymphocyte. The binding attachment occurs through an interaction of the viral glycoprotein gp120/gp41 and the CD4 receptor complex on the cell surface. (*Courtesy of* Eric Hunter, PhD.)

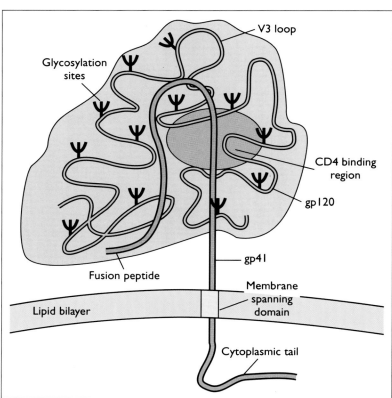

FIGURE 2-17 Envelope glycoprotein complex of HIV-1. The gp41 fragment (*purple*) consists of a cytoplasmic tail and a hydrophobic membrane-spanning domain and is joined with the larger gp120 component (*blue line*) via a fusion domain. The gp120 glycoprotein has several glycosylation sites and hypervariable loops (*eg*, V3), which lead to antigenic variation between viral strains. The CD4-binding region (*red*) is located toward the center of the complex and consists of components from both the gp120 and gp41 fragments. (*Adapted from* Hahn BH: Viral genes and their products. *In* Broder S, Merigan TC, Bolognesi D (eds): *Textbook of AIDS Medicine.* Baltimore: Williams & Wilkins; 1994:21–44; with permission. Moore JP, Jameson BA, Weiss RA, Sastentar QJ: The HIV–cell fusion relation. *In* Bentz J (ed): *Viral Fusion Mechanisms.* Boca Raton, FL: CRC Press; 1993:233–289.)

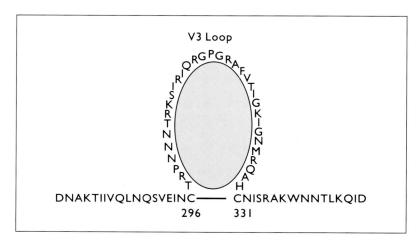

FIGURE 2-18 V-loop regions in *env* and antigenic variation. Within the envelope gene, there are regions that are highly variable and others that are more conserved. Within the variable regions are a series of loops (V-loops), which contain hypervariable regions. Differences in these regions result in a high degree of antigenic variation between strains. The V3 loop is one of the more important hypervariable regions. The loop begins with cystine-to-cystine disulfide bonds at positions 296 and 331; the remaining amino acids form a loop between the cystine groups. At the tip of the V3 loop is a GPGRAF region, which is a particularly important antigenic determinant. (*Courtesy of* Eric Hunter, PhD.)

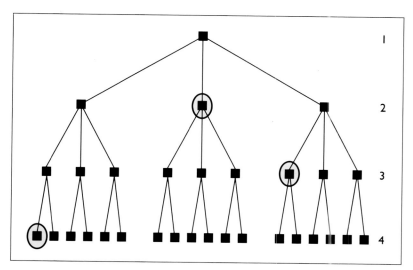

FIGURE 2-19 Genotype selection in HIV infection. Antigenic variation is a hallmark of HIV infection. It is believed that an individual is initially infected with a single genotype. However, this virus rapidly evolves over a period of weeks into a complex mixture of highly related, yet genetically distinct, viral variants. This slide represents the evolution of a family of viruses in an infected patient from a single genotype (*top of tree*) into the typical genetic quasi-species of HIV-1. At any given timepoint, a predominant genotype can be identified in either the plasma or peripheral blood mononuclear cells; however, other variants continue to exist simultaneously. Changes in selective pressure, due to either the immune response or the initiation of antiretroviral therapy, shift the population of viral variants such that another genotype becomes the most prevalent (represented by circled variants at a given timepoint). (Saag MS, Hahn BS, Gibbons J: Extension variation of HIV-1 *in vivo. Nature* 1988, 334:440–444.)

DIAGNOSIS OF HIV-1 INFECTION

Methods for diagnosing HIV-1 infection

Method	Product measured
Culture in PBMCs	Infectious virus (as measured by RT activity or p24 antigen)
Antibody detection techniques	
ELISA	Anti-HIV antibody or p24 antigen
Western blot	Anti-HIV antibody
Polymerase chain reaction (PCR)	Proviral DNA Transcribed cDNA
Quantitative-competitive PCR (QC-PCR)	Viral RNA or DNA
Branched-chain DNA amplification (bDNA)	"Labeled" viral RNA

FIGURE 2-20 Methods for diagnosing HIV-1 infection. Many methods are available to detect HIV in patients. The most direct is to culture HIV via co-cultivation of patient peripheral blood mononuclear cells (PBMCs) with stimulated PBMCs from uninfected donors. Under the proper conditions, this *in vitro* culture system results in an explosive viral infection, leading to the production of millions of virions. The culture is read as positive by detecting either reverse transcriptase (RT) activity or p24 antigen in the virus culture supernatant. Due to the technical difficulty and expense of performing viral culture, other techniques have been developed to detect the presence of HIV infection. Many of these techniques rely on detection of the antibody response to HIV rather than detection of the virus itself. The two most commonly employed antibody tests are the enzyme-linked immunosorbent assay (ELISA) and the Western blot test, both of which are highly sensitive (> 99%) tests. Newer techniques for detecting HIV include PCR, QC-PCR, and bDNA, but their roles in clinical staging and predicting progression of HIV disease remain undefined.

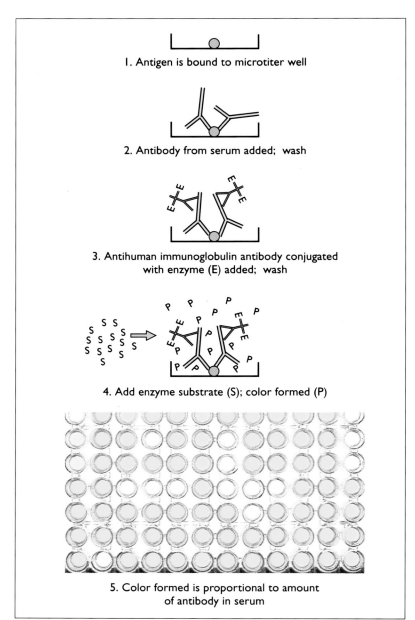

1. Antigen is bound to microtiter well

2. Antibody from serum added; wash

3. Antihuman immunoglobulin antibody conjugated with enzyme (E) added; wash

4. Add enzyme substrate (S); color formed (P)

5. Color formed is proportional to amount of antibody in serum

FIGURE 2-21 ELISA antibody test. The ELISA test is based on the capture of anti-HIV-specific antibodies by viral antigens that are coated on a microwell (*1*). Once the antibody binds to the HIV antigens, a washing procedure is performed (*2*) followed by incubation with a goat antihuman immunoglobulin antibody that is conjugated with an enzyme (*3*). The goat antihuman antibody binds tightly and specifically to any human antibody that has bound to HIV antigen, and after a washing procedure, an enzyme substrate is added, which is cleaved by the enzyme to form a product that yields a color (*4*). The relative amount of color present in the well (*5*) is proportional to the amount of human anti-HIV antibody present in the patient's sera. (Saag MS: AIDS testing now and in the future. *In* Sande MA, Volberding PA (eds): *Medical Management of AIDS*, 4th ed. Philadelphia: W.B. Saunders; 1994: in press. *Figure adapted from* Brock TD, Madigan MT: *Biology of Microorganisms*, 5th ed. Englewood Cliffs, NJ: Prentice Hall; 1988:454; with permission.)

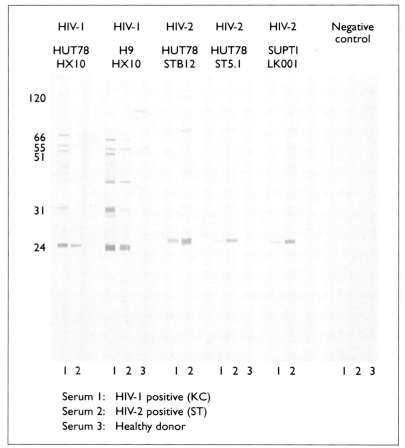

Serum 1: HIV-1 positive (KC)
Serum 2: HIV-2 positive (ST)
Serum 3: Healthy donor

FIGURE 2-22 Western blot. A representative Western blot of both HIV-1 and HIV-2 using different cell lines to express the virus (HUT 78, H9, or sup T1). Serum from an HIV-1–positive patient, an HIV-2–positive patient, and an unidentified healthy donor are represented in *lanes 1, 2,* and *3* of each Western preparation, respectively. (*Courtesy of* Beatrice Hahn, MD.)

I. Tissue culture for HIV yields cellular lysate (proteins)

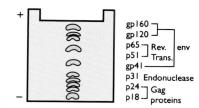

2. Mixture subjected to polyacrylamide gel electrophoresis; proteins separate by MW

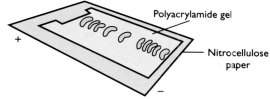

3. Transfer the separated proteins from the gel to nitrocellulose paper; cut into strips

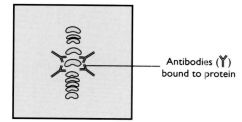

4. Nitrocellulose paper containing blotted proteins is incubated with patient sera; if antibody is present, it recognizes and binds to a specific protein

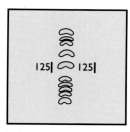 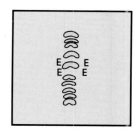

5. Add marker to bind to antigen–antibody complexes, either radiolabeled protein (*left*) or antibody-containing conjugated enzyme (*right*)

 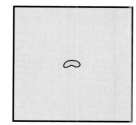

6. Develop blot by either exposing blot to x-ray film (*left*) or adding substrate of enzyme (*right*); dark spot appears where antibody bound to antigen on blot

FIGURE 2-23 Western blot. The Western blot antibody test works on the same principle as ELISA, *ie*, capturing antibody with HIV-specific antigens. In contrast with the ELISA, the antigens on the Western blot are separated on a polyacrylamide gel (*2*) and transferred to nitrocellulose paper (*3*). The nitrocellulose paper is cut into strips, which are incubated with the patient's sera (*4*). If antibody is present, it binds specifically at the point where the antigen migrated. This allows accurate determination of the specific antigen against which the antibody is targeted. (Saag MS: AIDS testing now and in the future. *In* Sande MA, Volberding PA (eds): *Medical Management of AIDS*, 4th ed. Philadelphia: W.B. Saunders; 1994:in press. *Figure adapted from* Brock TD, Madigan MT: *Biology of Microorganisms*, 5th ed. Englewood Cliffs, NJ: Prentice Hall; 1988:492; with permission.)

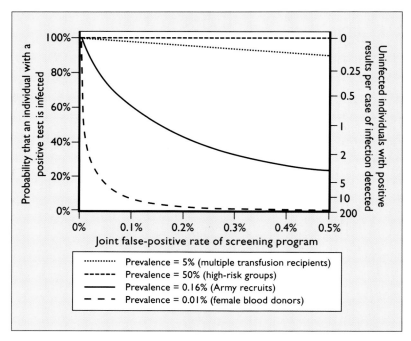

Figure 2-24 Positive predictive value of ELISA and Western blot. Although the sensitivity and specificity of the ELISA and Western blot tests are high, the positive predictive value of the two tests, even when used in combination, depends on the population of patients being tested. If the prevalence of HIV infection is high (*eg*, intravenous drug users from the inner city), the probability that an individual with a positive test is truly infected remains at 100% even when the joint false-positive rate is 0.5%. Conversely, if the prevalence of HIV infection is very low (0.01%), such as with female blood donors, even a joint false-positive rate of 0.02% will lead to at least half of the individuals who test positive having a false-positive test. This concept is a critically important one to consider when making decisions about universal testing. (*From* Meyer UB, Paulker SG: Screening for HIV: Can we afford the false-positive rate? *N Engl J Med* 1987, 317:238–241; with permission.)

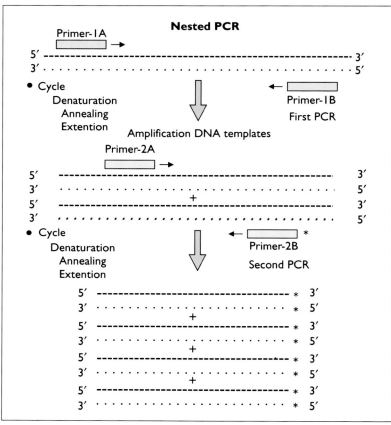

Nested PCR

Figure 2-25 Polymerase chain reaction (PCR). The PCR techniques have recently been applied to detection of HIV viral genomes. PCR can be used to detect integrated proviral DNA obtained from cells or RNA in plasma or cells after the RNA is converted to cDNA by reverse transcription. The principle of PCR is to use homologous primers that bind at the 5′ ends of defined regions of both strands of DNA. The primers are usually 20–30 base pairs in length and, with the use of the unique enzyme Taq polymerase, will yield a product that duplicates the HIV genome. Through a series of cycles consisting of denaturation (in which the double-stranded DNA is converted to single-strands through heat), annealing (in which the strands come back together but with the incorporation of primers at the specific target location), and extension (in which the Taq polymerase converts the DNA into new product), the PCR results in a doubling of the initial genetic material. By repeating the cycle 30 times, the original target is amplified at 2^{30}, leading to easier detection. The concept of nested PCR uses a second set of primers (2A and 2B) that fall within the region of DNA product amplified by the first set of primers. This can increase the sensitivity of the PCR technique substantially. (Saiki RK, Gelfand DH, Stoffel S, *et al.*: Primer directed enzymatic amplification of DNA with a thermostatic DNA polymerase. *Science* 1988, 239:487–491.)

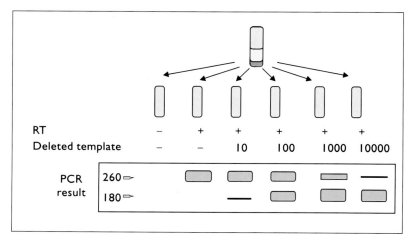

Figure 2-26 Quantitative-competitive PCR (QC-PCR). This method employs a competitor RNA fragment that has an 80–base pair deletion within the PCR-amplified region. In this example, the PCR fragment from the patient sample is 260 base pairs long, whereas the competitor fragment is 180 base pairs long. To each well, an equal amount of patient-derived viral RNA is added. To each well, increasing amounts of the competitor are added in serial 10-fold increments. A control well is also maintained in which no RNA from either patient or competitor is added. The more competitor RNA that is added, the weaker the signal becomes from the patient's sample. Where there is equivalence (in this case, 100 copies/mL), this indicates the amount of virus that is present in the patient's sample. (*Figure courtesy of* J. Lifson, MD. Piatek M, Saag MS, Yank LC, *et al.*: High levels of HIV-1 in plasma during all stages of infection determined by competitive PCR. *Science* 1993, 259:1749–1754.)

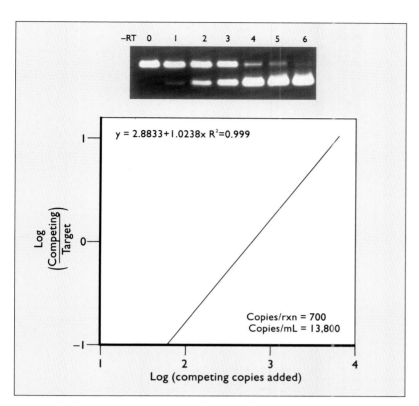

FIGURE 2-27 Quantitative competitive PCR. Representative results from an experiment using QC-PCR demonstrates the decreasing bands from the patient with increasing bands from the competitor as more competitor RNA is added. A linear relationship between the log amount of competing copies added versus the log of the competing target sequence signal leads to the ability to create a line where the point of equivalence can be determined. The point of equivalence indicates the relative amount of virus present originally in the patient's sample. (*Courtesy of* J. Lifson, MD.)

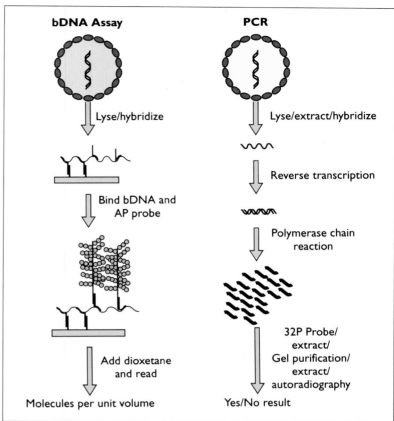

FIGURE 2-28 Branched-chain DNA amplification (bDNA). A new technique to detect the presence of viral RNA from patient material is the bDNA assay. As opposed to PCR amplification, whereby the actual viral product is amplified, the bDNA assay captures the viral RNA that is present with specific capture probes and then applies detector probes, which emit a signal. By amplifying the signal, as opposed to the viral RNA itself, the technique allows the viral copy to become detectable and quantifiable based on the amount of relative signal present. (*Courtesy of* Chiron Laboratories.)

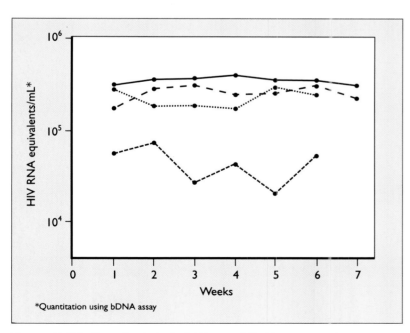

FIGURE 2-29 Branched-chain DNA amplification assay. A representative experiment shows the stability of RNA levels as measured by bDNA from four patients who had weekly blood samples drawn while not on antiretroviral therapy. Similar findings have been noted with PCR methodologies. (*Courtesy of* Chiron Laboratories.)

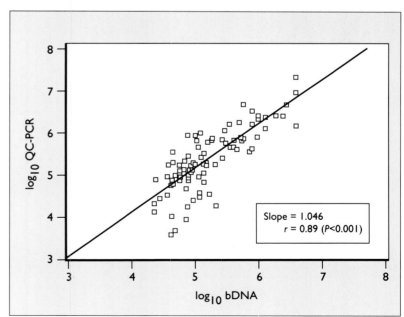

FIGURE 2-30 Correlation between QC-PCR and bDNA results. Although QC-PCR and bDNA are designed to detect viral RNA through different mechanisms (amplification of viral genome versus amplification of signal once the RNA is captured), there is a strong correlation between the values measured by the two tests. In samples evaluated in a blinded fashion, the values show a linear relationship with a slope of 1.046 and an r-value of 0.89 ($P > 0.001$).

PATHOGENESIS AND NATURAL HISTORY

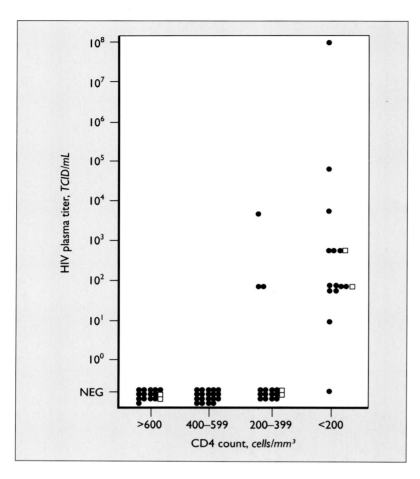

FIGURE 2-31 Plasma viremia. Viral burden as measured by plasma viremia increases with advanced stages of disease. In patients with higher CD4+ counts (> 400/mm^3), HIV is very difficult to culture from plasma. However, as the disease progresses and the CD4+ counts drop below 300, viral titers of 1:1000 and 1:10,000 are common. It is unclear whether this increase in culturable virus at late stages of disease is due to increased levels of viral replication, decreased ability to clear free virus from plasma, or both. (*From* Saag MS, Crain MJ, Delker WD, *et al.*: High level viremia in adults and children infected with HIV-1. *J Infect Dis* 1991, 164:72–80; with permission.)

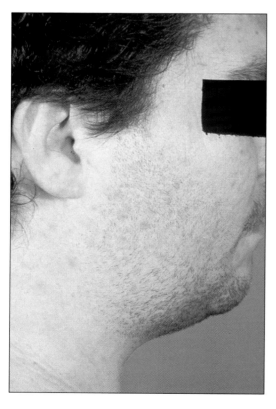

FIGURE 2-32 Seroconversion skin rash. Two to 4 weeks after initial infection with HIV-1, approximately 40% of patients develop an acute mononucleosis-like illness often associated with a faint, erythematous skin rash, which can be quite fleeting. Detailed virologic studies of individuals at the time of seroconversion have led to important insights into HIV pathogenesis.

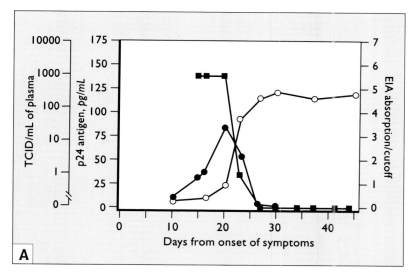

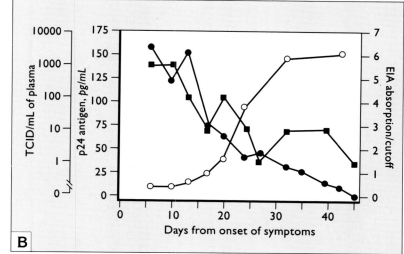

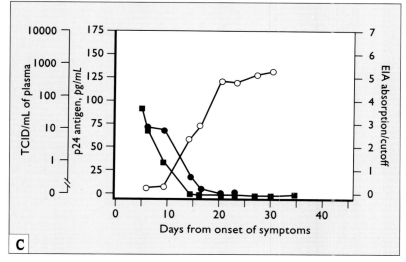

FIGURE 2-33 Seroconversion and viremia. Seroconversion profiles from three patients followed from the time of presentation with the acute seroconversion syndrome. In each patient panel, the *open-circle line* represents the ELISA absorbance value, the *solid-circle line* represents p24 antigen value, and the *solid-box line* represents the titer of culturable free virus in plasma. For each patient, as the immune system response is established, the level of both free virus in plasma and p24 antigen drops precipitously coincident with the development of an effective immune response. For patients A and C, the drop in plasma viral burden is quite rapid; however, for patient B, it is a bit more prolonged. (*From* Clark SJ, Saag MS, Delker WD, *et al.*: High titers of cytopathic virus in plasma of patients with symptomatic HIV-1 infection. *N Engl J Med* 1991, 324:954–960; with permission.)

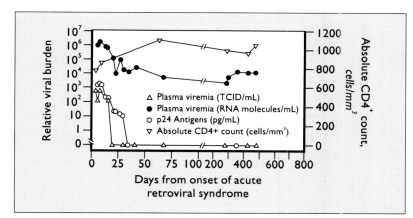

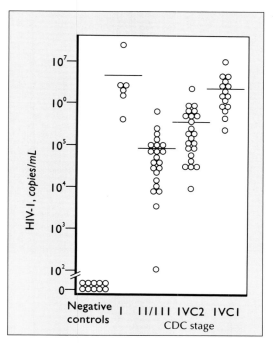

FIGURE 2-34 Viral replication profile. A representative patient from the time of acute seroconversion with serial CD4+ count measurements, p24 antigen, culturable free virus in plasma, and plasma viremia measured via QC-PCR. Coincident with the development of an effective immune response, the levels of p24 antigen and culturable free virus in plasma drop to undetectable levels within 20–30 days after seroconversion. In contrast, although the viral burden as measured by QC-PCR drops by over 100-fold, the levels do not approach the undetectable range and remain in the 1000 to 10,000 range over the course of the next year. These data indicate that viral replication is an ongoing process throughout the period of clinical latency and underscores the increased sensitivity of QC-PCR methods over standard p24 antigen or plasma culture assays. (*Courtesy of* Jeff Lifson, MD.)

FIGURE 2-35 Plasma viremia vs CDC stage of disease. Levels of quantitative free virus in plasma were measured by QC-PCR for patients with acute seroconversion (stage I), asymptomatic infection (stage II/III), advanced symptomatic disease (stage IVC2), or AIDS (stage IVC1). All negative control patients who were evaluated had no detectable virus in the plasma. There was a 100-fold difference between the patients with acute seroconversion vs asymptomatic infection, a roughly 10-fold increase as the patients developed more symptomatic disease, and an additional 10-fold increase as they developed AIDS-defining illnesses. (*Courtesy of* Jeff Lifson, MD.)

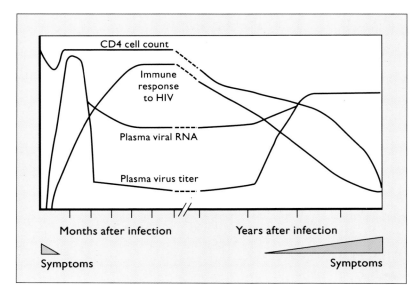

FIGURE 2-36 Hypothetical course of HIV infection in adults. High levels of plasma viremia as measured by either culturable free virus from plasma or plasma RNA titer decrease dramatically as the immune system response is established after acute seroconversion. Over time, as the CD4+ cell count begins to decline, the level of viral burden begins to increase coincident with the development of symptomatic HIV disease. (*Courtesy of* HIV Information Network.)

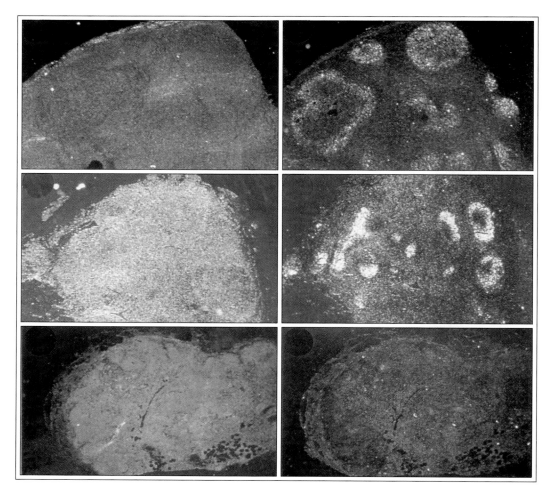

FIGURE 2-37 Lymph node destruction. Lymph nodes were evaluated from patients with early HIV disease (*top row*), intermediate-stage disease (*middle row*), and advanced-stage disease (*lower row*). The righthand column shows *in situ* hybridization detection of virus within the lymph nodes at the different stages of disease. In early-stage disease, a large amount of virus is present and is well organized around germinal centers. As the disease advances, the level of viral burden within the lymph node actually decreases and becomes more disorganized. By advanced stage of disease, virus is still present within the lymph node, but the relative viral burden is substantially less than that in early disease and virtually no residual normal nodal architecture remains. (*From* Pantaleo G, Graziosi C, Demarest JF, *et al.*: HIV-1 infection is active and progressive in lymphoid tissue during the clinically latent stage of disease. *Nature* 1993, 362:355–358; with permission.)

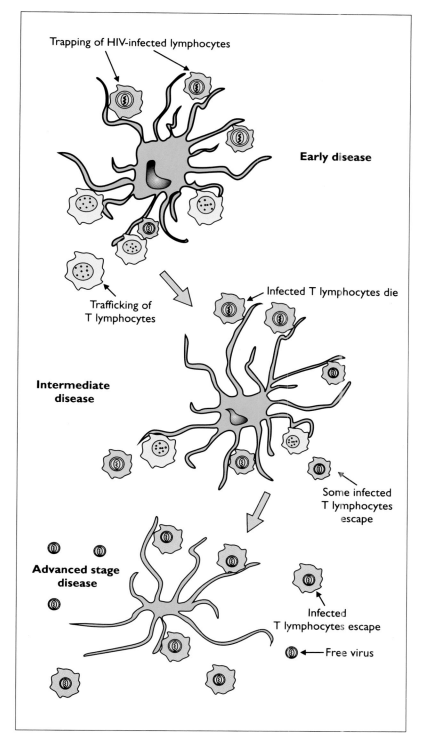

Trapping of HIV-infected lymphocytes

Early disease

Trafficking of T lymphocytes

Infected T lymphocytes die

Intermediate disease

Some infected T lymphocytes escape

Advanced stage disease

Infected T lymphocytes escape

Free virus

FIGURE 2-38 Lymph node destruction. The follicular dendritic cell in the lymph node serves as a filter for circulating lymphocytes. In early disease, most T lymphocytes are uninfected, yet the close proximity of infected and uninfected cells results in enhanced opportunity for the infection of new cells. As the disease progresses, many of the infected cells trapped by the follicular dendritic cell die, and the organization of the lymph node deteriorates, resulting in a higher proportion of infected circulating T lymphocytes and higher viral burden in the plasma. (*Figure adapted from* Fauci AS: Multifactorial nature of human immunodeficiency virus disease: Implications for therapy. *Science* 1993, 262:1011–1018; with permission.)

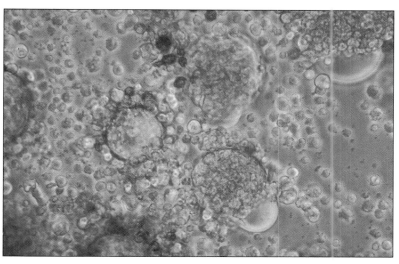

FIGURE 2-39 Syncytium formation. As HIV infection progresses, the phenotype of the predominant viral species may change from a virus that does not cause clumping of cells in tissue culture (non-synctium-inducing virus NSI), to a virus that readily causes syncytium formation (SI phenotype). Certain cell lines are more susceptible to syncytium induction, such as the MT2 cell or, as depicted here, the Sup T1 cell. Note the confluence of infected cells into ballooning syncytia throughout the tissue culture. Although the conversion from NSI to SI phenotype has been associated with more rapid disease progression, the actual role that an SI phenotype virus plays in causing a more rapid decline of CD4+ cell counts remains unclear.

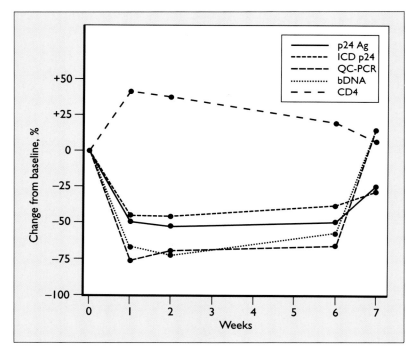

FIGURE 2-40 Virologic response to antiretroviral therapy. Nucleoside antiretroviral therapy has been shown to increase survival and delay disease progression. The application of surrogate markers, such as the CD4+ count, p24 antigen, and viral RNA markers of QC-PCR and bDNA, are beginning to be used to determine the relative activity of antiretroviral drugs. This figure depicts the percent change from baseline over 6 weeks when zidovudine therapy is initiated. Therapy is stopped at week 6, and the patient receives no antiretroviral therapy between weeks 6 and 7. Note the dynamic decrease in viral burden as measured by QC-PCR and bDNA within 1 week of therapy and a sharp rebound after withholding drug for just 1 week. Also, note the strong concordance between the decrease in viral burden as measured by plasma RNA values and the reciprocal increase in CD4+ cell counts.

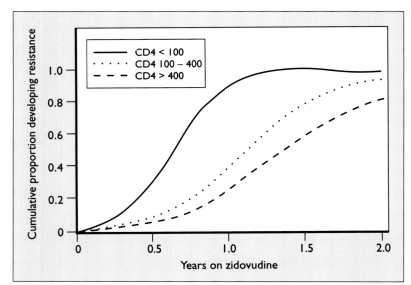

FIGURE 2-41 Development of antiretroviral resistance. One limitation to antiretroviral therapy is the development of resistant strains of HIV, which leads to reduced effectiveness of the drugs. Resistance occurs more rapidly and more profoundly among individuals who have lower CD4+ counts than those with intermediate or early infection. These data suggest that resistance occurs more rapidly in patients with advanced disease due, at least in part, to more rapid viral turnover and a less effective immune response. (*From* Richmann DD, Grimes JM, Lagakos SW, *et al.*: Effect of stage of disease and drug dose on zidovudine susceptability of isolates of human immunodeficiency virus. *J Acquir Immune Defic Syndr* 1990, 3:743–746; with permission.)

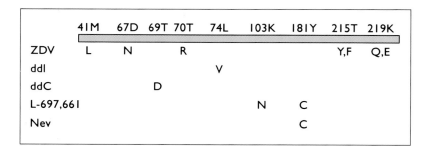

FIGURE 2-42 Resistance-conferring mutations have been identified for virtually all antiretroviral agents in clinical practice. Amino acid changes at positions 41, 67, 70, 215, and 219 confer resistance to zidovudine, whereas mutations at amino acid 74 lead to reduced susceptibility to didanosine (ddI). Changes at amino acid 69 have been associated with reduced susceptibility to zalcitibine (ddC). The nonnucleoside reverse transcriptase inhibitors L-697,661 and nevirapine (Nev) have shown marked changes in susceptibility when amino acid changes occur in position 103 and 181 (L-697,661) or positions 181, 188, and 190 (nevirapine).

SELECTED BIBLIOGRAPHY

Hahn BH: Viral Genes and Their Products. *In* Broder S, Merigan TC, Bolognesi D (eds): *Textbook of AIDS Medicine*. Baltimore: Williams & Wilkins; 1994:21–44.

Saag MS: AIDS Testing: Now and in the Future. *In* Sande MA, Volberding PA (eds): *The Medical Management of AIDS*. 4th ed. Philadelphia: W.B. Saunders; 1994, in press.

Moss AR, Bacchetti P: Natural History of HIV Infection. *AIDS* 1989, 3:55–61.

CHAPTER 3

Host Response

Hedy Teppler
G. Diego Miralles
Kent J. Weinhold

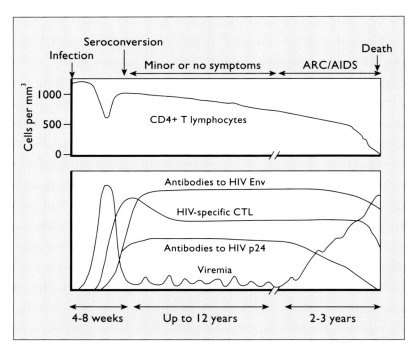

FIGURE 3-1 Natural history of HIV infection and the immune response. Acute HIV infection is associated with a steep but transient decrease in the number of circulating CD4+ T cells, followed by a slower gradual loss over many years of latent disease. Initial viremia leads to seeding of virus throughout the body. With the development of immune responses to the virus, especially HIV-specific cytotoxic T cells (CTL), there is containment of the plasma viremia. HIV-specific antibodies are detectable only after the viremia has declined, suggesting that control of the viremia is due to the cytotoxic effector cells, rather than antibodies. Antibodies to HIV envelope are detectable within months after the acute infection and their levels remain elevated, whereas anti-p24 antibody levels decline in later stages of disease. The period of clinical latency may last 12 years or longer, during which few or no symptoms are present. Viremia during the clinical latency is at a low or undetectable level, although active viral replication persists within lymphoid tissue. Changes in the immune response and/or the virus itself lead to a resurgence of viral replication and viremia, progressive immune dysfunction, and the clinical signs and symptoms of HIV disease. (*Adapted from* Weiss RA: How does HIV cause AIDS? *Science* 1993, 260:1273–1279; with permission.)

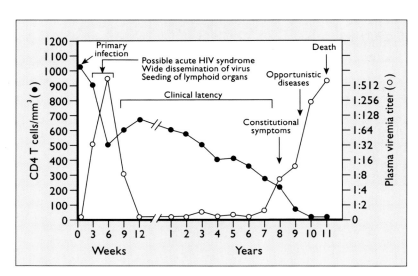

FIGURE 3-2 Typical clinical course of HIV infection. After initial infection with HIV, there is wide dissemination of virus and seeding of lymphoid tissues throughout the body, accompanied by a transient decline in CD4+ T-lymphocyte counts. This decline may be associated with the acute HIV illness. With the onset of the immune response, plasma viremia declines dramatically. During the period of clinical latency, there are few or no symptoms and low levels of virus detectable by quantitative culture. However, despite low levels of viremia, viral RNA may be detected at this and all stages of infection. Ultimately, viral replication escapes the control of the immune system. Increasing viremia is associated with decreasing CD4+ T-lymphocyte counts and progressive immune dysfunction. This leads to the constitutional symptoms of AIDS-related complex (ARC) and later to the opportunistic diseases characteristic of AIDS. (*From* Pantaleo G, Graziosi C, Fauci AS: The immunopathogenesis of human immunodeficiency virus infection. *N Engl J Med* 1993, 328:327–335; with permission.)

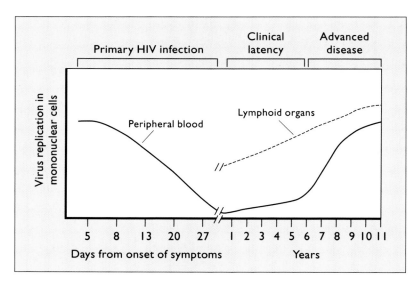

FIGURE 3-3 HIV replication in lymphoid tissue vs peripheral blood. In primary HIV infection and advanced disease, high level of viremia is present. However, during the period of clinical latency, little or no virus is detectable by culture of the peripheral blood, yet active viral replication continues in lymphoid tissues at all stages of disease. (*Adapted from* Fauci AS: Multifactorial nature of human immunodeficiency virus disease: Implications for therapy. *Science* 1993, 262:1011–1018; with permission.)

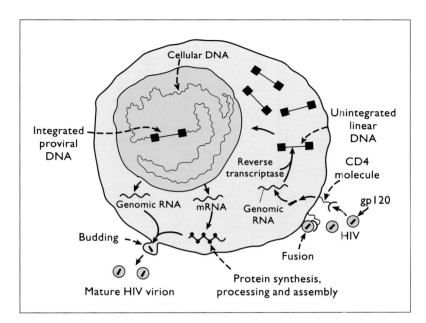

FIGURE 3-4 The life cycle of HIV. HIV infection of a susceptible cell proceeds in a series of steps, including viral attachment and entry, reverse transcription, integration, activation, protein synthesis, processing, assembly, and budding. Many of these steps are potential targets for antiviral therapy. HIV replication results in subsequent dissemination of virus to many tissues and organs. (*From* Fauci AS: The human immunodeficiency virus: Infectivity and mechanisms of pathogenesis. *Science* 1988, 239:617; with permission.)

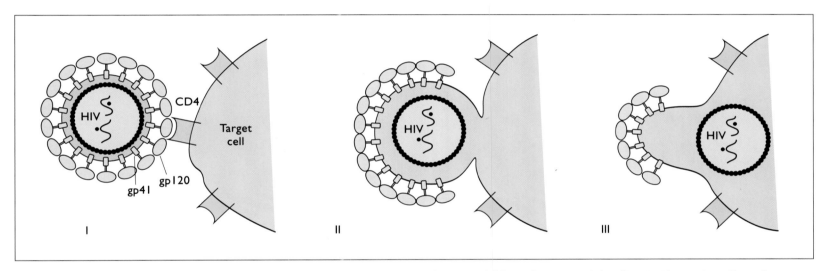

FIGURE 3-5 CD4 receptor for HIV entry. HIV gains entry to CD4+ cells in a two-step process. The viral envelope component gp120 first binds with cell CD4, followed by fusion, which involves the viral glycoprotein gp41. The CD4–gp120 interaction has a greater binding affinity than the interaction of CD4 with its natural ligand, the class II major histocompatibility complex (MHC) molecule. After entry of the viral capsid into the cell, the subsequent steps of the viral life cycle proceed, leading to the maturation of new virions. With translation and posttranslational processing, viral proteins are expressed on the surface of the infected cell, which may allow recognition of infected cells by the effector mechanisms of host defense. (*Adapted from* Levy J: HIV pathogenesis and long-term survival. *AIDS* 1993, 7:1402, with permission.)

A. CD4+ cells infected by HIV
CD4+ T lymphocytes Monocyte/macrophages Microglia in CNS Follicular dendritic cells

B. Other cell types reportedly infected by HIV	
Langerhans' cells of the skin Megakaryocytes Astrocytes and oligodendro- cytes Endothelial cells Colorectal cells	Cervical cells Retinal cells Renal epithelia Pulmonary macrophages Transformed B cells

FIGURE 3-6 Cell types infected by HIV. **A** and **B**, The majority of the cell types demonstrated to be infected *in vivo* with HIV are CD4+ (*panel 6A*), but certain CD4- cell types have been infected *in vitro* (*panel 6B*). Microglia are of monocyte/macrophage lineage and are CD4+. CD4- cells are infected via alternate entry receptors, such as galactosyl ceramide (Gal-C), Fc receptors, and complement receptors. The significance of these findings is as yet uncertain. In some cases, tissue monocyte/macrophages may have been the infected cell type. This suggests that infected blood monocytes may transport the infection to various tissues as the cells migrate and differentiate into fixed tissue macrophages.

IMMUNE RESPONSE TO HIV

Humoral immune response

Binding antibodies
Neutralizing antibodies
  Type-specific
  Group-specific
Antibodies with role in ADCC
  Protective
  Pathogenic
Enhancing antibodies

FIGURE 3-7 Humoral immune response. Antibodies to HIV usually appear within 2–12 weeks of primary infection and are directed toward products of *gag, pol,* and *env* genes, as well as to smaller regulatory proteins. Binding antibodies are useful for diagnosis of HIV infection but do not have a defined role in host defense. Potentially protective antibodies are neutralizing antibodies, which may be type- or group-specific, and those which assist in antibody-dependent cellular cytotoxicity (ADCC), in which antibodies cooperate with cellular effectors to eliminate infected cells. However, because ADCC may kill uninfected cells, these antibodies are potentially pathogenic as well (*see* Fig. 3-13). Levels of antibodies that mediate ADCC are highest in the early stages of HIV infection. Enhancing antibodies are also potentially pathogenic, because they can facilitate cell entry via an alternate entry mechanism and lead to increased viral replication.

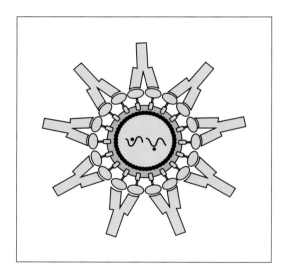

FIGURE 3-8 Neutralizing antibodies. Neutralizing antibodies are defined *in vitro* as antibodies that inhibit the infectivity of HIV by interacting with the viral envelope. Group-specific antibodies are capable of neutralizing many viral strains, whereas type-specific antibodies neutralize only a given strain. For vaccine development, it would be optimal to elicit group-specific neutralizing antibodies to confer protection against many strains of HIV.

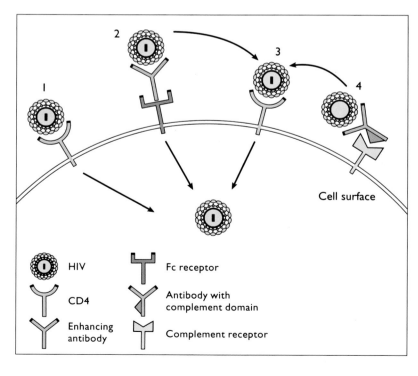

FIGURE 3-9 Enhancing antibodies. Conventionally, HIV infects cells by binding directly to CD4 (*1*). However, antibodies that enhance infection have been identified in flavivirus infections. At defined concentrations (usually subneutralizing levels), these antibodies allow entry of virus into cells by an alternate receptor-mediated mechanism, such as the Fc or complement receptor, so that infection (and possibly viral replication) is greater in the presence of antibody than in its absence. In the case of HIV, enhancing antibodies have been reported that utilize the Fc and complement receptors for entry (*2* and *4*, respectively). Alternatively, it has been proposed that these alternate receptors simply facilitate entry by shuttling bound virus to nearby CD4 molecules for entry (*3*). However, these findings have been observed only *in vitro*, and their significance in the pathogenesis of HIV infection is unknown. (*Adapted from* Bolognesi D: Do antibodies enhance the infection of cells by HIV? *Nature* 1989, 340:431–432; with permission.)

Cellular immune response

Antigen-specific effector cells
  CD4+ T-helper lymphocytes
  CD4+ class II MHC-restricted CTL
  CD8+ class I MHC-restricted CTL
  CD8+ T-cell–mediated suppression
Nonspecific effector cells
  Antibody-dependent cellular cytotoxicity
  Natural killer cells

Figure 3-10 Cellular immune response. Of the HIV-specific T-cell responses, CD4+ helper and cytotoxic T cells have been described, but their significance is unclear. It appears that CD8+ cytotoxic T cells (CTL) play an important role in the containment of viral burden. CD8+ CTL have been demonstrated *in vivo* in peripheral blood, lung, and cerebrospinal fluid, and their activity declines in the later stages of HIV disease. CD8+ viral suppressor T cells have been demonstrated to inhibit viral replication *in vitro* through the production of soluble factors that have not been characterized. This activity is not major histocompatibility complex (MHC)-restricted. Antibody-dependent cellular cytotoxicity (ADCC) refers to the ability of natural killer cells, which are not MHC-restricted or antigen-specific, when in the presence of anti-HIV antibodies, to bind to and kill HIV-infected target cells *in vitro*. Natural killer cells alone also have the ability to kill HIV-infected target cells *in vitro*.

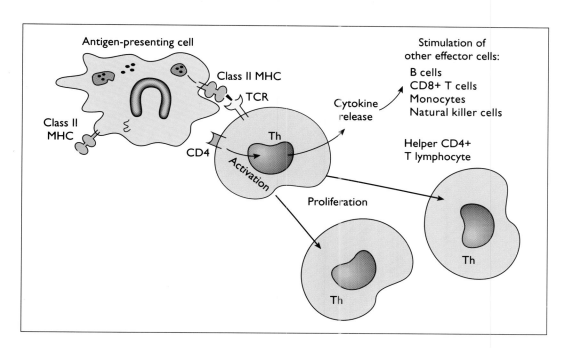

Figure 3-11 CD4+ T-helper responses. Antigen-presenting cells present antigen in the context of the MHC class II molecule to CD4+ T cells. The CD4+ T-helper cell (Th) response plays a central role in regulating cellular and humoral immunity. This response leads to proliferation and cytokine secretion, which may stimulate other effector cells, including CD4+ and CD8+ T lymphocytes, B lymphocytes, natural killer cells, and monocytes. (TCR—T-cell receptor.)

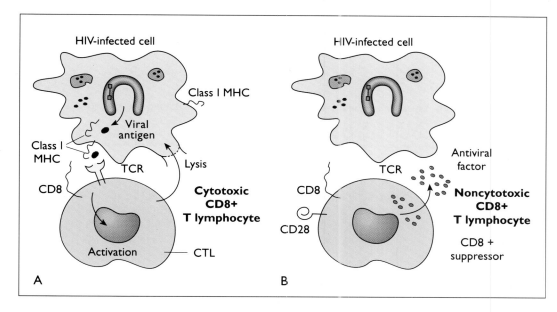

Figure 3-12 CD8+ T-cell responses. CD8+ T cells may inhibit HIV by two mechanisms. **A,** Direct killing of HIV-infected cells by HIV-specific cytotoxic T lymphocytes (CTL) occurs when these cells recognize HIV antigen presented by infected cells in the context of the MHC class I molecule and then cause lysis. **B,** In the second mechanism, noncytotoxic "viral suppressor" CD8+ T lymphocytes inhibit HIV replication in infected cells by the secretion of soluble suppressor factors. These suppressor factors have been shown to operate at the level of viral transcription but otherwise have not been well characterized. This interaction is not MHC-restricted and is mediated by CD8+ T cells, which also bear the CD28 antigen. This antiviral suppression does not lead to suppression of CD4+ T-cell activation or proliferation. (TCR—T-cell receptor.)

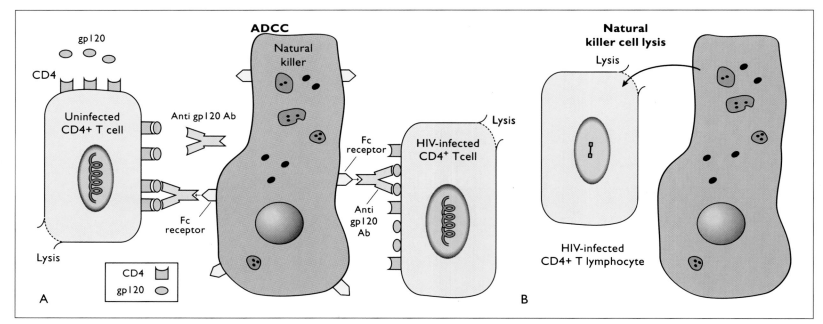

FIGURE 3-13 Natural killer cell responses. **A**, Antibody-dependent cellular cytotoxicity (ADCC) is a form of cellular immunity mediated by natural killer cells. HIV-specific antibodies can form complexes with whole virions or, as illustrated, with envelope components of HIV. These HIV components, such as gp120, may be expressed on the surface of an infected cell (*right cell*) or, in soluble form, may bind to the surface of an uninfected CD4⁺ cell (*left cell*). Natural killer cells effect cell lysis when their surface Fc receptors bind to the constant Fc portion of these antibodies. Therefore, although the antibody responsible is HIV-specific, the effector cell is not. Because ADCC can kill both infected and innocent bystander uninfected cells, its effect may be protective or pathogenic. **B**, Natural killer cells also can kill HIV-infected cells in the absence of antibody.

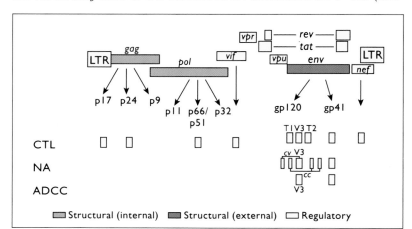

FIGURE 3-14 Antigenic determinants recognized during HIV-1 infection. Cytotoxic T lymphocytes (CTL) from infected patients recognize numerous determinants encoded by *env*, *gag*, and *pol* structural genes as well as within *vif* and *nef* regulatory elements. Neutralizing antibodies (NA) are directed against several envelope determinants including the principal neutralizing domain within the third hypervariable region (V3) and gp120 as well as several conformational conserved (cc) and variable (cv) epitopes. Neutralization determinants have also been identified within gp41. Antibody-dependent cellular cytotoxicity (ADCC) is specific for multiple epitopes within both gp120 and gp41. (*From* Karzon DT: Preventive vaccines. *In* Broder S, Merigan TC, Bolognesi (eds): *Textbook of AIDS Medicine*. Baltimore: Williams and Wilkins; 1994:671; with permission.)

HIV-INDUCED IMMUNE DEFECTS

CD4⁺ T-cell abnormalities

CD4⁺ T-cell numerical decline
 ↓ proliferative response to mitogens
 ↓ secretion of cytokines
Intrinsic CD4⁺ T-cell defects
 ↓ response to recall antigens (early)
 ↓ response to alloantigens (mid)
 ↓ response to mitogens (late)
 ↓ expression of IL-2 receptor
Aberrant cytokine secretion
  ↓ production of IFN-γ, IL-2
  ↑ production of IL-4, IL-10

FIGURE 3-15 HIV-induced CD4+ T-cell defects. HIV infection results in multiple abnormalities of CD4⁺ T-cell function, even before cell numbers decline. These abnormalities include a hierarchical loss of proliferative responses to antigen, alloantigen, and mitogen over the course of infection, as well as abnormal patterns of cytokine secretion. (IL—interleukin; IFN—interferon.)

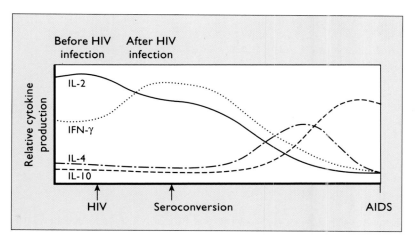

FIGURE 3-16 CD4⁺ T-cell cytokine production. *In vitro* studies of CD4⁺ cells from patients with HIV infection suggest that the usual pattern of cytokine secretion is altered by infection. Before HIV infection, interleukin-2 (IL-2) and interferon-γ (IFN-γ) are the predominant cytokines produced, and relatively little IL-4 and IL-10 are made. In early disease, less IL-2 and IFN-γ are produced, and later their production falls even further, whereas IL-4 and IL-10 production increases. It is possible that other immune cells are partially responsible for these changes in cytokine production, because other immune cells can produce cytokines (*eg*, macrophages in the case of IL-10). (*Figure from* Levy J: HIV pathogenesis and long-term survival. *AIDS* 1993, 7:1402; with permission. Clerici M, Shearer GM: A Th1 to Th2 switch is a critical step in the etiology of HIV infection. *Immunol Today* 1993, 14:107–111.)

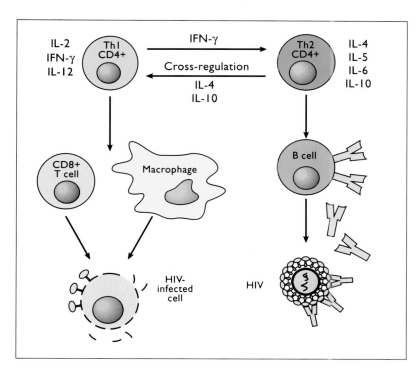

FIGURE 3-17 Th1 and Th2 type responses. T-helper subset populations Th1 and Th2 have been identified in animals and humans based on the pattern of cytokines secreted after stimulation *in vitro*. In this model, the Th1 subset favors a cellular immune response by secreting cellular activators, such as IL-2, IFN-γ, and IL-12. The Th2 subset favors a humoral response, including IL-4, IL-5, IL-6, and IL-10, and causes activation of B cells leading to antibody formation. A recent hypothesis proposes a competitive balance between these subsets based on the change in patterns of cytokine production in cells of patients with HIV infection. This model suggests that the Th1-predominant pattern favoring cellular immunity is normal and perhaps protective, whereas a Th2-predominant pattern develops in association with progressive of HIV disease and may be predictive of disease progression. It may be possible to influence the type of Th response by administering cytokines that favor the Th1 phenotype (IL-2 or IL-12), inhibiting cytokines that favor the Th2 phenotype (IL-4 and IL-10), or using vaccine strategies to elicit Th1 rather than Th2 responses. (*Figure adapted from* Cohen J: T cell shift: Key to AIDS therapy? *Science* 1993, 262:175, with permission. Clerici M, Shearer GM: A Th1 to Th2 switch is a critical step in the etiology of HIV infection. *Immunol Today* 1993, 14:107–111.)

CD8⁺ T-cell abnormalities

Decreased class I MHC-restricted CTL (including HIV-specific responses)
Expression of activation markers, such as HLA-DR, CD38
Loss of IL-2 receptor (CD25) expression
Loss of clonogenic potential

FIGURE 3-18 CD8⁺ T-cell abnormalities. Although CD8⁺ T-cell numbers may increase in the early stages of HIV infection, functional abnormalities are present, including increased expression of activation markers and impaired effector function. Some of these abnormalities may be related to a lack of CD4⁺ T-cell help.

B-cell abnormalities

Chronic B-cell activation
  Spontaneous B-cell proliferation
  Polyclonal hypergammaglobulinemia
Intrinsic defect in antigen- and mitogen-induced B-cell proliferation
Decreased numbers of circulating B cells
Activation and clonal deletion of VH3⁺sIg⁺ cells
Increased Epstein-Barr virus related B-cell lymphomas

FIGURE 3-19 B-cell abnormalities. B cells are not infected with HIV *in vivo* with HIV, but their functional abnormalities include spontaneous proliferation, resulting in the commonly observed hypergammaglobulinemia. Despite chronic activation, there is impairment of the B-cell response to antigenic and mitogenic stimulation. These abnormalities are due in part to dysregulation of cytokines that stimulate B cells, such as IL-4, IL-5, IL-6, and IL-10.

Monocyte/macrophages in HIV infection

Infected via CD4 receptor
Noncytopathic infection
Potential resevoir for HIV
Potential vehicle for dissemination of HIV to brain, lung, and
  bone marrow

FIGURE 3-20   Role of monocyte/macrophages in HIV infection. Monocyte/macrophage infection occurs via the CD4 receptor, which is expressed on the cell membrane, although in smaller quantities than on the CD4+ T lymphocyte. Infection does not cause cell lysis, which allows for viral persistence. Because monocytes migrate from the blood into tissue and differentiate into tissue macrophages, they may serve as a vehicle for transporting virus to a variety of tissues. Normal cell numbers and many normal functions are maintained.

Monocyte/macrophages functions in HIV infection

Functions intact
  Phagocytosis
  Superoxide production
  Antimicrobial activity (to certain pathogens)
  Antifungal activity
  Antitumor activity
  Tumor necrosis factor production
  ADCC

Functional defects
  Chemotaxis
  C3R-mediated clearance, FcR function
  IL-1 production, oxidative burst response
  Antigen presentation
  Antimycobacterial activity

FIGURE 3-21   Monocyte/macrophage function in HIV infection. Monocytes and macrophages are both antigen-presenting cells that stimulate T- and B-lymphocyte responses. In addition, they are primary effector cells in the cellular immune system and have an extensive array of antimicrobial, antifungal, chemotactic, and secretory functions, including the production of proinflammatory cytokines. Many of these functions are preserved in HIV infection, whereas others are impaired. Some of these abnormalities may be due to the lack of appropriate inductive signals, such as IFN-γ, from CD4+ T cells. Perhaps among the most important of functional impairments is the decreased killing of mycobacteria, such as *Mycobacterium tuberculosis* and *M. avium* complex, both of which are intracellular pathogens that cause opportunistic disease in HIV infection. There are conflicting reports regarding the effect of HIV on peripheral blood dendritic cells (DC), which are more potent antigen-presenting cells than monocyte/macrophages. Certain studies suggest HIV infection leads to impairment of the ability of peripheral blood DC to stimulate T cell responses to antigens, whereas others have found no effect or increased DC function after exposure to HIV. (C3R—complement 3 receptor; FcR—Fc receptor.)

Monocyte/macrophage lineage cells in other systems

System	Infected cell types
CNS	Macrophages
	Microglia
Bone marrow	Monocyte precursors
Lungs	Alveolar macrophages

FIGURE 3-22   Monocyte/macrophages in other systems. In the central nervous system (CNS), most infected cells are of monocyte lineage, *ie*, macrophages or resident microglia. Direct HIV infection of these cells or the immune response to HIV may be related to the development of meningoencephalitis, dementia, and other CNS syndromes seen in HIV infection. HIV infection of monocyte precursors in the bone marrow may have a role in hematologic abnormalities. In addition, infected pulmonary alveolar macrophages have been demonstrated *in vivo*. Cells of monocytic origin may contribute to pathogenesis either by transmission of virus to various tissue sites and/or by aberrant cytokine production.

Natural killer cell defects

Not infected by HIV
Some subsets of NK cells diminished in early disease
Impaired function, even in early disease
Addition of IL-2 *in vitro* improves defective NK cell activity

FIGURE 3-23   Natural killer cell defects. Natural killer (NK) cell function is abnormal in HIV infection, with decreased cell numbers in some subsets. Impaired function, possibly due to certain viral products that suppress NK activity, leads to decreased cell killing and persistence of HIV-infected cells. Also, cytokine dysregulation may contribute to NK cell dysfunction, because the addition of IL-2 can augment NK cell function *in vitro*. NK cells from HIV-infected individuals can mediate ADCC activity.

Proposed mechanisms of CD4⁺ T-cell depletion and dysfunction

Direct viral cytopathic effects
Single cell killing
Syncytium formation
HIV-specific immune responses (HIV-specific CTL, ADCC, NK cell killing)
Autoimmune mechanisms
Anergy
Superantigen-induced deletion or anergy
Apoptosis
Thymic dysfunction

FIGURE 3-24 CD4+ T-cell defects. Multiple mechanisms have been proposed for CD4⁺ T-cell depletion and dysfunction. Direct destruction of cells due to HIV infection and viral-specific immune responses has been described, at least *in vitro*. Autoimmunity may include gp120 mimicry of MHC class II epitopes or anti–class II antibodies, which have cross-reactivity to gp120. Anergy refers to a state of CD4⁺ T cells that is quiescent and nonresponsive but viable; this anergic state may be due to inappropriate cell signaling by the CD4–gp120 interaction. Superantigen stimulation can lead to anergy or deletion of multiple subsets of CD4⁺ T cells, either by lytic infection or apoptosis. Apoptosis is a mechanism of programmed cell death or cell suicide, which may be induced by a number of signaling mechanisms including the gp120–CD4 interaction, cytokines such as tumor necrosis factor-α (TNF-α) and superantigen or standard recall antigen. The thymus plays an important role in normal T-cell development, and within the thymus, immature CD4⁺ T-cell precursors are susceptible to HIV infection. Thymic dysfunction therefore contributes to CD4⁺ T-cell depletion either by direct HIV infection of precursor cells or by failure of T-cell development due to an abnormal thymic microenvironment.

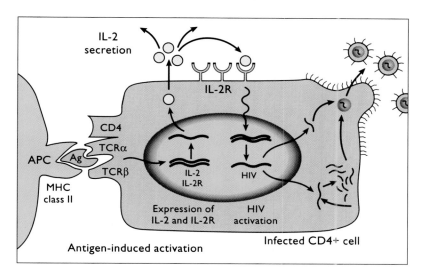

FIGURE 3-25 Single cell killing of CD4+ T cells. Antigen induction of HIV-infected CD4⁺ cells can activate viral replication and lead to cell lysis. The interaction of antigen (Ag) presented by an antigen-presenting cell (APC) in the context of MHC class II with the T-cell receptor (TCR) and CD4 molecule results in cellular activation. As a result, synthesis of IL-2 and IL-2 receptor (IL-2R) is upregulated. Cellular activation results in induction of HIV replication with production of new virions. CD4⁺ cell lysis and dysfunction may result from toxic or suppressive effects of virus and viral products on the infected cell, or lysis of the cell can be due to viral budding and release.

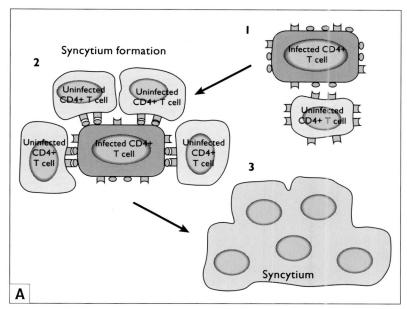
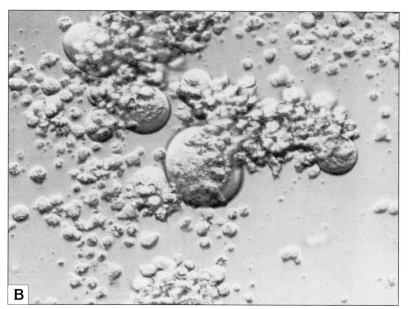

FIGURE 3-26 Syncytium formation. **A,** Syncytium formation is an *in vitro* phenomenon, which describes the fusion of an infected cell with uninfected cells. This is generally regarded as a two-step process: the initial binding of gp120 to CD4 (*shown*), followed by the interaction between the fusogenic domain of gp41 and the plasma membrane of the uninfected cell (*not shown*). It is unclear whether this occurs *in vivo*, but viral strains that cause syncytium formation *in vitro* have been associated with increased virulence

and disease progression *in vivo*. **B,** Light micrograph demonstrates formation of syncytia between HIV-infected cells and uninfected cells. The large cells resembling balloons are the syncytia. (*Photograph courtesy of* Dr. Cecil Fox, Bethesda MD. Fauci AS: Immunology of AIDS and HIV infection. *In* Mandell GL, Douglas RG Jr, Bennett JE (eds): *Principles and Practice of Infectious Diseases*, 3rd ed. New York: Churchill Livingstone; 1990: 1049; with permission.)

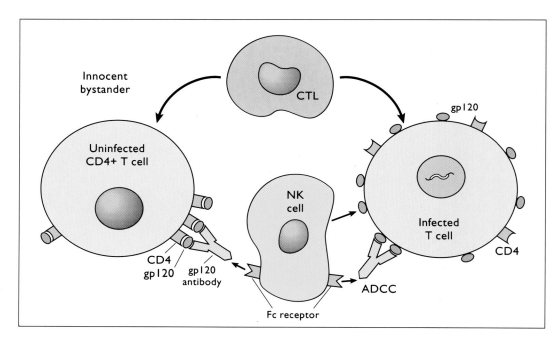

FIGURE 3-27 HIV-specific immune responses can kill uninfected and infected cells. Immune responses to HIV, such as CTL and NK cell-mediated killing with or without ADCC, may confer protection by eliminating HIV-infected cells. However, these mechanisms may also contribute to immune dysfunction by eliminating uninfected "innocent bystander" cells. Soluble viral components, such as gp120, bind to CD4 molecules on infected or uninfected T cells and monocytes, and viral products or whole virus may bind to dendritic cells and follicular dendritic cells. HIV-specific antibody binds to these complexes and assists in the destruction of these cells by ADCC. Alternatively, HIV-specific CTLs have been shown to lyse uninfected CD4+ cells that have bound soluble gp120. All these responses have been demonstrated *in vitro*, but their significance *in vivo* is unclear.

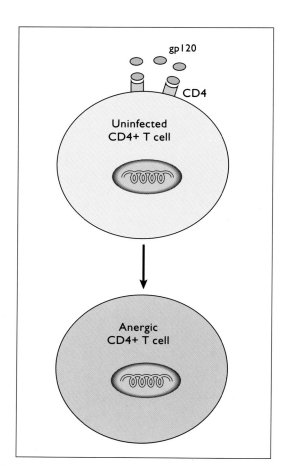

FIGURE 3-28 gp120-Induced anergy. The interaction of gp120 with CD4 may result in the induction of anergy, or a nonresponsive state of the CD4+ T cell, leading to dysfunction without cell lysis.

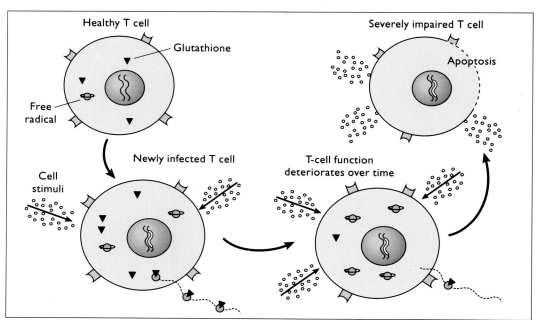

FIGURE 3-29 Gluthathione depletion and free radical damage. In one model of HIV immunopathogenesis, apoptosis may be set in action by the uncontrolled action of free radicals. Free radicals are highly reactive oxygen metabolites, which are produced in cells in the course of the normal inflammatory response, *eg*, on stimulation by tumor necrosis factor (TNF) secreted from macrophages acutely infected with HIV. Gluthathione is an antioxidant molecule normally present in cells, which neutralizes free radicals before they can cause cellular damage and transports them out of the cell. As CD4+ T-cell function declines, continued production of free radicals overwhelms the glutathione stores of the cell. The cell, no longer protected from free radical damage, cannot respond normally to stimuli. Ultimately, the severely damaged cell becomes nonfunctional, may signal other cells to die, and may itself commits suicide by apoptosis. (Staal FJP, Anderson MT, Staal GEJ, *et al.*: Redox regulation of signal transduction: Tyrosine phosphorylation and calcium influx. *Proc Natl Acad Sci U S A* 1994, 91(9):3619–3622. *Figure adapted from* Angier N: Theory tested on why body's defenses go haywire in AIDS. *New York Times* 1993; May 3:C3.)

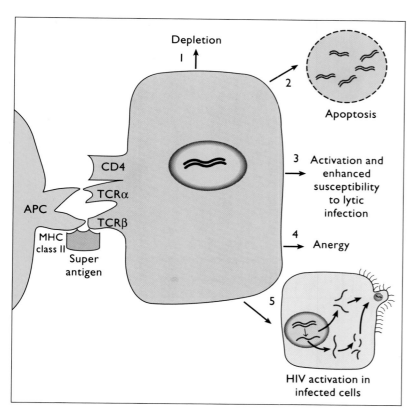

FIGURE 3-30 Superantigen-mediated CD4+ T-cell depletion or anergy. Conventional antigens bind in the groove of the MHC class II molecule and interact with the highly variable regions of the T-cell receptor (TCR). Superantigens are usually products of microbial origin, which can bind at separate, more conserved sites on the T-cell receptor. In this way, superantigen can bind to and activate large subsets of CD4+ T cells (1% to 10% of the total) in comparison with conventional antigenic peptides, which bind only a very small proportion ($< 1/10^5$) of total T cells. It has been hypothesized that this superantigen interaction may lead to the preferential depletion of certain CD4+ T-cell subsets, either directly (1), as a second signal in apoptosis (2), through activation of the cells and subsequent enhanced susceptibility to lytic HIV infection (3), or through induction of anergy (4). None of these mechanisms requires the cell to be HIV-infected. Alternatively, the effect of superantigen on infected CD4+ cells may be to activate viral replication with subsequent cell lysis (5). (APC—antigen-presenting cell.)

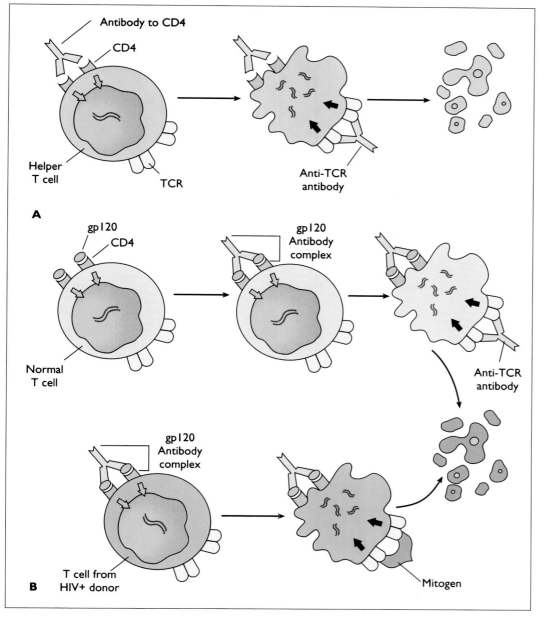

FIGURE 3-31 HIV-induced apoptosis. **A,** Apoptosis is a particular mechanism of cell death in which the cell actively fragments and is phagocytosed without associated inflammatory responses. The hallmarks of apoptosis are DNA fragmentation and formation of membrane blebs. During immunologic development, apoptosis allows the clonal deletion of autoreactive T cells in the thymus. Apoptosis also has been postulated as one of the mechanisms responsible for CD4 cell depletion in HIV infection. In normal CD4 cells, simultaneous activation of CD3 and CD4 receptors leads to T-cell proliferation. However, when CD4 activation precedes T-cell receptor (TCR) stimulation, the T cell undergoes cell death by apoptosis. (Gougeon ML: *Science* 1993, 260:1269–1270. *Figure adapted from* Cohen JJ: Apoptosis: The physiologic pathway of cell death. *Hosp Pract* 1993, (Dec):35; with permission.) **B,** If T cells from uninfected individuals are crosslinked with gp120/anti-gp120 and then their TCR is stimulated by anti-TCR, mitogens, or superantigens, they also undergo apoptosis. The same findings have also been confirmed in peripheral blood mononuclear cells from HIV-infected individuals. These findings suggest that circulating CD4 cells from infected individuals are primed to die by apoptosis upon signals that would otherwise mediate proliferation. The role of this process in CD4 cell depletion *in vivo* remains unknown. (Ameisen JC: Programmed cell death and AIDS: From hypothesis to experiment. *Immunol Today* 1992, 13:388.)

Skin test anergy in HIV infection

DTH skin responses depend on disease stage
Loss of DTH responses is an independent predictor of disease
  progression
Underlying mechanisms
    gp120 coating of CD4 receptors
    Downregulation of CD4 in infected cells
    Cytokine dysregulation

FIGURE 3-32 An anergic state is characterized by lack of delayed-type hypersensitivity responses (DTH) and represents a qualitative abnormality of CD4 cells. It is one of the earliest clinical signs of immune dysfunction during HIV infection, and it has been shown to be an independent predictor of progression to AIDS. The underlying mechanisms probably involve gp120-CD4 interactions and the downregulation of the CD4 receptor in cells infected by HIV. (Blatt SP, *et al.*: Delayed-type hypersensitivity skin testing predicts progression to AIDS in HIV infected patients. *Ann Intern Med* 1993, 119:177–184.)

CYTOKINES IN HIV INFECTION

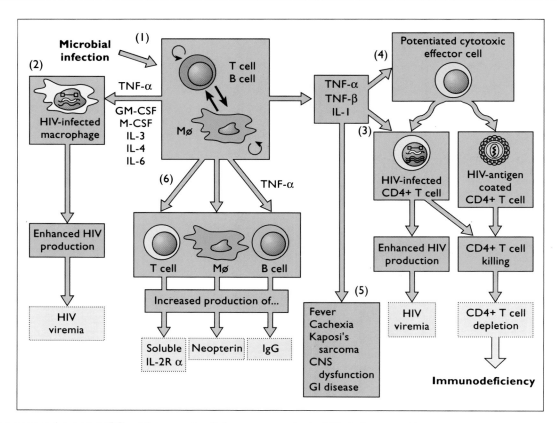

FIGURE 3-33 Cytokine networks and AIDS pathogenesis. Cytokines involved in regulating the immune system may contribute to the pathogenesis of AIDS, as outlined in this model. (*1*) Following microbial infection (*eg*, with HIV), cytokines such as tumor necrosis factors-α and -β (TNF-α, TNF-β), granulocyte-macrophage colony-stimulating factor (GM-CSF), macrophage colony-stimulating factor (M-CSF), and interleukins (IL) 1, 3, 4, and 6, which have stimulatory effects on HIV, are produced by various types of cells, including T cells, B cells, and macrophages (Mø). In addition, IL-2 (induced by IL-1) activates T cells, which will produce TNF-α, TNF-β, IL-3, and IL-4. (*2*) In macrophages infected by HIV, the cytokines TNF-α, GM-CSF, M-CSF, IL-3, IL-4, and IL-6 stimulate HIV production, which may increase the HIV burden in the body. (*3*) In T cells infected by HIV, TNF and IL-1 enhance the replication of HIV, and TNF selec-

tively kills infected cells, causing HIV viremia and CD4+ T-cell depletion. (*4*) TNF and IL-1 potentiate cytotoxic effector functions, which will kill not only infected CD4+ T cells but also uninfected CD4+ T cells coated with HIV antigen, resulting in CD4+ T-cell depletion and immunodeficiency. (*5*) Increased TNF levels can result in clinical features observed in AIDS. (*6*) TNF-α augments the production of soluble IL-2Rα; immunoglobulin G (IgG) and neopterin from T cells, B cells, and macrophages, respectively. Production of neopterin and IgG may be stimulated by IFN-γ and IL-6, respectively, which are induced by TNF-α. Laboratory findings detected in the development of AIDS are represented by the *green boxes*. (*Adapted from* Matsuyama T, Kobayashi N, Yamamoto N: Cytokines and HIV infection: Is AIDS a tumor necrosis factor disease? *AIDS* 1991, 5:1405–1417, with permission.)

Cytokine regulation of HIV expression and regulation

Cytokine	Target cells(s)	Effect
Bulk supernatant	T,M	↑
IL-1	T,M	↑
IL-2	T	↑
IL-3	M	↑
IL-4	T,M	↑↓
IL-6	M	↑
IL-10	M	↑↓
IL-13	M	↓
TNF-α, TNF-β	T,M	↑
TGF-β	T,M	↑↓
M-CSF	M	↑
GM-CSF	M	↑
IFN-α, IFN-β	T,M	↓
IFN-γ	M	↑↓

FIGURE 3-34 Cytokine regulation of HIV expression. Many cytokines have been tested under a variety of *in vitro* conditions for their effect on HIV replication and expression. The most potent inducers of HIV replication are tumor necrosis factor (TNF)-α, TNF-β, and interleukin (IL)-6. Potent inhibitors of HIV replication are interferon (IFN)-α and IFN-β. Several cytokines, such as IL-4 and transforming growth factor (TGF)-β, have dual effects on HIV expression. Target cells, either T lymphocytes (T) or monocytes/macrophages (M), are cell types in which the effect was observed. (*Adapted from* Fauci AS: Multifactorial nature of human immunodeficiency virus disease: Implications for therapy. *Science* 1993, 262:1011–1018; with permission. Matsuyama T, Kobayashi N, Yamamoto N: Cytokines and HIV infection: Is AIDS a tumor necrosis factor disease? *AIDS* 1991, 5:1405–1417.) (M-CSF—monocyte colony-stimulating factor; GM-CSF—granulocyte-macrophage colony-stimulating factor.)

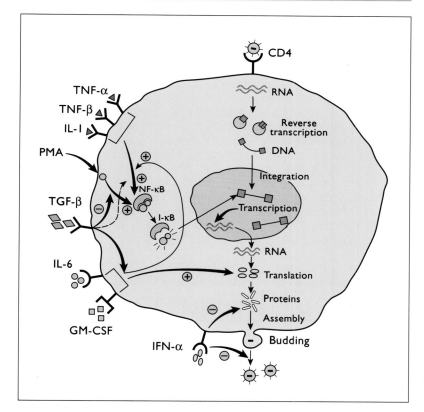

FIGURE 3-35 Mechanisms of cytokine effects on HIV expression. The effects of several cytokines on transcriptional and posttranscriptional control of HIV expression are shown. Among cytokines with HIV-inducing effects, TNF-α, TNF-β, and IL-1, each interacting with a specific receptor, can activate HIV expression by acting on the transcriptional factor, nuclear factor-κB (NF-κB), to dissociate from its inhibitor (I-κB). The activated NF-κB ordinarily acts on cellular genes to initiate gene transcription in uninfected cells, but in infected cells it interacts with specific binding sites in the HIV long terminal repeat (LTR) promoter region to activate HIV expression (*see* Fig. 3-34). GM-CSF also can enhance viral replication in macrophages but may require a binding site in the HIV LTR that is distinct from the NF-κB binding site. IL-6 appears to enhance viral expression by a posttranscriptional effect. Among cytokines with inhibitory effects on HIV expression, transforming growth factor β (TGF-β) may suppress viral expression by inhibiting transcription and can downregulate the activating effects of stimuli such as IL-6 and phorbol myristate acetate (PMA, a mitogen). IFN-α inhibits viral protein synthesis in acutely infected cells as well as viral assembly and budding in chronically infected cells. (Poli G, Fauci AS: The effect of cytokines and pharmacologic agents on chronic HIV infection. *AIDS Res Hum Retroviruses* 1992, 8:191–197. *Figure adapted from* Fauci AS: The immune response to HIV infection. *In* Paul W (ed): *Fundamentals of Immunology*, 3rd ed. New York: Raven Press; 1993:1386; with permission.)

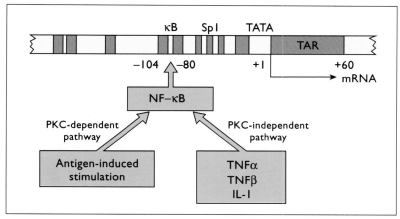

FIGURE 3-36 Transcription factor NF-κB and HIV replication. The regulatory region in the long terminal repeat (LTR) region of the HIV genome contains NF-κB binding sites (κB). NF-κB is a DNA-binding protein located in the cytosol, which is usually complexed to its inhibitor I-κB. In the course of normal immune activation, stimulation of the cell by various agents such as antigens, mitogens, and cytokines causes induction of the activated form of NF-κB, which requires its dissociation from I-κB. In infected cells, activated NF-κB binds to specific regions in cellular genes and results in the initiation of gene transcription. However, the HIV LTR also contains NF-κB binding sites, and in HIV-infected cells, binding of NF-κB to κB can activate HIV replication. By distinct pathways, antigens, mitogens (such as phorbol ester), and cytokines (such as TNF-α, TNF-β, and IL-1) can activate NF-κB and may induce HIV expression. (PKC—protein kinase C.) (*Adapted from* Matsuyama T, Kobayashi N, Yamamoto N: Cytokines and HIV infection: Is AIDS a tumor necrosis factor disease? *AIDS* 1991, 5:1405–1417, with permission.)

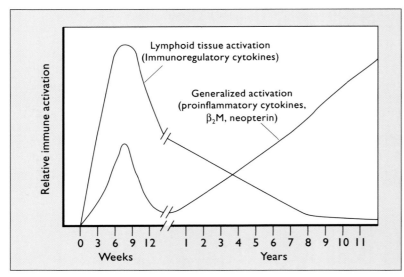

Possible clinical manifestions of cytokine dysregulation

Clinical manifestation	Possible cytokine mediators
Kaposi's sarcoma	IL-1, IL-6, TNF-α
CNS disorders	TNF-α, IL-1, TGF-β, others?
Chronic diarrhea and malabsorption	TNF-α, others?
HIV wasting	TNF-α, others?
Aphthous ulceration of upper GI tract	TNF-α
HIV-associated nephropathy	??

FIGURE 3-37 Immune (cytokine) activation in HIV infection. Increasing evidence suggests that immune (cytokine) activation plays a role in HIV immunopathogenesis. Early in infection, there is activation of the lymphoid tissues (*see* Figs. 3-38 and 3-39) and a detectable but limited period of generalized immune activation. Later in the course of infection, the lymphoid activation wanes as lymphoid tissue is gradually destroyed, but at this stage there is progressive generalized immune activation with increased proinflammatory cytokine secretion (such as TNF-α), and increased serum markers of immune activation (such as neopterin and β_2-microglobulin, β_2M). Certain proinflammatory cytokines, including TNF-α, may have a role as endogenous cofactors in activation of HIV replication. (*Adapted from* Fauci AS: Multifactorial nature of human immunodeficiency virus disease: Implications for therapy. *Science* 1993, 262:1016, with permission.)

FIGURE 3-38 Possible clinical manifestations of cytokine dysregulation. Various cytokines may be involved in producing the clinical features observed in AIDS. Kaposi's sarcoma cells *in vitro* grow in response to cytokines such as IL-1, IL-6, and TNF-α. Marked CNS dysfunction may occur in the absence of major histopathologic changes, and some *in vitro* models suggest IL-1, TNF-α, TGF-β, and other cytokines or neuropeptides may be involved in CNS dysfunction. Chronic diarrhea and malabsorption are often observed in the absence of demonstrable pathogens and may be due to direct HIV infection of gut cells or to cytokines elaborated by infected gut macrophages or lymphoid tissue cells. HIV wasting may occur in the absence of diarrhea, is associated with markers of immune activation, and may be mediated by proinflammatory cytokines. Aphthous ulceration of the gastrointestinal (GI) tract occurs without demonstrable pathogens. Early reports suggest inhibitors of TNF-α, such as thalidomide, may be useful in the treatment of these ulcers, indicating a possible pathogenic role for TNF-α in this syndrome. Preliminary reports suggest HIV-associated nephropathy may be responsive to treatment with corticosteroids, which are broadly immunosuppressive, suggesting there is an immune or inflammatory component to this syndrome as well.

SYSTEMIC AND TISSUE CONSEQUENCES OF HIV INFECTION

Thymic dysfunction in HIV infection

Thymic precursor cells express CD4 and can be infected
T-cell maturation disrupted
Thymic epithelial cell maturation and function disrupted
Thymic microenvironment destroyed

FIGURE 3-39 Thymic dysfunction. Although a functional thymus is commonly assumed *not* to be necessary in adults, thymic function may be particularly important in the setting of HIV infection in which progressive T-cell depletion occurs. The profound thymic destruction that occurs in late stages of HIV infection may impair the ability to generate functional T cells, even if adequate thymic precursor cells are present.

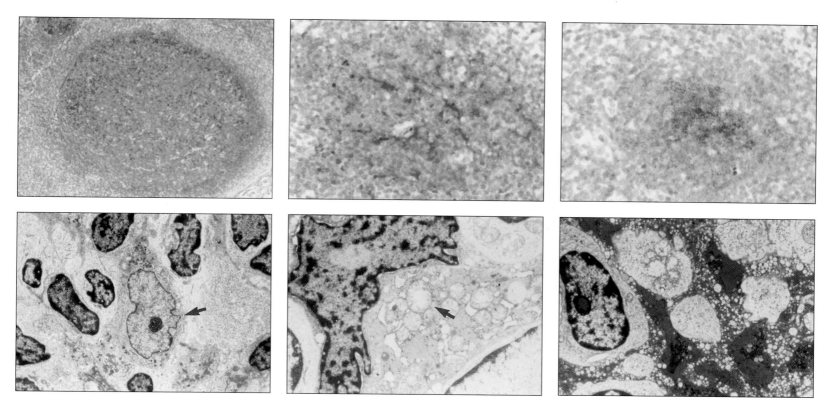

FIGURE 3-40 Lymphoid architecture during the course of infection. Early in the course of HIV infection, there is lymphoid hyperplasia, followed later in disease by gradual involution and destruction of lymphoid architecture. These changes are associated with the destruction of the follicular dendritic cell (FDC) network. Electron microscopy (in the *lower panels*) shows healthy FDCs in early disease with subsequent dissolution of the FDC as disease progresses. Consequently, the abilities of the FDC to present antigen in the generation of an immune response and to trap virus are impaired. With the loss of this trapping function, virus spills over into the circulation and viremia increases. (*From* Fauci A: Multifactorial nature of human immunodeficiency virus disease: Implications for therapy. *Science* 1993, 262:1011–1018; with permission.)

Lymphoid tissue in HIV pathogenesis
Reservoir of virus
Site of viral replication at all stages of disease
Trapping or filtering effect of free virions by FDC
Site for exposure of susceptible cells to large quantities of virus

FIGURE 3-41 The role of lymphoid tissue in HIV pathogenesis. The importance of lymphoid tissue in HIV pathogenesis centers on its role in the clearance of virus in primary infection, in generation of immune responses, and also as a reservoir for virus and site of active viral replication throughout the course of disease. Follicular dendritic cells (FDCs) are critical in trapping virus and in generating the immune response, but they also may play a role in transmission of HIV to susceptible T cells, which traffic through the lymphoid tissue. (Pantaleo G, Graziosi C, Demarest JF, *et al.*: HIV infection is active and progressive in lymphoid tissue during the clinically latent stage of disease. *Nature* 1993, 362:355–358. Embretson J, Zupancic M, Ribas JL, *et al.*: Massive covert infection of helper T lymphocytes and macrophages by HIV during the incubation period by AIDS. *Nature* 1993, 362:359–362.)

A. Autoimmune manifestations: clinical
Arthritis
Reiter's syndrome
Systemic lupus erythematosus-like syndrome
Rash
Glomerulonephritis
Cottonwool spots
Polymyositis
Sjögren's syndrome
Anemia
Thrombocytopenia
Coagulopathies
Neuropathies and possibly other neurologic manifestations
Diminished glutathione levels

FIGURE 3-42 Autoimmune manifestations in HIV infection. A wide variety of autoimmune manifestations are apparent in HIV disease. **A,** The clinical syndromes are reported in up to 50% of persons with HIV infection, especially early in disease when there is immune activation. These include syndromes typical of other autoimmune rheumatologic and hematologic diseases. Diminished glutathione levels may lead to increased risk of oxidative damage due to a number of potential insults. *(continued)*

B. Autoimmune manifestations: Laboratory

Antibodies to lymphocytes, platelets, and neutrophils
Antinuclear and anticytoplasmic antibodies
Antibodies to albumin, immunoglobulin, and other serum
  proteins
Antibodies to MHC class II molecules may interfere with anti-
  gen-presenting cell function
Lupus anticoagulant

FIGURE 3-42 *(continued)* **B.** Laboratory abnormalities, however, can be present even in the absence of clinical autoimmune disease. Abnormal antibody production is common and is likely due to the generalized activation of B lymphocytes.

IMMUNE-BASED THERAPIES

Rationale for immune-based therapies

Restore immune competence
Inhibit host-derived cofactors of viral replication
Inhibit host mechanisms that cause complications of HIV
  disease
Improve immunity for treatment/prevention of opportunistic
  complications

FIGURE 3-43 Rationale for immune-based therapies. Given the modest benefit afforded by currently available antiretroviral therapies and the increasing understanding of the immunopathologic aspects of HIV disease, interest is growing in therapeutic strategies that target the immune response. These therapies include the obvious aim of restoring overall immune function and of interrupting the host-derived mechanisms, which may contribute to viral pathogenesis, but also novel strategies to improve immunity for the treatment and prevention of opportunistic infections and neoplasms that characterize AIDS.

Restore immune competence

Improve CD4+ T-cell numbers
  Inhibit apoptosis
  Restore glutathione levels
Cellular therapies
  Transplantation of stem cells
  Transfusion of peripheral blood lymphocytes
  Ex vivo expansion of lymphocyte subsets
Replace deficient cytokines, *ie*, IL-2, IFN-γ
Enhance anti-HIV immune response
  Passive or active immunization

FIGURE 3-44 Restoring immune competence. A number of strategies are being investigated for their potential to restore overall immune competence. These interventions broadly aim to improve cell numbers and function and include inhibition of CD4+ T-cell destruction, replacement of lymphoid cells by stem cell or mature lymphocyte transfer, expansion of CD8+ cytotoxic T cells (unselected or HIV-specific) *ex vivo* with subsequent transfer back to the patient, replacement of deficient cytokines such as IL-2, and enhancement of anti-HIV immunity by passive or active immunization.

Targeting host factors in pathogenesis

Inhibit host-derived cofactors of viral replication
  Inhibit proinflammatory cytokines, such as TNF-α and IL-6
    In primary infection
    As stimulated by opportunistic infections (such as tuberculosis)
Inhibit host mechanisms that cause complications of HIV
  disease
Role for immunosuppression?

FIGURE 3-45 Targeting host factors in pathogenesis. It may be possible to interrupt the cycle in which HIV infection causes expression of host-derived factors that may stimulate viral replication, such as the proinflammatory cytokines. Possible agents under study include pentoxifylline and thalidomide, which inhibit TNF-α. The presence of immune activation in HIV infection and the utility of corticosteroids in certain conditions, such as moderate to severe *Pneumocystis carinii* pneumonia, immune thrombocytopenia, severe aphthous ulcers, and rheumatologic complications of HIV disease, suggest a possible role for immunosuppression in some situations.

Improve immunity for treatment/prevention of opportunistic complications

Passive immunization
  Specific neutralizing antibodies
Active immunization
  Better adjuvants(?)
Cytokines
Cytokine antagonists

FIGURE 3-46 Improve immunity for treatment or prevention of opportunistic infections. In general, treatment of opportunistic infections in HIV infection must be continued for life because cure or sterilization is not achieved and recurrences are frequent despite current maximal therapy. It may be possible to use immune-based therapeutics to improve their treatment or prevention. Strategies under investigation include the adjunctive use of specific neutralizing monoclonal antibodies in the treatment of certain opportunistic infections such as cytomegalovirus disease, the identification of better adjuvants for active immunization, and the adjunctive administration of cytokines or cytokine inhibitors in certain opportunistic processes.

Vaccines in HIV infection

Issues
  Prophylactic vs therapeutic
  Neutralizing antibody vs CTL responses
Active immunization
  Recombinant HIV subunit
  Live vector HIV subunit(s)
  Attenuated HIV
  Killed HIV
Passive immunization with anti-HIV Ig

FIGURE 3-47 Vaccines in HIV infection. In light of alarming epidemiologic trends worldwide, an effective immunization strategy for HIV is urgently needed. Vaccines are being studied both for prevention of new infections and as therapy to improve anti-HIV immune responses after infection has occurred. It is not yet clear whether the generation of neutralizing antibodies or HIV-specific cytotoxic T lymphocytes (CTLs), or both, is needed for effective immunization in either the prophylactic or therapeutic strategies. Another major issue concerns the timing of large-scale studies, primarily for prophylactic vaccines, given the lack of a single clear "best" strategy at present. A number of vaccine preparations being studied include recombinant HIV subunits such as gp120 or gp160 vaccines produced in various prokaryotic and eukaryotic expression systems (eg, bacteria, yeast, insect, and mammalian cells). Live vector vaccines, which express one or more HIV subunits are also being studied, alone and in combination with recombinant subunit vaccines. Attenuated vaccine is a particular problem in light of HIV's nature as a retrovirus, which must integrate into the host genome; this approach has the potential risk of HIV reverting to a pathogenic phenotype after integration has occurred. Killed whole virus is another strategy in clinical trials. In addition, passive immunization of infected persons with anti-HIV immunoglobulin (Ig) has suggested some clinical benefit.

SELECTED BIBLIOGRAPHY

Rosenberg Z, Fauci A: Immunology of HIV Infection. *In* Paul WE (ed): *Fundamental Immunology*, 3rd ed. New York: Raven Press, 1993.

Weiss R: How does HIV cause AIDS? *Science* 1993, 260:1273–1279.

Matsuyama T, Kobayashi N, Yamamoto N: Cytokines and HIV infection: Is AIDS a tumor necrosis factor disease? *AIDS* 1991, 5:1405–1417.

Pantaleo G, Graziosi C, Fauci AS: The immunopathogenesis of human immunodeficiency virus infection. *N Engl J Med* 1993, 328:327–335.

Fauci A: Multifactorial nature of human immunodeficiency virus disease: Implications for therapy. *Science* 1993, 262:1011–1018.

CHAPTER 4

Classification and Spectrum

Gregory J. Dore
David A. Cooper

SURVEILLANCE DEFINITIONS

A. 1982 Surveillance definition of AIDS

Cryptosporidiosis
Pneumocystis carinii pneumonia
Strongyloidosis
Toxoplasmosis
Candidiasis (esophageal)
Cryptococcosis
Mycobacterium avium
Mycobacterium kansasii
Cytomegalovirus
Herpes simplex virus
Progressive multifocal leukoencephalopathy
Kaposi's sarcoma
Lymphoma

B. 1985 Revised surveillance definition of AIDS

The above diseases plus the following with laboratory evidence of HIV infection:
    Histoplasmosis (disseminated)
    Candidiasis (bronchi, lungs)
    Isosporiasis
    Non-Hodgkin's lymphoma
    Kaposi's sarcoma (in persons ≤ 60 yrs)
    Lymphoid interstitial pneumonitis (children)

C. 1987 Revised surveillance definition of AIDS

All of the above diseases plus the following with laboratory evidence of HIV infection:
    Multiple pyogenic bacteria (children < 13 years)
    Coccidioidomycosis
    HIV encephalopathy
    Mycobacterium tuberculosis (extrapulmonary)
    HIV wasting syndrome
    Recurrent salmonella bacteremia
Presumptive diagnoses of:
    Candidiasis (esophageal)
    Cytomegalovirus (eyes)
    Kaposi's sarcoma (all)
    Mycobacteriosis (disseminated)
    Pneumocystis carinii pneumonia
    Toxoplasmosis (brain)
    Lymphoid interstitial pneumonitis

D. 1993 Revised surveillance definition of AIDS

All of the above diseases plus the following with laboratory evidence of HIV infection:
    Mycobacterium tuberculosis (lungs)
    Recurrent bacterial pneumonia
    Invasive cervical cancer

FIGURE 4-1 Surveillance definition of AIDS. The first cases of AIDS were identified in 1980 and reported in the medical literature in 1981. In 1982, a case definition was published by the US Centers for Disease Control (CDC). This surveillance definition required the reliable diagnosis of a disease that was moderately predictive of a defect in cell-mediated immunity in the absence of known causes of immune deficiency. **A.** The diseases that were indicative of AIDS were specified and included ten opportunistic infections, two cancers, and progressive multifocal leukoencephalopathy. (Centers for Disease Control: Update on acquired immunodeficiency syndrome (AIDS)—United States. *MMWR* 1982, 31:507–508, 513–514.) **B, C,** and **D.** Since the isolation in 1983–84 of HIV-1, the causative virus of AIDS, there have been three revisions of the surveillance definition of AIDS, in 1985, 1987, and 1993, with the addition of several further diseases. (Centers for Disease Control: Revision of the case definition of acquired immunodeficiency syndrome for national reporting—United States. *MMWR* 1985, 34:373–375. Centers for Disease Control: Revision of the CDC surveillance case definition for acquired immunodeficiency syndrome. *MMWR* 1987, 36(suppl 1S):3S–15S. Centers for Disease Control: 1993 Revised classification system for HIV infection and expanded surveillance case definition for AIDS. *MMWR* 1992, 41[RR-17]:1–19.)

A. 1993 Revised classification system for HIV infection and expanded AIDS surveillance case definition for adults and adolescents ≥ 13 years of age*

	Clinical categories		
CD4⁺ T-cell categories	**(A)** Asymptomatic, acute (primary) HIV, or PGL	**(B)** Symptomatic, not (A) or (C) conditions	**(C)** AIDS-indicator conditions
(1) ≥ 500/μL	A1	B1	C1
(2) 200–499/μL	A2	B2	C2
(3) < 200/μL AIDS-indicator T-cell count	A3	B3	C3

*HIV-infected persons classified in A3, B3, or any C cell meet the 1993 AIDS surveillance case definition.

B. Category B conditions

Bacillary angiomatosis
Candidiasis, oropharyngeal (thrush)
Candidiasis, vulvovaginal
Cervical dysplasia
Cervical carcinoma *in situ*
Constitutional symptoms
Hairy leukoplakia, oral
Herpes zoster (shingles)
Idiopathic thrombocytopenic purpura
Listeriosis
Pelvic inflammatory disease
Peripheral neuropathy

FIGURE 4-2 1993 revised classification for HIV/AIDS. The CDC in 1993 revised the classification system for HIV infection to emphasize the clinical importance of the CD4⁺ T-lymphocyte count in the categorization of HIV-related clinical conditions. Consistent with the 1993 revised classification system, the CDC also expanded the AIDS surveillance case definition to include all HIV-infected persons who have < 200 CD4⁺ T lymphocytes/μL or a CD4⁺ T-lymphocyte percentage of total lymphocytes of < 14%. This expansion adds three clinical conditions—pulmonary tuberculosis, recurrent pneumonia, and invasive cervical cancer—and retains the 23 clinical conditions in the AIDS surveillance case definition published in 1987 (*see* Fig. 4-1C). **A,** The expanded AIDS surveillance case definition. Persons with AIDS-indicator conditions (category C) as well as those with CD4⁺ T-lymphocyte counts < 20/μL (categories A3 or B3) became reportable as AIDS cases in the United States and territories, effective 1 January 1993 (PGL—persistent generalized lymphadenopathy). **B,** Category B conditions are listed. Category C includes the clinical conditions listed in the AIDS surveillance case definition (*see* Figs. 4-1A–D). (CDC: 1993 revised classification system for HIV infection and expanded surveillance case definition for AIDS among adolescents and adults. *MMWR* 1992, 41[RR-17]:1–19.)

PRIMARY HIV INFECTION

Clinical manifestations of primary HIV-1 infection

General
Fever
Pharyngitis
Lymphadenopathy
Arthralgia
Myalgia
Lethargy/malaise
Anorexia/weight loss

Neuropathic
Headache/retro-orbital pain
Meningoencephalitis
Peripheral neuropathy
Radiculopathy
Brachial neuritis
Guillain-Barré syndrome
Cognitive/affective impairment

Dermatologic
Erythematous maculopapular rash
Diffuse urticaria
Desquamation
Alopecia
Mucocutaneous ulceration

Gastrointestinal
Oral/oropharyngeal candidiasis
Nausea/vomiting
Diarrhea

FIGURE 4-3 Clinical manifestations of primary HIV-1 infection. The main clinical features of primary HIV-1 infection reflect both the lymphocytopathic and neurologic tropism of HIV-1. Patients typically present with an illness of acute onset characterized by fever, lethargy, malaise, myalgias, headaches, retro-orbital pain, photophobia, sore throat, lymphadenopathy, and maculopapular rash. Meningoencephalitis may also occur. The time from exposure to HIV-1 until the onset of the acute clinical illness is typically 2–4 weeks. The clinical illness lasts 1–4 weeks. This acute clinical illness associated with seroconversion for HIV-1 has been reported in 53% to 95% of cases. (Pedersen C, Lindhart BO, Jensen BL, *et al.*: Clinical course of primary HIV infection: Consequences for subsequent course of infection. *BMJ* 1989, 299:154–157. Tindall B, Barker S, Donovan B, *et al.*: Characterization of the acute clinical illness associated with human immunodeficiency virus infection. *Arch Intern Med* 1988, 148:945–949.)

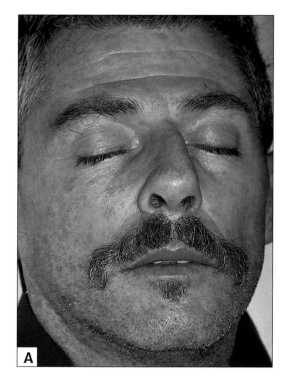

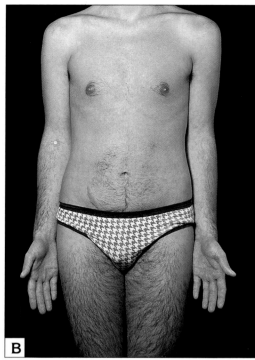

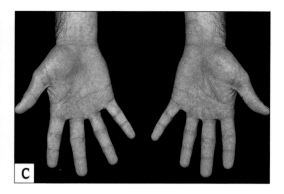

FIGURE 4-4 Characteristic rash in primary HIV-1 infection. The most frequent dermatologic evidence of primary HIV-1 infection is an erythematous, nonpruritic, maculopapular rash. This rash is generally symmetric, with lesions 5–10 mm in diameter. **A, B,** and **C,** It primarily affects the face (*panel 4A*) or trunk (*panel 4B*), but it can also affect the extremities, including the palms (*panel 4C*) and soles, or can be generalized.

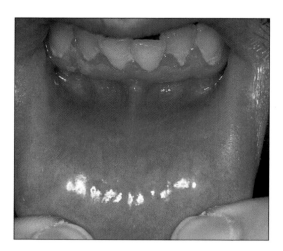

FIGURE 4-5 Mucocutaneous inflammation in primary HIV-1 infection. Mucocutaneous inflammation and ulceration are distinctive features of primary HIV-1 infection. Inflammation of the buccal mucosa and gingiva is common, and ulceration has been reported at these sites as well as the palate and esophagus. The ulcers are generally round or oval and sharply demarcated, with surrounding mucosa that appears normal. (Gaines H, von Sydow, Pehrson PO, *et al.*: Clinical picture of primary HIV infection presenting as a glandular-fever-like illness. *Br Med J* 1988, 297:1363–1368. Hulsebosch HJ, Claessen FAP, van Ginkel CJW, *et al.*: Human immunodeficiency virus exanthem. *J Am Acad Dermatol* 1990, 23:483–486. Rabeneck L, Popovic M, Gartner S, *et al.*: Acute co-infection with human immunodeficiency virus (HIV) and esophageal ulcers. *JAMA* 1990, 263:2318–2332.)

A. Immunologic responses to primary HIV-1 infection

Humoral
Immune complex formation
Neutralizing antibodies
Antibodies that mediate ADCC

Cellular
Lymphopenia (CD4+ and CD8+) followed by lymphocytosis (predominantly CD8+) and inversion of CD4+:CD8+ ratio

Cytokines and cell products
Increased interferon-α
Increased neopterin
Increased β_2-microglobulin

FIGURE 4-6 Immunologic responses to primary HIV-1 infection. Following HIV infection, there is a short but intense period of viral replication, as demonstrated by the ease of viral isolation and high levels of serum HIV p24 antigen. The frequency with which HIV can be isolated decreases following seroconversion, and serum levels of HIV p24 decrease to undetectable levels. This viral clearance is associated with resolution of clinical symptoms and signs. **A,** Increased levels of interferon-α, neopterin, and β_2-microglobulin detected in blood and cerebrospinal fluid reflect activation of the cellular immune system. (ADCC—antibody-dependent cell-mediated cytotoxicity.) *(continued)*

B. Serologic markers in primary HIV infection

HIV p24 antigen
  Appears within 1–18 days of infection
Anti-HIV IgM response
  Appears within 2 weeks of infection
  Peaks at 2–5 weeks
  Undetectable at 3 months

FIGURE 4-6 *(continued)* **B,** In persons with symptomatic primary HIV infection, specific HIV antibodies are usually detectable with the first few weeks of onset of the acute illness. HIV p24 antigen can be detected in both the serum and cerebrospinal fluid in the period prior to seroconversion and has been detected in blood as early as 24 hours after onset of the acute illness. (Albert J, Gaines H, Sonnerborg A, *et al.*: Isolation of human immunodeficiency virus (HIV) from plasma during primary HIV infection. *J Med Virol* 1987, 23:67–73. von Sydow M, Gaines H, Sonnerborg A, *et al.*: Antigen detection in primary HIV infection. *BMJ* 1988, 296:238–240. Cooper DA, Imrie AA, Penny R: Antibody response to human immunodeficiency virus following primary infection. *J Infect Dis* 1987, 115:1113–1118.)

DIFFERENTIAL DIAGNOSIS

Differential diagnoses of primary HIV-1 infection

Epstein-Barr virus mononucleosis
Cytomegalovirus mononucleosis
Toxoplasmosis
Rubella
Viral hepatitis
Secondary syphilis
Disseminated gonococcal infection
Primary herpes simplex virus infection
Other viral infection
Drug reaction

FIGURE 4-7 Differential diagnoses of primary HIV-1 infection. Although originally described as "mononucleosis-like" and still described as such in the CDC classification system of HIV-1 disease, symptomatic primary HIV-1 infection is a distinct and recognizable clinical syndrome. (Centers for Disease Control: Classification system for human T-lymphotropic virus type III/lymphadenopathy-associated virus infection. *MMWR* 1986, 35:334–339. The skin rash associated with primary HIV-1 infection is a valuable differential diagnostic aid. Skin eruptions are rare in patients with Epstein-Barr virus infection (unless antibiotics have been given), toxoplasmosis, and cytomegalovirus infection and do not affect the palms and soles in patients with rubella. Mucocutaneous ulceration is a fairly distinctive finding because it is unusual in most of the other differential diagnoses.

Clinical factors differentiating Epstein-Barr virus (EBV) mononucleosis from primary HIV-1 infection

Primary HIV-1 infection	EBV mononucleosis
Acute onset	Insidious onset
Little or no tonsillar hypertrophy	Marked tonsillar hypertrophy
Enanthema on hard palate	Enanthema on border of both hard and soft palates
Exudative pharyngitis uncommon	Exudative pharyngitis common
Mucocutaneous ulcers common	No mucocutaneous ulcers
Rash common	Rash rare
Jaundice rare	Jaundice (8%)
Diarrhea possible	No diarrhea

FIGURE 4-8 Primary HIV-1 infection vs Epstein-Barr virus (EBV) mononucleosis. Although serologic testing for HIV-1 and EBV usually provides the definitive diagnosis, clinicians should be aware that false-positive tests for heterophile antibodies may occur during primary HIV-1 infection. (Gaines H, von Sydow M, Pehrson PO, Lundbergh P: Clinical picture of primary HIV infection presenting as a glandular fever-like illness. *BMJ* 1988, 297:1363–1368.)

ASSOCIATED CLINICAL CONDITIONS SEEN IN PRIMARY HIV-1 INFECTION

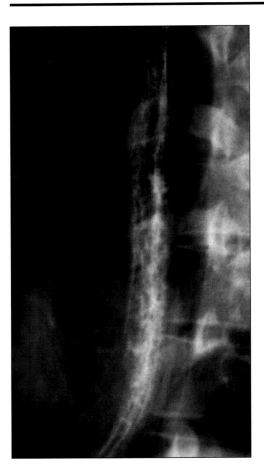

FIGURE 4-9 Esophageal candidiasis. Esophageal candidiasis is one of the opportunistic infections listed in the CDC clinical definition of AIDS and is the most frequently reported opportunistic infection in patients with AIDS after *Pneumocystis carinii* pneumonia. Several cases of esophageal candidiasis in association with primary HIV infection have been reported. In this radiograph, the barium swallow shows loss of the normal mucosal pattern throughout the length of the esophagus, consistent with an erosive esophagitis induced by severe candidal infection. Esophageal candidiasis during primary HIV infection is associated with a transient but severe decrease in the percentage and absolute number of CD4+ cells and with an increase in the absolute number of CD8+ cells. It is important that cases of primary HIV infection are not misdiagnosed as AIDS on the basis of opportunistic infections associated with such transient immunodepression. (Cilla G, Trallero EP, Furundarena JR, *et al.*: Esophageal candidiasis and immunodeficiency associated with acute HIV infection. *AIDS* 1988, 2:399–400. Tindall B, Hing M, Edwards P, *et al.*: Severe clinical manifestations of primary HIV infection. *AIDS* 1989, 3:747–749.)

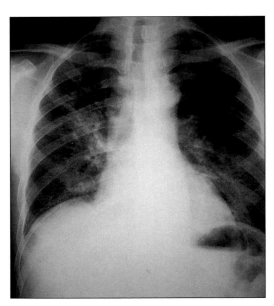

FIGURE 4-10 *Pneumocystis carinii* pneumonia. *P. carinii* pneumonia (PCP) is one of the opportunistic infections listed in the CDC clinical definition of AIDS and the most frequently reported. However, it has also been recently described as developing during symptomatic, primary HIV-1 infection. These cases all occurred within 2 weeks of the onset of symptoms of primary HIV infection and were associated with profound CD4 lymphopenia, but all regained normal CD4+ counts and percentages within 4 months and had been followed for between 29 and 48 months after the episodes of PCP with no signs or symptoms of progression to AIDS. (Vento S, Di Perri G, Garofano T, *et al.*: *Pneumocystis carinii* pneumonia during primary HIV-1 infection. *Lancet* 1993, 324:24–25.) The chest radiograph demonstrates bilateral abnormal shadowing most prominent in the perihilar regions with no evidence of pleural effusions or mediastinal lymphadenopathy. This appearance is consistent with PCP.

SPECTRUM OF HIV DISEASE

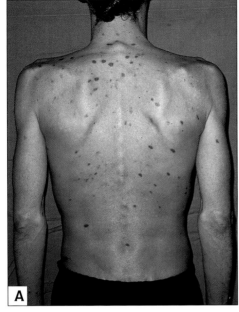
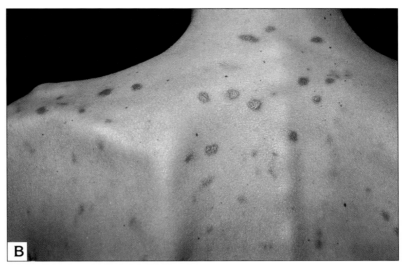

FIGURE 4-11 HIV wasting syndrome. Wasting is an extremely common and almost inevitable consequence of HIV infection. Its causative factors include reduction in nutrient intake, such as through anorexia or malabsorption; disturbances in metabolism, such as protein wasting, fever, and hypermetabolic states; and other medical conditions including endocrine disturbances. The rapid breakdown of protein associated with the development of opportunistic infections and malignancies in AIDS patients is difficult to reverse even with aggressive alimentation including total parenteral nutrition. Nutritional assessment and adequate alimentation, along with evaluation for and management of underlying opportunistic infections and malignancies (such as Kaposi's sarcoma as seen in this patient), are important to minimize loss of muscle mass. Antiretroviral therapy may also have a role in maintenance of weight in the earlier stages of HIV infection. (Kotler DP: *Gastrointestinal and Nutritional Manifestations of Aids.* New York: Raven Press; 1991. *Gastrointestinal and Nutritional Manifestations of AIDS.* New York: Raven Press; 1991. Kotler DP, Tierney AR, Culpepper-Morgan JA, *et al.*: Effect of home total parenteral nutrition upon body composition in patients with AIDS. *JPEN* 1990, 14:454–458.)

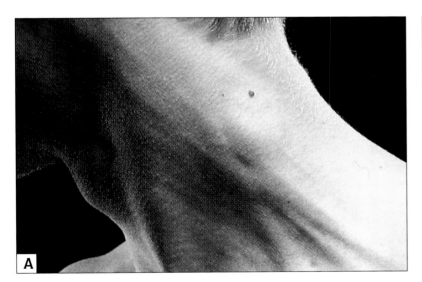
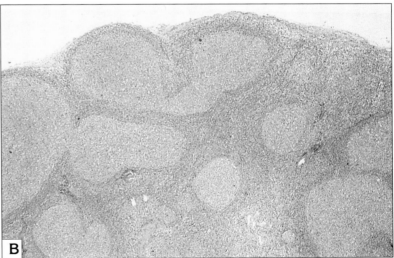

FIGURE 4-12 Lymphadenopathy. Persistent generalized lymphadenopathy (PGL) and its association with progression to AIDS were described prior to the discovery of HIV as their common causal agent. **A,** PGL is defined as palpable lymphadenopathy (lymph node enlargement of ≥ 1 cm) at two or more extrainguinal sites persisting for > 3 months in the absence of a concurrent illness or condition other than HIV infection to explain the findings. It appears that PGL and associated B-cell activation may be caused by the polyclonal B-cell stimulation by infectious agents such as herpesviruses and HIV. **B,** On histologic examination, lymph nodes affected by PGL show extensive follicular hyperplasia, although this finding is seen in lymphadenopathy of other causes as well. *(continued)*

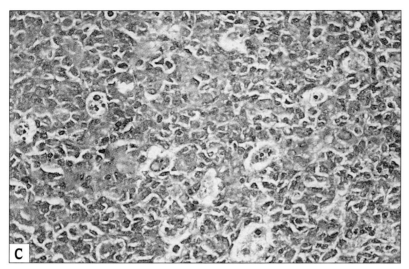

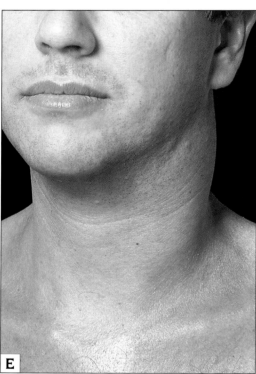

FIGURE 4-12 *(continued)* **C,** On high magnification, the reactive center of a lymph node demonstrates irregularly nucleated small and large lymphoid cells (centrocytes) and blast cells. **D,** As PGL progress, the lymph nodes show follicular depletion, which is considered a poor prognostic sign with rapid progression to AIDS (*all panels*, hematoxylin-eosin stain). **E,** It is important to distinguish the lymphadenopathy of PGL from other causes, such as mycobacterial infection, both typical and atypical (as seen in *panel 12E*); other infections including cytomegalovirus, toxoplasmosis and syphilis; malignancies, in particular non-Hodgkin's lymphoma and Kaposi's sarcoma; and drug reactions. In a patient with either asymmetrical or rapidly expanding lymphadenopathy, causes other than PGL should be considered (Centers for Disease Control: Persistent, generalized lymphadenopathy among homosexual males. *MMWR* 1982, 31:249–250. Centers for Disease Control: Classification system for human T-lymphotropic virus type III/lymphadenopathy-associated virus infections. *MMWR* 1986, 35:334–339. *Panels 12A–D from* Farthing CF, Brown SE, Staughton RCD: *A Colour Atlas of AIDS and HIV Disease*, 2nd ed. London: Wolfe Medical Publications, Ltd; 1988: 29; with permission.)

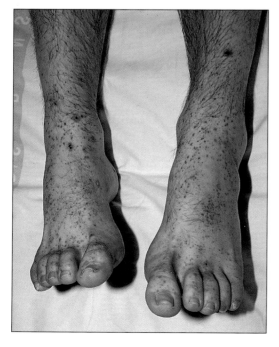

FIGURE 4-13 HIV vasculitis. This patient demonstrates cutaneous vasculitis, which occurred prior to the development of an AIDS-defining illness. A wide range of inflammatory vascular diseases have been described in patients infected with HIV at all stages of the illness. These have included necrotizing arteritis, polyarteritis nodosa, Henoch-Schönlein purpura, and drug-induced hypersensitivity vasculitis. The systemic vasculitis seen in HIV-infected patients most commonly involves the skin, peripheral nerves, skeletal muscles, and central nervous system. (Gherardi R, Belec L, Mhiric C, *et al.*: The spectrum of vasculitis in human immunodeficiency virus-infected patients. *Arthritis Rheum* 1993, 36:1164–1174.)

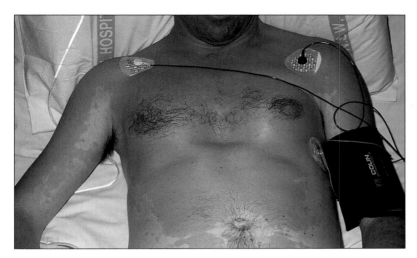

FIGURE 4-14 Adverse drug reactions. A severe adverse reaction developed in this patient following orally administered ciprofloxacin. Patients with HIV infection have a higher incidence of adverse drug reactions than the immunocompetent population. The most common agent implicated is trimethoprim-sulfamethoxazole, due to its widespread use for prophylaxis against *P. carinii* pneumonia and toxoplasmic encephalitis. Reactions to trimethoprim-sulfamethoxazole include an increased incidence of fever, rash, and leukopenia. Cutaneous eruptions vary from a mild maculopapular rash to severe mucocutaneous inflammation and Stevens-Johnson syndrome. Mild gastrointestinal toxicity is probably the most common adverse reaction and is often transient.

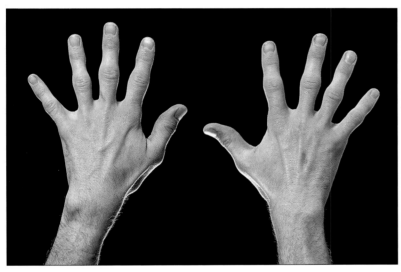

FIGURE 4-15 HIV polyarthritis. A symmetric polyarthritis involving the small joints of both hands developed prior to the onset of an AIDS-defining illness in this patient. In a prospective study, the musculoskeletal system was found to be involved in 70% of patients with HIV infection, with active arthritis developing in 24%. Although arthralgias are the most common manifestation, other associated disorders appear to be reactive arthritis, including Reiter's syndrome, psoriatic arthritis, Sjögren's syndrome, polymyositis, and necrotizing vasculitis. Oligoarthritis affecting the lower limbs appears to be the most common form of arthritis, but an inflammatory polyarthritis in HIV patients has been increasingly recognized in populations such as Africans in Zimbabwe, where rheumatologic disorders are uncommon. (Berman A, Espinoza LR, Diaz JD, *et al.*: Rheumatic manifestations of human immunodeficiency virus infection. *Am J Med* 1988, 85:59–64. Seifert M: *The Rheumatology of HIV Infection* (Topical Reviews, no. 11). Arthritis and Rheumatism Council for Research, Jan 1989. Davis P, Stein M, Latif S, Emmanuel J: HIV and polyarthritis. *Lancet* 1988, i:936.)

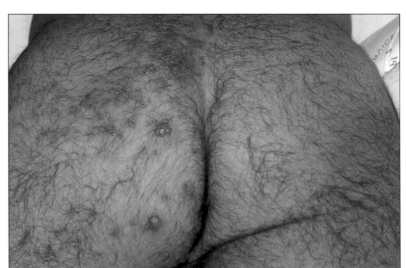

FIGURE 4-16 Herpes zoster. Herpes zoster is common in both the asymptomatic period of HIV disease and in AIDS. Although the course of herpes zoster is usually uneventful, it may be complicated by persistent postherpetic neuralgia and dissemination, both cutaneous and less commonly visceral. HIV-infected patients not only develop herpes zoster more frequently than immunocompetent hosts but also can experience more than one episode in a relatively short period of time, an uncommon occurrence in immunocompetent hosts. Herpes zoster is considered to be a category B condition in the classification system for HIV infection if there are at least two distinct episodes or more than one dermatome is involved. (Melbye M, Grossman RJ, Goedert JJ: Risk of AIDS after herpes zoster. *Lancet* 1987, i:728–730. Ryder JW, Croen K, Kleinschmidt-de Masters BK, *et al.*: Progressive encephalitis three months after resolution of cutaneous zoster in a patient with AIDS. *Ann Neurol* 1986, 19:182–188. Dolin R, Reichman RC, Mazur MH, *et al.*: Herpes zoster and varicella infections in immunosuppressed patients. *Ann Intern Med* 1978, 89:375–388.

SELECTED BIBLIOGRAPHY

Tindall B, Barker S, Donovan B, *et al.*: Characterization of the acute clinical illness associated with human immunodeficiency virus infection. *Arch Intern Med* 1988, 148:945–949.

Albert J, Gaines H, Sonnerborg A, *et al.*: Isolation of human immunodeficiency virus (HIV) from plasma during primary HIV infection. *J Med Virol* 1987, 23:67–73.

Cooper DA, Gold J, Maclean P, *et al.*: Acute AIDS retrovirus infection: Definition of a clinical illness associated with seroconversion. *Lancet* 1985, i:537–540.

Tindall B, Hing M, Edwards P, *et al.*: Severe clinical manifestations of primary HIV infection. *AIDS* 1989, 3:747–749.

Centers for Disease Control and Prevention: 1993 revised classification system for HIV infection and expanded surveillance case definition for AIDS among adolescents and adults. *MMWR* 1992, 41[RR-17]:1–19.

CHAPTER 5

Cutaneous Manifestations

Alvin E. Friedman-Kien

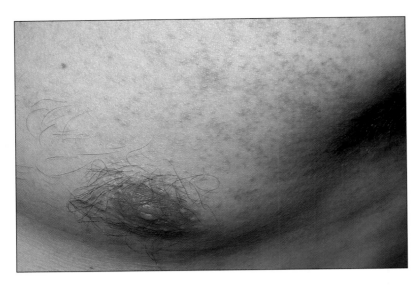

FIGURE 5-1 Acute seroconversion rash of HIV infection. A flulike illness often occurs within 3–8 weeks after exposure to HIV, which is usually associated with a mild morbilliform exanthem. The skin rash is characterized by a generalized erythematous macular and papular eruption, usually involving the trunk and extremities, which may be mildly pruritic. The acute illness of HIV infection may last for a few days to 1 week with spontaneous resolution. The exanthematous rash resembles the eruption seen with other viral illnesses such as rubella or may mimic an allergic drug eruption. In most patients, an asymptomatic latency period ensures for several years after the acute HIV infection subsides, until various HIV-related opportunistic infections or neoplasms develop as the patient becomes progressively immunodeficient.

SUPERFICIAL FUNGAL INFECTIONS OF THE SKIN AND MUCOUS MEMBRANES

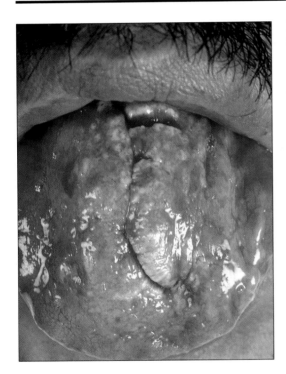

FIGURE 5-2 Candidiasis. "Thrush" (moniliasis), due to *Candida albicans* (yeast, *Monilia*), is one of the most common fungal infections occurring on the tongue and oral mucosa in HIV-infected individuals. This condition is characterized by white to yellowish mucoid patches located on the tongue and buccal, pharyngeal, or gingival mucosa. When candida infection involves the corners of the mouth (cheilitis), fissures and inflammation result. The plaques of "thrush" are easily scraped off with a wood tongue depressor or spoon and, when smeared on a glass slide and stained with KOH, reveal the typical hyphae of *C. albicans*. Candidiasis of the tongue and mucosal surfaces may become severely inflamed with erosions that cause significant discomfort, interfering with eating and speech. Invasive candidiasis of the esophagus is painful and causes great difficulty in swallowing. Antifungal agents such as clotrimazole, amphotericin, ketoconazole, and fluconazole are effective in providing temporary alleviation of this mucosal infection, but it unfortunately tends to recur frequently in the immunocompromised host. Long-term prophylaxis with these drugs is commonly used to prevent thrush and other fungal infections in the HIV-infected host.

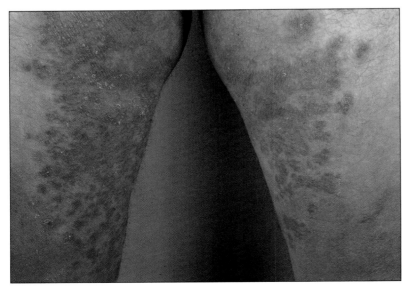

FIGURE 5-3 Candidiasis of the glabrous skin, including the intertriginous areas, is frequently observed with the development of large, itchy, moist, sometimes scaly red areas of inflammation with tiny satellite lesions surrounding the border. The groin, gluteal cleft, and axillae are frequently infected.

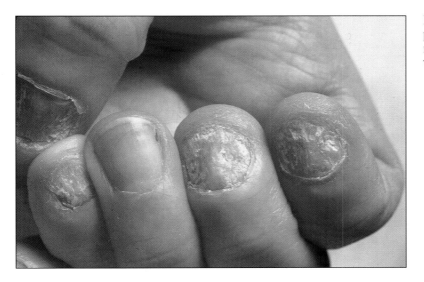

FIGURE 5-4 Candidal infection of the periungual tissue, known as paronychia, is characterized by swelling, erythema, and tenderness, sometimes with a purulent discharge around the nails. When the nails are involved, they become brittle, thickened, and opaque.

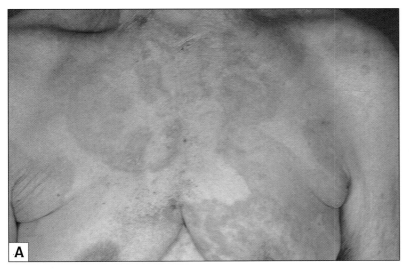

A

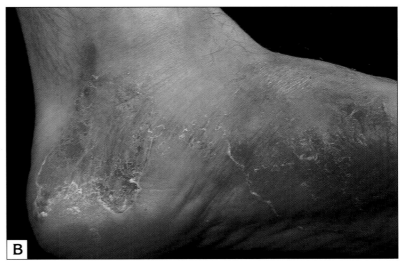

B

FIGURE 5-5 A and **B**, Tinea infections of the skin and nails with dermatophytes such as *Trichophyton rubrum* or *T. tonsurans* are more severe in HIV-infected hosts, frequently causing widespread pruritic, scaly, erythematous eruptions of the skin known as tinea corporis (*panel 5A*) or feet (tinea pedis, *panel 5B*). These eruptions especially occur on the webs between the fingers and toes, on the soles of the feet, and in the folds of the skin. In patients with AIDS, recurrences are very common. Various topical and systemic antifungal medications may provide temporary relief, but prolonged topical administration or much higher doses are usually required than are needed to quell these infections in immunocompetent individuals.

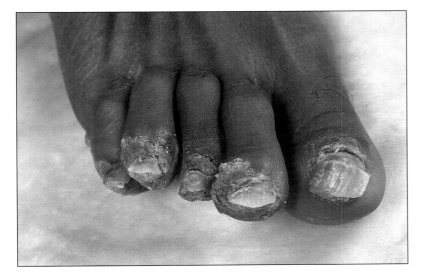

FIGURE 5-6 Onychomycosis. Tinea infections of the nails usually cause marked thickening and discoloration with opacification of several nails in these patients. Although topical antifungal preparations are not useful, systemic antifungal agents such as Lamisil, fluconazole, and itraconazole are effective treatment for fungal infections of the nails. In general, those patients who are prone to such fungal infections tend to have rather extensive involvement of their skin and nails, which is resistant to the conventional forms of treatment.

SEBORRHEIC DERMATITIS

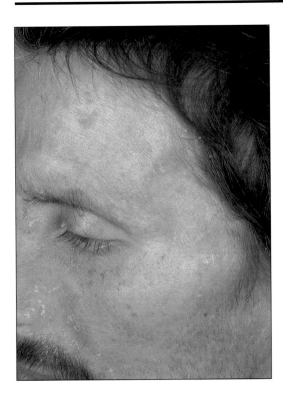

FIGURE 5-7 Seborrheic dermatitis is frequently seen in HIV-positive individuals. It is characterized by moderate to severe scaling and erythema usually involving the scalp and face and often seen in a "butterfly" distribution over the cheeks, nose, and eyebrow regions. The skin behind the ears, neck, chest, axillae, and groin may be involved as well. As with most HIV/AIDS-related skin disorders, seborrheic dermatitis is often more exaggerated and resistant to the traditional treatment regimens, including antiseborrheic tar shampoos and topical steroid creams. Seborrheic dermatitis tends to be recurrent or persistent in these patients. Antifungal agents, such as ketoconazole cream or shampoo are often effective in the treatment of seborrhea. It has been suggested that the fungus *Pityrosporon ovale*, commonly found on the skin, may play a role in the pathogenesis of seborrheic dermatitis.

SYSTEMIC FUNGAL INFECTIONS

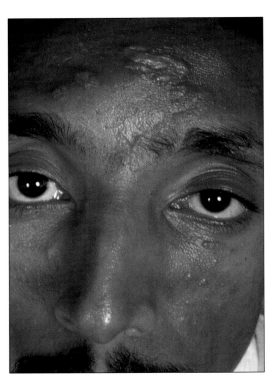

FIGURE 5-8 Cryptococcosis. The fungus *Cryptococcus neoformans* often causes meningitis in patients with AIDS. Systemic spread of this infection with skin involvement is occasionally seen. The cutaneous lesions of cryptoccis are usually characterized by multiple, discrete, flesh- to red-colored papules, varying in size from 1–6 mm. The cryptococcal skin lesions are usually disseminated or found in clusters, and they often are slightly umbilicated, sometimes resembling the lesions of molluscum contagiosum. Immediate biopsy and fungal cultures of any suspicious skin lesions should be performed to ascertain the correct diagnosis, especially in those patients with HIV disease who develop new skin eruptions associated with central nervous system symptoms (*eg*, sudden or gradual memory loss, disorientation, and personality changes). The organism can be cultured readily from the spinal fluid or skin lesion and identified histologically in skin biopsies. Prompt initiation of systemic treatment with antifungal drugs such as fluconazole may be life-saving. In AIDS patients with low peripheral blood CD4+ lymphocyte counts, prophylaxis with antifungal medications is standard therapy.

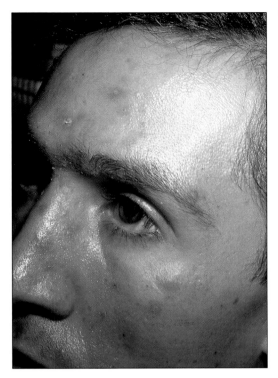

FIGURE 5-9 Histoplasmosis. A systematic fungal infection due to *Histoplasma capsulatum* is also seen in patients with AIDS, who may develop widespread, slightly tender, red, nodular skin lesions. The patient shown here had a latent pulmonary histoplasmosis infection acquired in childhood, which became reactivated and disseminated with progression of his underlying immunodeficiency.

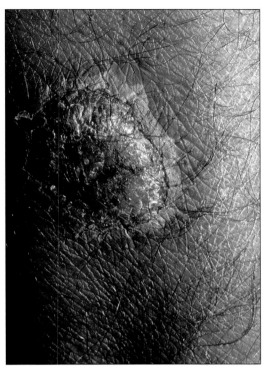

FIGURE 5-10 Blastomycosis. In patients with AIDS, unusual systemic fungal infections, such as blastomycosis and sporotrichosis, are seen and may cause similar inflammatory skin lesions. The astute physician should immediately perform a biopsy and culture for any suspicious or peculiar skin lesions to determine the possible presence of infectious agents in order to initiate appropriate systemic therapy. This HIV-seropositive patient suddenly developed numerous, 1- to 2-cm, indurated tender plaques on his skin associated with an acute febrile illness with pulmonary and neurologic symptoms. The illness proved to be due to North American blastomycosis. Biopsy specimens of the granulomatous skin lesions were found to contain the encapsulated intracellular organisms, which took several weeks to grow in the laboratory. On the basis of histologic diagnosis, treatment was begun and probably saved the patient's life.

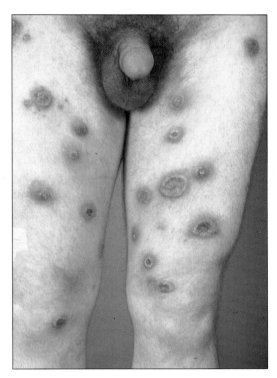

FIGURE 5-11 Sporotrichosis. A patient who worked as a horticulturist and who was known to be HIV-positive for several years, sustained cuts on his hand from rose thorns. Within a few days, he developed local inflammation on his left hand along with lymphangitis extending up his arm and axillary lymphadenopathy. By the next week, multiple large, tender, nodular red lesions developed all over his skin, and some of the lesions became ulcerated. A biopsy of one of these lesions revealed a granuloma with the organism of *Sporotrichum* readily detectable in the tissue. A culture was also taken, which was positive for *Sporotrichum* several weeks later.

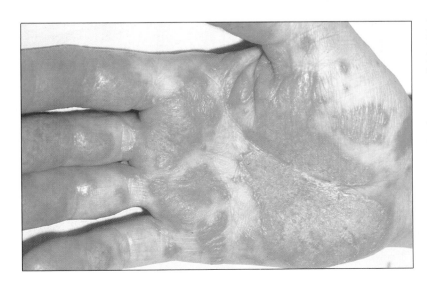

FIGURE 5-12 Reiter's syndrome. Reiter's syndrome is characterized by a severe and debilitating form of psoriasis associated with polyarthritis, iritis, and urethritis. This condition has been reported to be more prevalent in patients with HIV infection and AIDS. It involves extensive psoriatic plaques and generalized erythroderma with marked scaling of the skin, including the palms and soles (keratoderma blennorrhagicum). Systemic methotrexate, sometimes used for the treatment of severe psoriasis or Reiter's syndrome in otherwise healthy patients, can be dangerous in AIDS patients in whom this agent may further suppress their already compromised immune system.

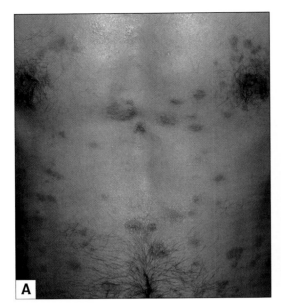
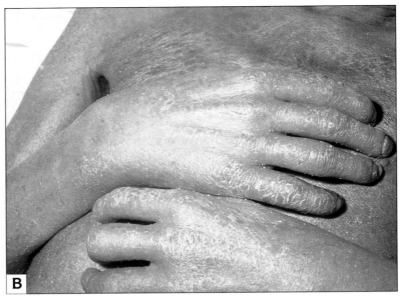

FIGURE 5-13 Psoriasis. Those AIDS patients who have a prior history of psoriasis often experience a worsening of the symptoms of this condition as their HIV disease progresses. Some HIV-infected patients who have never had psoriasis may suddenly develop this condition. **A**, Psoriasis in the HIV-infected host tends to be more severe, characterized by widely disseminated, thickened, salmon-colored plaques, with superimposed thick adherent and silvery scales located over the glabrous skin and scalp. **B**, Generalized, exfoliative psoriatic erythroderma may be seen in the HIV-infected host as well. "Psoriatic arthritis," usually involving the distal phalanges joints, may occur. The nails on the feet and hands are frequently "pitted" and thickened, and they take on a yellowish opaque color, which mimics onychomycosis. The vigorous use of topical tar preparations and high-potency topical steroid creams, as well as ultraviolet light or PUVA therapy, conventionally used for psoriasis, may only be partially effective in alleviating this condition in patients with HIV disease.

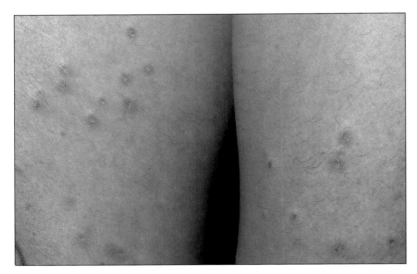

FIGURE 5-14 Generalized pruritus. Generalized, persistent itching of the skin of undetermined etiology is often seen in HIV-infected patients. Widespread lichenification, excoriations, and hyperpigmentation of the skin develop, which respond poorly to antihistamines and topical steroid creams.

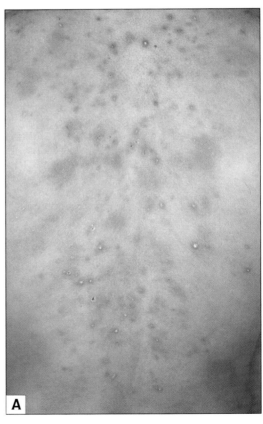

FIGURE 5-15 "Itchy red bump disease" (pruritic papular dermatoses of HIV disease) and eosinophilic pustular folliculitis. **A**, A common skin condition seen in HIV-infected persons is characterized by discrete "itchy red bumps," perifollicular papules that initially appear to be pustular or acneiform but rapidly become excoriated. This rash is most frequently seen on the chest, back, and face but may be widespread on other parts of the body. An unrelenting pruritus is usually associated with this eruption. *(continued)*

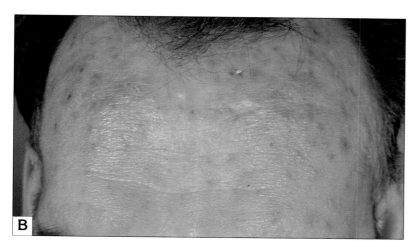

FIGURE 5-15 *(continued)* It may appear at any time during the course of disease in the HIV-infected host. **B,** A particular variant of the "itchy red bump disease" associated with HIV infection is known as *eosinophilic pustular folliculitis*. Histologically, biopsy specimens of these lesions show a perifollicular inflammatory infiltrate, which frequently includes an abundance of eosinophils surrounding the hairbulb; however, eosinophils are often not present in these papules. Treatment includes the use of various topical steroid creams or lotions containing 0.25% menthol and 0.25% phenol, which may provide temporary relief for the severe itching that accompanies these conditions. Various antihistamines and hydroxyzine (10–50 mg given every 4–6 hours) may be helpful and can provide temporary relief. About 30% to 60% of patients with this condition respond to the antifungal drug itraconazole (Sporanox, 200 mg three times daily), although there is no evidence that any fungal organism is involved in this condition.

VIRAL INFECTIONS

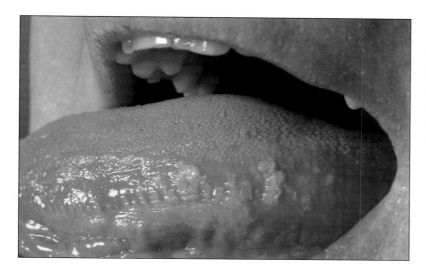

FIGURE 5-16 Oral hairy leukoplakia. The appearance of symptomatic verrucous white excrescences on the lateral margins of the tongue (hairy leukoplakia) is frequently seen in HIV-positive persons, often prior to the development of symptomatic HIV disease. These lesions are believed to be due to the Epstein-Barr virus, which is found to be present under electron microscopic examination. Occasionally, such lesions occur on the other mucosal surfaces of the mouth. The lesions clinically mimic "thrush" but are not readily scraped off as with oral candidiasis.

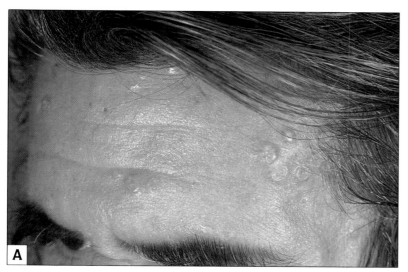

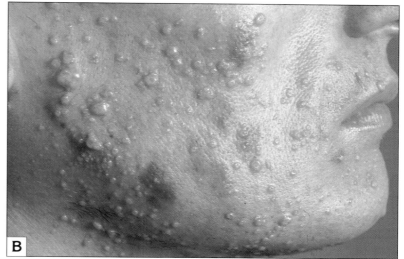

FIGURE 5-17 Molluscum contagiosum. Widespread papular skin lesions of molluscum contagiosum, which is due to the human poxvirus, are frequently seen in HIV-infected hosts, especially those with low CD4+ lymphocyte counts. **A** and **B,** The asymptomatic, "waxy," skin-colored to pink papules of molluscum contagiosum (*panel 17A*), which can vary in size from 1 mm to > 1 cm, are often found widely scattered on the skin or form localized clusters, sometimes coalescing into "giant" molluscum lesions (*panel 17B*). In the center of each papule is a slightly depressed crusted "core," which when squeezed exudes a "cheesy" white matter. Local destructive surgical treatments including curettage and electrocauterization are usually effective, although immunocompromised patients tend to develop new lesions throughout the course of their illness. The skin lesions of disseminated systematic fungal infections such as cryptococcosis may mimic molluscum contagiosum in AIDS patients.

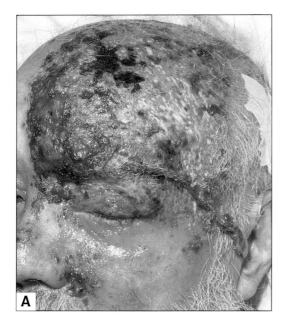
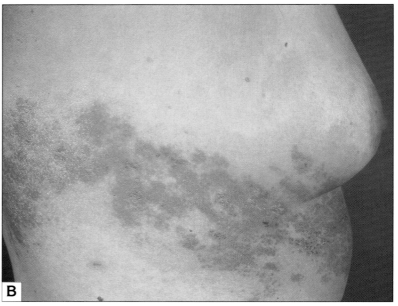

FIGURE 5-18 Herpes zoster ("shingles"). **A**, This skin eruption, common in HIV-infected hosts, is due to the reactivation of a latent varicella zoster virus infection of the cranial nerves, especially the trigeminal nerve (*panel 18A*) or the ganglia of the spinal nerves. Zoster is frequently seen in these patients prior to the onset of one or more opportunistic infections or the development of AIDS-related neoplasms, and it may serve as a harbinger or first sign of an underlying immunodeficiency. **B**, Herpes zoster is usually localized to involve one, or rarely two, adjacent neurodermatomes on the same side of the body. The prodromal symptoms of tingling, burning, and "shooting pains" usually precede or accompany the onset of local erythema and edema of the skin. Clusters of vesicles soon appear, which tend to coalesce and rapidly ulcerate. Superficial purulent crusts and scabs develop over the erosion and may last for several weeks. Residual scarring and hyperpigmentation often occur after healing at the involved area of skin. The sooner the condition is diagnosed and antiviral therapy is begun, the better will be the prognosis. High doses of acyclovir (800 mg five times a day for about 2 weeks) is recommended. Early initiation of treatment tends to arrest the progression and severity of the eruption and the associated pain symptoms, perhaps reducing the likelihood of postherpetic neuralgia that often persists indefinitely after resolution of the acute infection. Rarely, patients with AIDS may experience more than one episode of "shingles" over the course of their illness, usually involving different neurodermatomes.

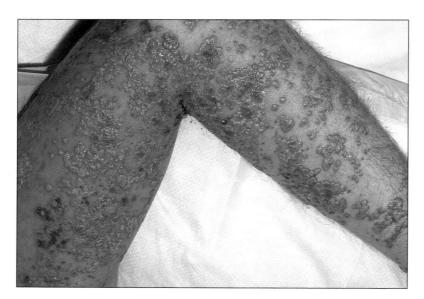

FIGURE 5-19 Disseminated herpes zoster. Disseminated zoster has also been seen in AIDS patients, resembling the widespread vesicular skin eruptions of chicken pox and sometimes associated with fever and with neurologic and visceral organ involvement. Intravenous acyclovir is often required to treat the more severe, disseminated varicella/zoster infection.

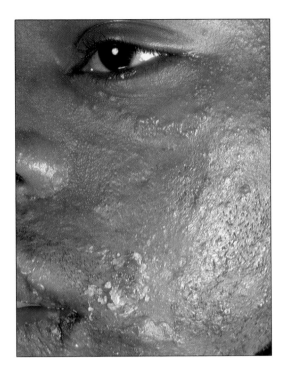

FIGURE 5-20 Herpes simplex. Recurrent infection with herpes simplex virus, types 1 or 2, is due to reactivation of a latent infection of different nerves. These localized infections most often involve the lips, oral mucosa, eye, nose, genitalia, or perianal regions. However, any site on the glabrous skin may also be affected. Occasionally, more than one mucocutaneous location may be involved simultaneously or at different times in the HIV-infected individual. Recurrent herpetic infections in HIV-infected patients tend to occur frequently, are often more severe, and are persistent for longer periods than in healthy individuals. Painful clusters of tiny vesicles develop and coalesce to form blisters that soon break, leaving painful ulcerations that often become secondarily infected with bacteria causing purulent crusts over the sores. Treatment with acyclovir (200–400 mg five times a day for up to 14 days) is usually effective in reducing the severity and longevity of recurrent episodes.

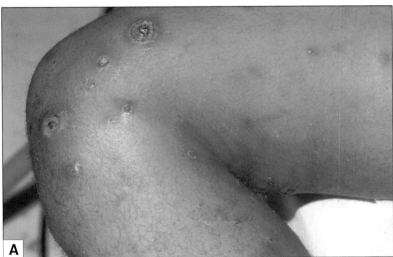

A

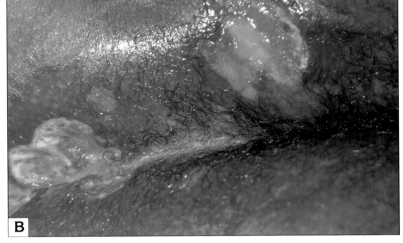

B

FIGURE 5-21 Disseminated herpes simplex. In some patients, dissemination of herpes simplex infection occurs with widespread vesicular eruptions of the skin and internal organ involvement. **A,** Such patients are usually very ill with high fever, nausea, vomiting, malaise, and headaches due to herpetic encephalitis. Long-term prophylaxis with acyclovir (200–400 mg three times daily) often prevents reactivation of latent herpes simplex infections. **B,** However, persistent infections with acyclovir-resistant strains

of the virus are now being seen with increasing frequency among immunocompromised patients, in whom the ulcerations gradually develop and last for several months creating unsightly lesions and considerable discomfort. Acyclovir-resistant strains of the herpes simplex virus may be sensitive to another antiviral agent, foscarnet, (given intravenously, 60 mg/kg every 8 hours daily for about 2 weeks). Patients receiving phosphonoformate must be well-hydrated and carefully monitored to avoid potential renal toxicity.

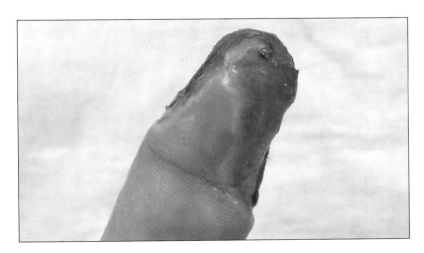

FIGURE 5-22 Herpetic "felon" (whitlow). Herpes simplex virus infection involving the fingertip, known as either a herpetic "felon" or herpetic "whitlow," is usually exquisitely painful and can be so severe as to cause total destruction of the distal phalanx in the immunocompromised patient. Intravenous acyclovir or phosphonoformate may be helpful in these cases.

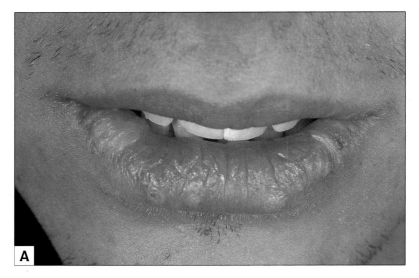

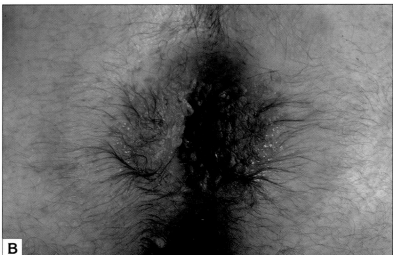

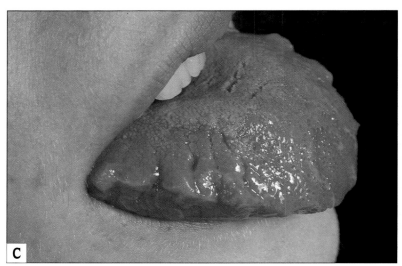

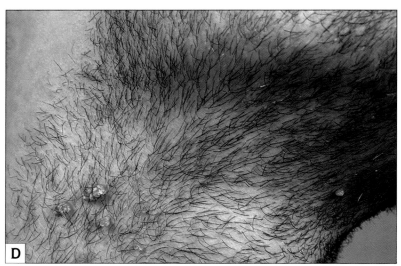

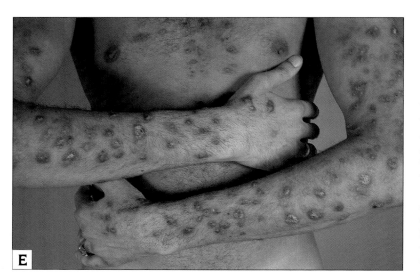

FIGURE 5-23 Human papillomavirus infections. Various kinds of warts involving the skin and mucous membranes are due to different strains of the human papillomaviruses. **A**, Common warts (verrucae vulgares), flat warts (verrucae planae, *panel 23A*), filiform warts, plantar warts, and anogenital warts (condylomata acuminata) are frequently seen in patients with HIV disease, in whom warts tend to be more widespread and larger in growth than in immunocompetent persons. **B**, Warts involving the anogenital region are especially exuberant, often developing a cauliflower configuration. **C** and **D**, Warts may also develop on the tongue (*panel 23C*) and oral mucosa; myriad flat and filiform warts may develop on the face, especially on the bearded area (*panel 23D*); and common warts may occur anyplace on the feet and the periungual regions of the fingers and toes. **E**, Cases of extensive large warts developing widely over the skin have also been seen in HIV-infected patients. In general, all types of warts in these patients tend to be resistant to treatment. The conventional forms of treatment include the topical application of caustic chemical agents such as 50% trichloroacetic acid and/or 25% to 50% salicylic acid for verrucae vulgares and 50% podophyllum in benzoin for condylomata; however, treatment needs to be used at more frequent intervals than in immunocompetent patients. Destructive surgical methods, including electrocauterization or laser therapy, can also be used for treating the different types of mucocutaneous warts, although special precautions must be taken to avoid the aerosolization of the HIV present in the patient's blood that may occur during laser treatment.

PARASITIC INFESTATIONS

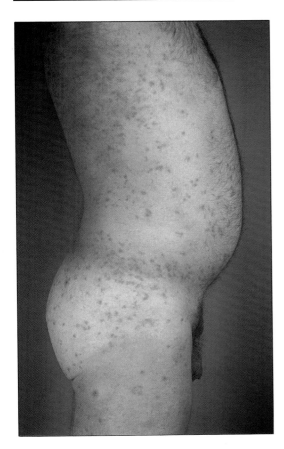

FIGURE 5-24 Scabies. Ectoparasitic infection of the skin with scabies tend to be more severe and widespread in patients who are immunocompromised. Widespread excoriated pruritic, tiny red papules develop that are usually more concentrated in the anogenital regions (especially the glans penis), wrist, axillae, waist, webs between the fingers, as well as the intertriginous folds. Microscopic examination of the scrapings or biopsy specimens from these papules reveal the presence of scabitic mites *Sarcoptes scabiei* and their eggs located within burrows in the epidermis. Repeated topical treatments with lindane (Kwell), crotamiton (Eurax), or permethrin (Elimite) will usually rid the host of infestation. The itchy red papules may persist for sometime despite adequate treatment, due to a localized delayed hypersensitivity reaction to the residual proteins from the killed parasites within the skin. In such cases, both the physician and patient often assume that the infestation has not been adequately treated. Such posttreatment reactions are effectively treated with an antihistamine and the topical application of topical steroid creams, until the symptoms subside.

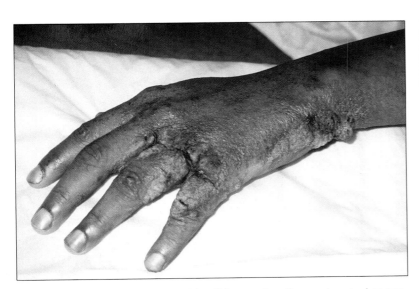

FIGURE 5-25 "Norwegian scabies." Long-standing untreated cases of severe scabies, known as *Norwegian scabies*, present with highly pruritic, thick, lichenified, hyperkeratotic plaques mostly seen in the skinfolds, fingerwebs, and sometimes the eyelid margins due to chronic, overwhelming mite infestation. Vigorous, repeated treatments with antiscabitic agents will eventually clean this unusual parasitic disease.

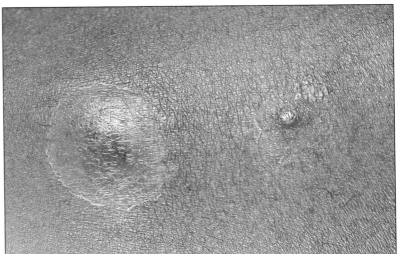

FIGURE 5-26 Cutaneous pneumocystosis. Dissemination of a pulmonary infection with *Pneumocystis carinii* rarely causes skin lesions in the immunocompromised host. Cutaneous papular lesions due to *P. carinii* have been seen in patients receiving aerosolized pentamidine as prophylaxis for pneumocystis pneumonia. The 2- to 6-mm papular skin lesions are flesh-colored to deep red and can resemble the lesion of molluscum contagiosum.

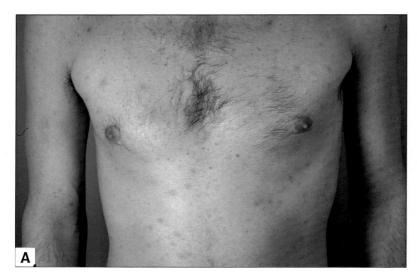

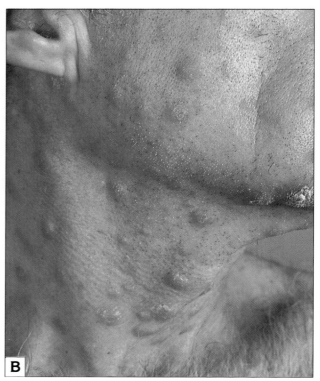

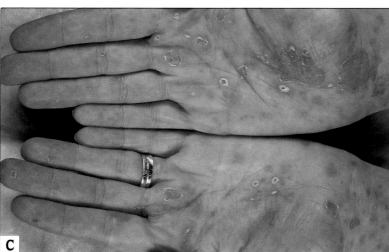

FIGURE 5-27 Syphilis. HIV-infected patients often give histories of multiple sex partners and various sexually transmitted diseases, especially syphilis. **A** and **B,** Although their previous episodes of syphilis had been adequately treated with antibiotics such as penicillin, a few patients will have reactivation of what seems to be latent syphilis, often manifested by a generalized skin rash typical of secondary syphilis. **C,** Sometimes, the rash involves the palms and soles. In some of these HIV-seropositive individuals, syphilis rapidly progresses to the more advanced tertiary-stage disease with mucocutaneous lesions and neurologic involvement.

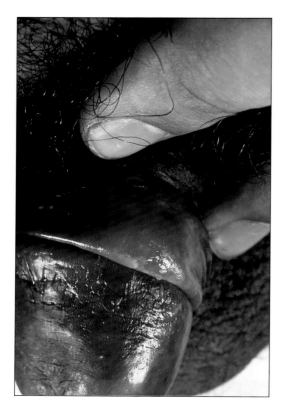

FIGURE 5-28 Primary chancre of syphilis. Some HIV-infected individuals who remain sexually active without observing proper "safe sex" precautions may present with primary chancres of syphilis. In the immunocompromised host with newly acquired syphilis, the disease may progress rapidly to the secondary and more advanced stages of disease during only a few months. Because of the patients' immunodeficiency, the standard serologic tests for diagnosing syphilis, such as the VDRL, rapid plasma reagin (RPR), and fluorescent treponemal antibody test (FTA), may not be reliable.

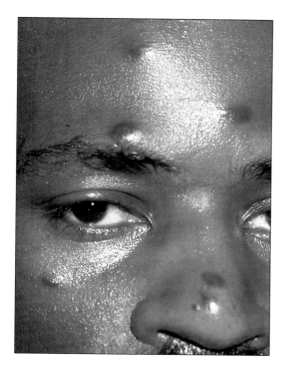

FIGURE 5-29 Bacillary epithelioid angiomatosis (BEA). BEA is an unusual infection characterized by multiple, tender, red vascular lesions of the skin and subcutaneous tissues caused by *Rochalimaea henselae*, a species of *Rickettsia* closely related to the organisms that cause "cat scratch" disease. This agent is sensitive to a variety of systemic antibiotics including erythromycin and tetracycline. The vascular proliferative lesions of BEA are most frequently seen in the skin but also occur subcutaneously and can involve the internal organs in patients with AIDS. These skin lesions may clinically resemble those of Kaposi's sarcoma, although histologically, BEA is similar to pyogenic granuloma rather than Kaposi's sarcoma. The causative organisms of BEA are readily detectable in specially stained tissue sections. The skin lesions of BEA can also mimic the skin eruption associated with verruca peruana due to infection with another bacteria, *Bartonella* sp. Because BEA can be fatal, early diagnosis and initiation of appropriate antibiotic treatment can be life-saving.

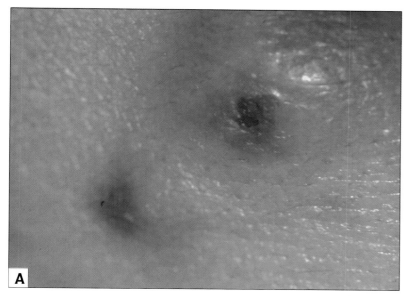

A

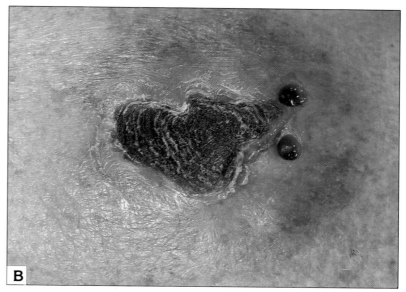

B

FIGURE 5-30 Mycobacterial infections of the skin. **A,** Mycobacteria such as *Mycobacterium tuberculosis* and *M. avium* complex usually cause systematic infections in AIDS patients. **B,** On occasion, granulomatous or abscesses of the skin due to these organisms can develop, which are tender, reddish-purple nodules that may be fluctuant and sometimes ulcerate. Special stains can be used to detect the mycobacteria in histologic specimens from these lesions; culture of mycobacteria usually takes several weeks to months. Patients with disseminated cutaneous mycobacterial infection generally have a poor prognosis.

HYPERSENSITIVITY REACTIONS

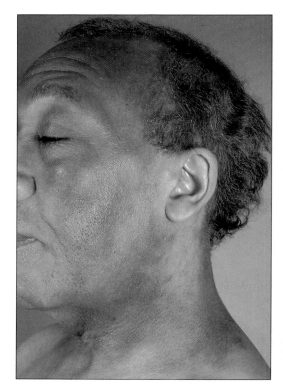

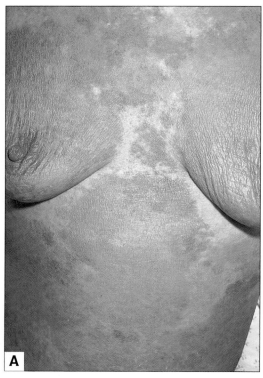

A

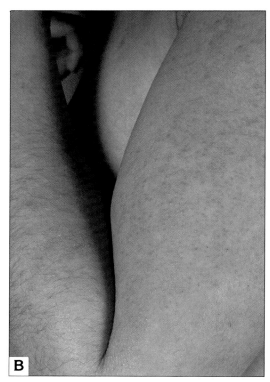

B

FIGURE 5-31 Photoallergic dermatitis. Patients with AIDS usually take a large variety of systemic medications, some of which can predispose to a phototoxic reaction, or photoallergic dermatitis can occur with various topical sensitizing agents, such as perfumes. Itchy erythema or eczematous patches and plaques appear on the light-exposed regions of the skin. Residual postinflammatory hyperpigmentation may develop and last for some time after the reaction has subsided. The ultraviolet spectrum is usually the cause of these light-sensitive reactions, but visible light may also be the cause in HIV-infected persons. The regular use of a sunscreen is helpful in preventing recurrences in such photosensitive individuals.

FIGURE 5-32 Drug eruptions. **A** and **B**, Remarkably, about 50% of HIV-infected patients have an increased propensity to developing an allergic reaction to trimethoprim-sulfamethoxazole (TSM—Bactrim, Septra), which is commonly used as both prophylaxis against and treatment of *Pneumocystis carinii* pneumonia (PCP), the most prevalent opportunistic infection associated with AIDS. A generalized skin rash usually develops within 7–10 days after therapy with TSM is started and is characterized by a highly pruritic, morbilliform, erythematous eruption, often associated with the fever. Desensitization to TSM, accomplished with a regimen of gradually escalating oral doses of the drug over an extended period, has been effective in inducing tolerance in some patients. The effort is worthwhile, because TSM is one of the most effective agents used for the prophylaxis and treatment of *P. carinii* pneumonia.

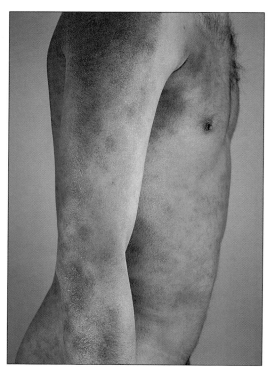

FIGURE 5-33 Hyperpigmentation. AIDS patients often develop unexplained hyperpigmentation and sometimes hypopigmentation, which are perhaps related to the multiplicity of medications and chronic inflammatory skin conditions to which the patients are prone.

ALOPECIA

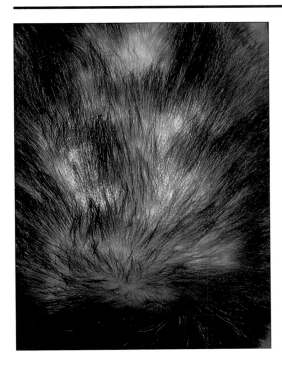

FIGURE 5-34 Alopecia. AIDS patients sometimes develop unexplained patchy alopecea, such as in this individual, perhaps due to nutritional deficiencies. After multiple infections and fevers, these patients often develop thinning of their scalp and body hair. Premature graying of the hair is frequently seen as well.

MALIGNANCIES

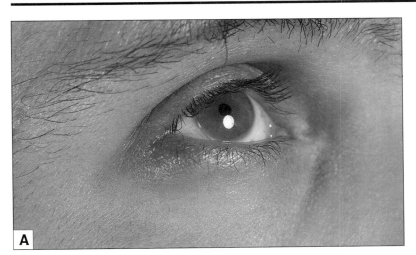

A

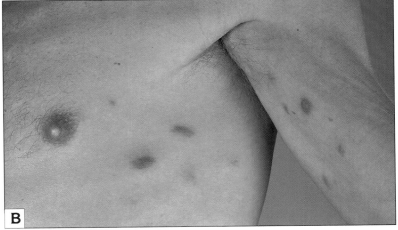

B

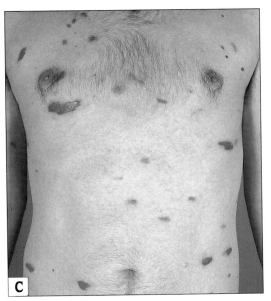

C

FIGURE 5-35 AIDS-related Kaposi's sarcoma. An aggressive and disseminated form of Kaposi's sarcoma is the most frequently reported neoplastic disorder associated with AIDS. Remarkably, 95% of all of the AIDS-related "epidemic" form of Kaposi's sarcoma occurring in North America, Europe, and Australia has been seen among homosexual or bisexual men, suggesting that in this population, Kaposi's sarcoma may be due to a sexually transmissible agent other than HIV. The Kaposi's sarcoma tumors are seen most often on the skin and mucosa as asymptomatic, pink to deep purple or dark brown, round to oval-shaped patches, which eventually become thickened plaques and nodular tumors. They appear as single lesions or in clusters, at the same or distant sites. **A**, A faint early patch-stage lesion, which resembles a bruise, can even occur in the lower eyelid area. **B** and **C**, Remarkably, in AIDS patients, the lesions almost always have a symmetric distribution over the skin along the lines of skin cleavage.

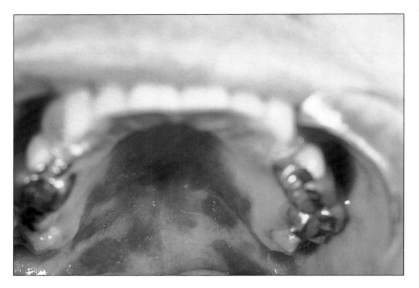

FIGURE 5-36 Oral Kaposi's sarcoma lesions are usually flat asymptomatic patches or plaques on the hard or soft palate. Nodular tumor lesions on the oral mucosa, including the pharynx, tongue, or gingival, can interfere with swallowing and speech. These lesions tend to ulcerate and bleed, become secondarily infected, and be very painful. Although usually asymptomatic, tumor lesions of the gastrointestinal tract may cause occasional bleeding.

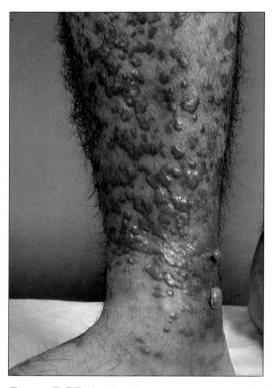

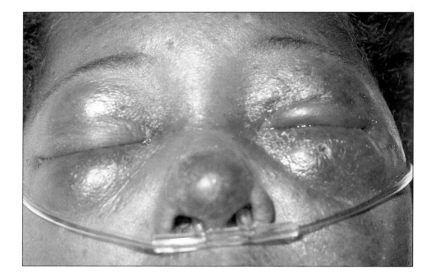

FIGURE 5-38 Individual mucocutaneous Kaposi's sarcoma lesions respond well to localized destructive treatments with laser, electro-cauterization, or liquid nitrogen cryotherapy. The administration of intralesional chemotherapeutic agents, including vinblastine, vincristine, adriamycin or interferon-α, have caused temporary regression of individual lesions. Kaposi's sarcoma is very sensitive to localized radiation therapy, although radiation of oral mucosal lesions tends to cause a particularly severe mucositis, associated with ulcerations, pain, and excessive dryness of the mouth, which makes eating and speaking difficult. In AIDS patients with a peripheral blood CD4+ lymphocyte count > 200/mm³, the use of systemic intramuscular injections of interferon-α in doses of up to 18 MU/d can also provide temporary remission of widespread Kaposi's sarcoma lesions. However, systemic interferon therapy causes adverse side effects, including transient flulike symptoms including fever and malaise. When treatment is discontinued the tumors usually recur. In patients with advanced disseminated disease, especially those with pulmonary involvement, severe swelling of the legs, or even the head and neck due to lymphatic involvement, systemic chemotherapy with such agents as vincristine, vinblastine, adriamycin, or etoposide, used as single agents or in various combinations, often provide remarkable, but temporary, regression of the tumors. These agents also have adverse side effects including bone marrow depression and alopecia. Adriamycin encapsulated in liposomes has been shown to cause fewer side effects.

FIGURE 5-37 As the disease progresses, the lymph nodes and visceral organs may also become involved. Progressive nodular tumors develop with invasion of the lymphatic system including lymph nodes, eventually causing chronic, debilitating, painful lymphedema, especially in the lower extremities. These cause bleeding and ulcerations of the skin, which often become secondarily infected. The terminally ill AIDS patient in Fig. 5-38 has Kaposi's sarcoma involving the head and neck with tumor involvment of the lymphatic system in the chest causing edema of the face. The patient also had Kaposi's sarcoma in his lungs. Pulmonary involvement eventually compromises breathing and may be life-threatening.

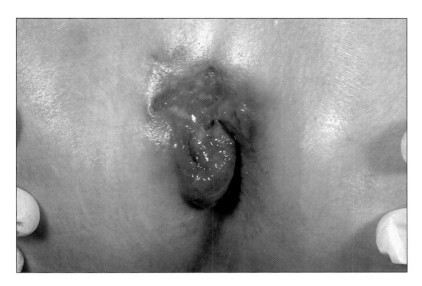

FIGURE 5-39 B-cell lymphoma of the skin. Patients with AIDS have an increased incidence of lymphomas, occurring in about 3% of the cases. On rare occasion, cutaneous lesions of lymphomas are seen; in this patient, a large nodular tumor suddenly developed, which proved to be a B-cell lymphoma of the skin, associated with a disseminated lymph node and eventually brain involvement.

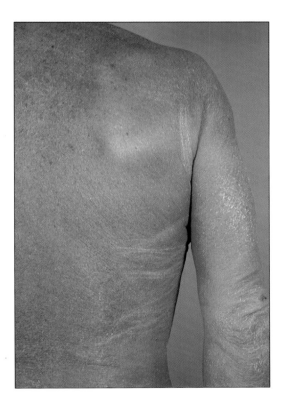

FIGURE 5-40 Cutaneous T-cell lymphoma (mycosis fungoides). A few patients with dual infections of HTLV-1 and HIV have been seen. These individuals present with severe generalized pruritus, chronic lichenification, and hyperpigmentation of their skin. Biopsies of the skin are not typically diagnostic of cutaneous T-cell lymphoma, because these individuals lack adequate T lymphocytes, which usually infiltrate the epidermal layers of the skin in this condition. Sézary cells may be detected in the peripheral blood lymphocytes or skin biopsy specimen by electron microscopy, and HTLV-1 may be cultured from the cells *in vitro* or detected by electromicroscopy of the peripheral blood lymphocytes. In most cases, serum antibodies to HTLV-1 are not present.

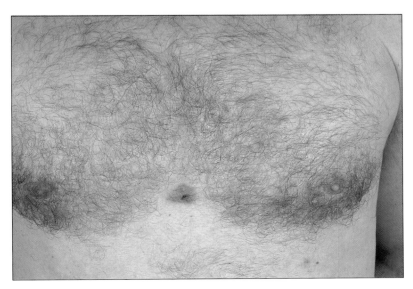

FIGURE 5-41 Basal cell carcinoma. Multiple basal or squamous cell carcinomas and malignant melanomas of the skin have been seen with increased frequency in AIDS patients. There is a tendency for these skin neoplasms to occur more often in those HIV-infected patients who have fair skin and previous excessive sun exposure. This 23-year-old HIV-positive man developed multiple basal cell carcinoma of his skin in a short time.

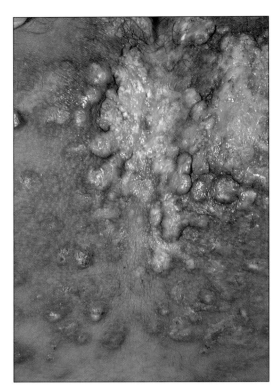

FIGURE 5-42 Squamous cell carcinoma. An increased prevalence of squamous cell carcinoma of the anorectal region has been seen among homosexual men with AIDS. This HIV-positive patient had suffered persistent condylomata acuminata of the perianal region for several years, which developed into squamous cell carcinoma of the anorectal region. He also had widespread verrucae vulgaris on his skin.

SELECTED BIBLIOGRAPHY

DeVita VT, Krigel R, Ostreicher R, *et al.*: *In* Friedman-Kien AE (ed.) *Color Atlas of AIDS*. W.B. Saunders Co: Philadelphia; 1989.

Cockerell CJ, Friedman-Kien AE: Cutaneous infections in patients with human immunodeficiency virus infection. *In* Leoung G, Mill J (eds.) *Opportunistic Infections in Patients with the Acquired Immunodeficiency Syndrome.* Marcel Dekker: New York; 1989.

Friedman-Kien AE, Farthing C: Hiv infection: A survey with special emphasis on mucocutaneous manifestations. *Semin Dermatol* 1990, 9:167–177.

Friedman-Kein AE (ed.): AIDS: Proceedings of a symposium held at the American Academy of Dermatology Forty-seventh Annual Meeting (also includes updated material from the Proceedings of the Forty-sixth Annual Meeting, December 1987, San Antonio, TX). *J Am Acad Dermatol* 1990, (*suppl*).

Buchbinder A, Friedman-Kein AE: Clinical aspects of Kaposi's sarcoma. *Semin Oncol* 1992, 4(5):867–874.

CHAPTER 6

Ophthalmic Manifestations

Janet L. Davis
Alan G. Palestine

ANTERIOR SEGMENT AND ADNEXAE

Molluscum Contagiosum

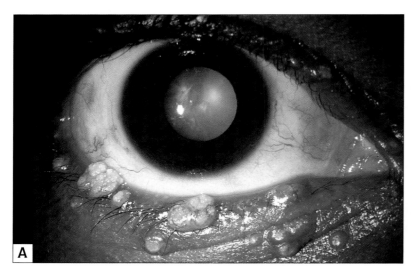

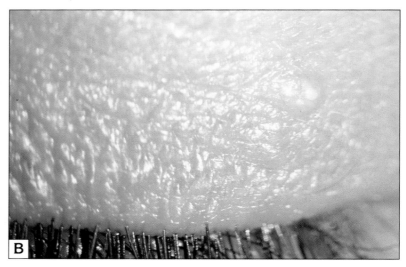

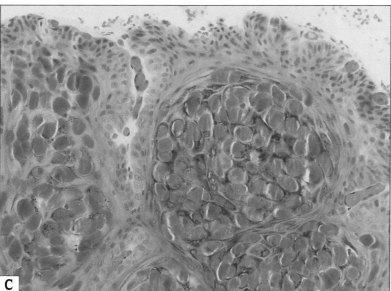

FIGURE 6-1 A, Molluscum contagiosum of the eyelid margin. Progressive infection of the eyelids and face with this large DNA pox virus is associated in HIV-infected patients with advanced stages of AIDS. (Schwartz JJ, Myskowski PL: Molluscum contagiosum in patients with human immunodeficiency virus infection: A review of twenty-seven patients. *J Am Acad Dermatol* 1992, 27:583–588.) Secondary keratoconjunctivitis can occur; epibulbar nodules are rare. Curettage, local excision, and cryotherapy can be attempted for eyelid margin lesions but recurrence is likely. (Robinson MR, Udell IJ, Garber PF, *et al.*: Molluscum contagiosum of the eyelids in patients with acquired immune deficiency syndrome. *Ophthalmology* 1992, 99:1745–1747). Recurrence may occur because of subclinical infection of epidermis up to 1.0 cm lateral to clinically visible lesions. **B,** Early lesion of molluscum contagiosum. Additional small lesions on the eyelid margin were producing symptoms and curettage was performed. **C,** Molluscum bodies from the small lesions in *Panel 1B.* Solid cores of molluscum bodies emerge through collars of stratified epithelium (hematoxylin and eosin, × 10). No recurrence was noted at 8 weeks after curettage. Curettage was probably successful in producing remission in this case because the lesions were small and few in number.

Herpes Zoster Ophthalmicus

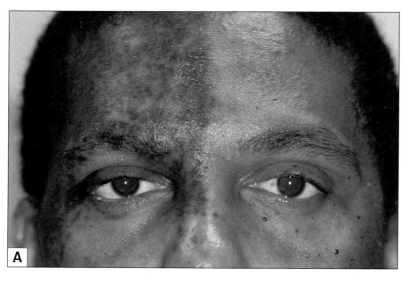

FIGURE 6-2 A, Herpes zoster ophthalmicus (HZO). A 38-year-old Haitian man was diagnosed with HIV infection after presenting with HZO. Intravenous acyclovir was begun 6 days after the vesicular eruption, and the skin lesions are shown healed 1 month after treatment. Punctate keratopathy and corneal anesthesia of the right eye developed, but elevated intraocular pressure was not documented. HZO in young adults may be a marker of early HIV infection or of AIDS. (Sandor EV, Millman A, Croxson TS, Mildvan D: Herpes zoster ophthalmicus in patients at risk for the acquired immune deficiency syndrome (AIDS). *Am J Ophthalmol* 1986, 101:153–155.) Complications such as optic neuritis and retinitis may be more common in the HIV-infected population. (Sellitti TP, Huang AJ, Schiffman J, Davis JL: Association of herpes zoster ophthalmicus with acquired immunodeficiency syndrome and acute retinal necrosis. *Am J Ophthalmol* 1993, 116:297–301.) Treatment with intravenous acyclovir has been recommended for patients in whom HIV-infection is suspected or confirmed. (*continued*)

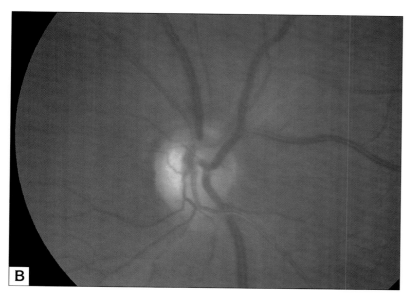

FIGURE 6-2 *(continued)* **B**, Two weeks after onset, while on acyclovir, the patient noted decreased vision in the right eye consistent with zoster-related retrobulbar optic neuritis. (Litoff D, Catalano RA: Herpes zoster optic neuritis in human immunodeficiency virus infection. *Arch Ophthalmol* 1990, 108:782–783.) The right optic nerve is cupped with pallor. The vision was counting fingers in a small temporal island. The left optic nerve was normal in appearance. Vision was 20/15.

Herpes Simplex Keratitis

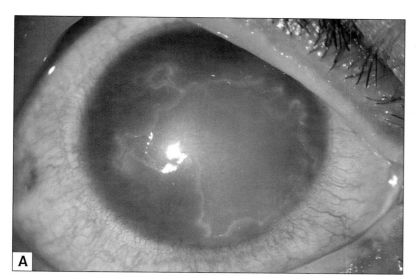

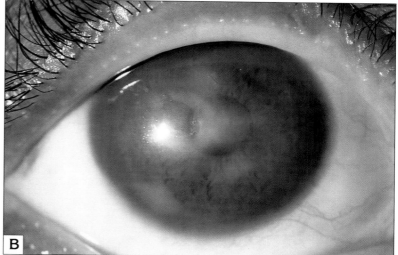

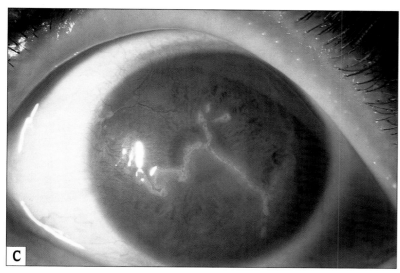

FIGURE 6-3 **A**, Herpes simplex keratitis. Nonhealing corneal ulcer of the right eye due to culture-positive herpes simplex I infection in a 15-year-old woman with AIDS dementia. Treatment with oral acyclovir, topical trifluridine, vidarabine, or idoxuridine for 2 months failed to sterilize the cornea. Interferon alfa-2A, 12 MU/mL, was given as a topical eye drop twice daily. **B**, Complete healing of the corneal ulcer after 3 weeks of treatment with interferon topical drops. (McLeish W, Pflugfelder SC, Crouse C, *et al.*: Interferon treatment of herpetic keratitis in a patient with acquired immunodeficiency syndrome. *Am J Ophthalmol* 1990, 109:93–95). **C**, Dendritic herpes simplex virus infection of the left cornea developed subsequently. Stromal scars and neovascularization from previous recurrences are seen. Frequent recurrences of dendritiform or geographic herpetic infections with prolonged healing times on topical antivirals may be typical for HIV infection. (Young TL, Robin JB, Holland GN, *et al.*: Herpes simplex keratitis in patients with acquired immune deficiency syndrome. *Ophthalmology* 1989, 96:1476–1479.)

Microsporidial Keratoconjunctivitis

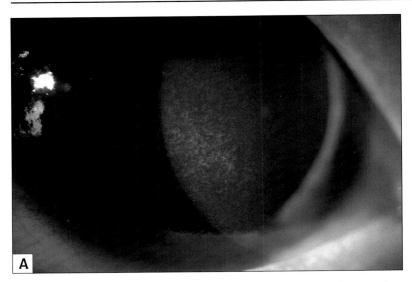

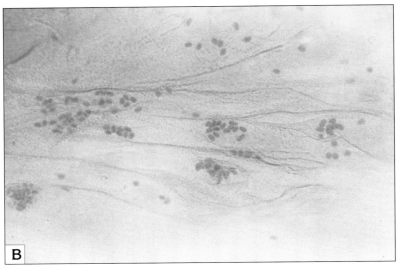

FIGURE 6-4 A, Microsporidial keratoconjunctivitis. Bilateral eye redness with foreign body sensation and a coarse punctate keratopathy was present. Vision was moderately reduced to 20/40. **B,** A smear of the cornea showed multiple microsporidial spores. Topical treatment with metronidazole (ready-to-use intravenous formulation) alleviated symptoms and reduced the amount of keratopathy. (Schwartz DA, Visvesvara GS, Diesenhouse MC, *et al.*: Pathologic features and immunofluorescent antibody demonstration of ocular microsporidiosis (*Encephalitozoon hellem*) in seven patients with acquired immunodeficiency syndrome. *Am J Ophthalmol* 1993, 115:285–292.)

Lymphogranuloma Venereum

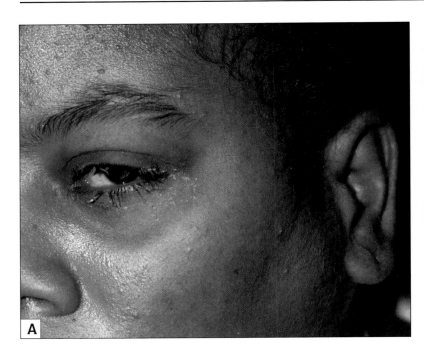

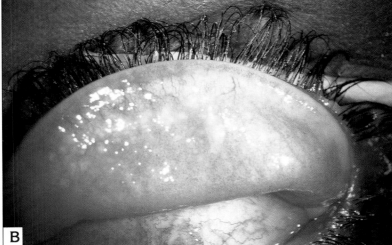

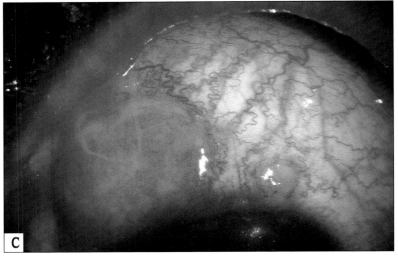

FIGURE 6-5 A, Lymphogranuloma venereum involving the eye. Submandibular and anterior cervical lymphadenopathy was present bilaterally in this 17-year-old with a 2-week history of eye pain, redness, and discharge. **B,** Papillary and follicular conjunctival reaction. McCoy cells inoculated with conjunctival scrapings formed cytoplasmic inclusions that stained with fluorescein-conjugated *Chlamydia trachomatis* monoclonal antibody, serovar L2. **C,** Exophytic lesion of the superior bulbar conjunctiva. A marginal corneal perforation with iris incarceration was present in the other eye. Treatment with oral tetracycline for 6 weeks resulted in resolution. (Buus DR, Pflugfelder SC, Schacter J, *et al.*: Lymphogranuloma venereum conjunctivitis with a marginal corneal perforation *Ophthalmology* 1988, 95:799–802.)

Bacterial Keratitis

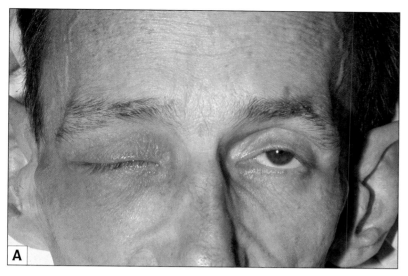 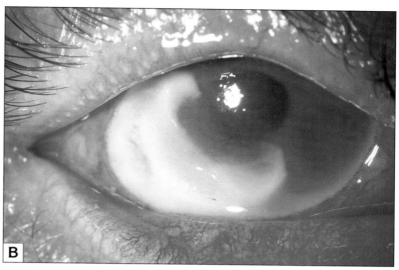

FIGURE 6-6 A, Pseudomonas sclerokeratitis. The patient presented with a 10-day history of pain and eyelid erythema and edema. **B,** The pseudomonas ulcer involved the peripheral cornea and extended into the sclera. Intensive topical and intravenous therapy with tobramycin and ceftazidime for 10 days as well as local cryotherapy failed to sterilize the eye. Progressive necrosis of the sclera with impending perforation occurred and enucleation was recommended. (Nanda M, Pflugfelder SC, Holland S: Fulminant pseudomonal keratitis and scleritis in human immunodeficiency virus-infected patients. *Arch Ophthalmol* 1991, 109:503–505.)

POSTERIOR SEGMENT

Cytomegalovirus Retinitis

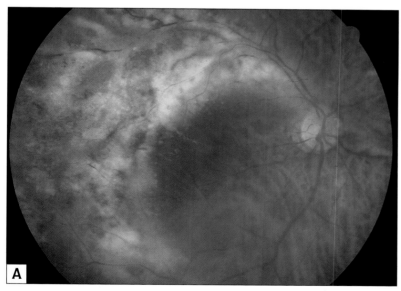 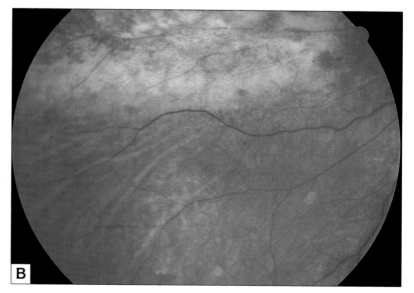

FIGURE 6-7 A, Classic ophthalmoscopic appearance of untreated cytomegalovirus (CMV) retinitis of the fulminant and edematous type. Fulminant retinitis is the more common appearance in the posterior pole. **B,** Classic appearance of indolent, granular CMV infection of the retinal periphery. Note the paucity of retinal hemorrhage. Small areas of central clearing are appearing due to spontaneous healing. Both the fulminant and indolent forms of untreated CMV retinitis show the characteristic small white "satellite" lesions just outside the borders of the confluent necrotizing retinitis. Recognition of "satellite" lesions is very helpful in distinguishing CMV retinitis from herpetic retinitis or toxoplasmosis.

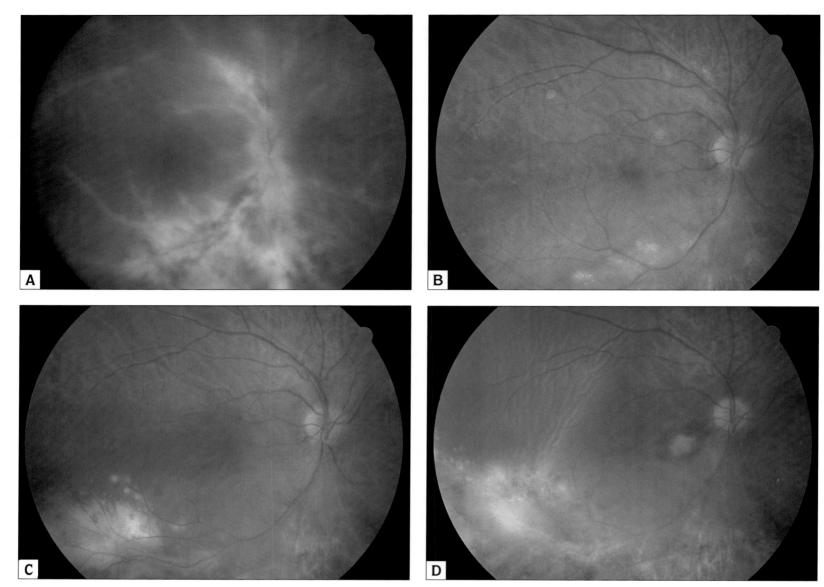

FIGURE 6-8 A, Fulminant, edematous CMV retinitis complicated by a mild vitreous reaction and diffuse periphlebitis or "frosted branch angiitis." (Spaide RF, Vitale AT, Toth IR, Oliver JM: Frosted branch angiitis associated with cytomegalovirus retinitis. *Am J Ophthalmol* 1992, 113:522–528.) **B,** Two months later, the retinitis is in remission on ganciclovir, 5 mg/kg daily. The retinal vessels now appear normal. The median time to complete response to medication is 31 ± 10 days. (Jabs DA, Enger C, Bartlett JG: Cytomegalovirus retinitis and acquired immunodeficiency syndrome. *Arch Ophthalmol* 1989, 107:75–80.) **C,** Recurrent retinitis with progression into new areas of retina is noted after 150 days of therapy. The median time to progression after treatment is started is 60 days. (The Ocular Complications of AIDS Study Group: Mortality in patients with the acquired immunodeficiency syndrome treated with either foscarnet or ganciclovir for cytomegalovirus retinitis. *N Engl J Med* 1992, 326:213–220.) **D,** Despite an increase in ganciclovir dose, the retinitis continued to progress and a new lesion appeared next to the optic nerve head. In addition, retinal detachment is now present in the temporal half of the retina due to hole formation in the area of active retinitis. Retinal detachment occurs in about 25% of patients with CMV retinitis. (Jabs DA, Enger C, Haller J, de Bustros S: Retinal detachments in patients with cytomegalovirus retinitis. *Arch Ophthalmol* 1991, 109:794–799.)

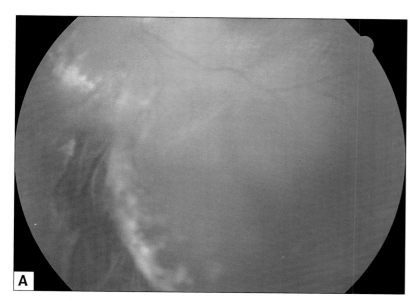

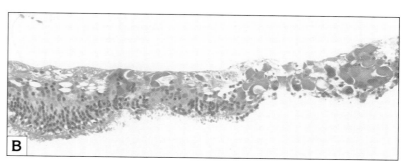

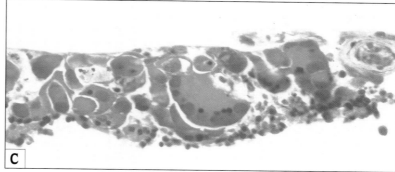

FIGURE 6-9 A, Active CMV retinitis at the border of a retinal tear and extensive retinal detachment. Although most detachments occur because of multiple, small holes at the border between normal and infected retina, large holes such as this one may form. Repair of such detachments is usually performed by vitrectomy surgery and injection of intraocular silicone oil. (Freeman WR, Friedberg DN, Berry C, *et al.*: Risk factors for development of rhegmatogenous retinal detachment in patients with cytomegalovirus retinitis. *Am J Ophthalmol* 1993, 116:713–720.) **B**, A biopsy specimen taken at the edge of a retinal hole from another case of CMV retinitis during retinal detachment repair shows relative preservation of the retinal architecture to the left of the frame. Cytomegalic inclusion cells replace the retina to the right of the frame (hematoxylin and eosin, × 20). **C**, High-power magnification of retinal cytomegalic inclusion cells (hematoxylin and eosin, × 40). In most cases, retinal biopsy is not needed to make a diagnosis of viral retinitis, but it can be useful in difficult cases. (Freeman WR, Wiley CA, Gross JG, *et al.*: Endoretinal biopsy in immunosuppressed and healthy patients with retinitis: Indications, utility, and techniques. *Ophthalmology* 1989, 96:1559–1565.)

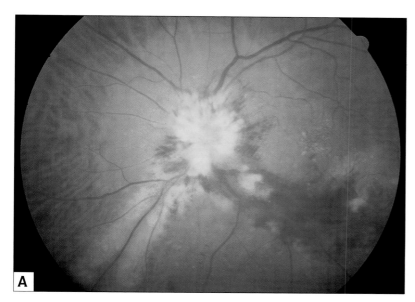

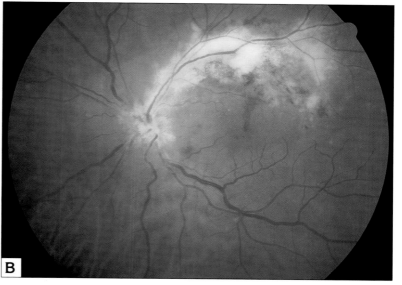

FIGURE 6-10 A, Cytomegalic optic neuritis. The papilla appears to be directly infected with CMV as there is severe visual loss to the counting fingers level and an afferent pupillary defect. There was no visual improvement despite treatment with antivirals. (Gross JG, Sadun AA, Wiley CA, Freeman WR: Severe visual loss related to isolated peripapillary retinal and optic nerve head cytomegalovirus infection. *Am J Ophthalmol* 1989, 108:691–698.) **B**, Superficial cytomegalic papillitis. Although ophthalmoscopically similar to *panel 10A*, CMV infection of the nerve appears to be superficial as the vision is only moderately impaired (20/40) and there is no afferent pupillary defect. With treatment, the papillitis cleared and vision returned to 20/20. (This photograph is less magnified than the one in *panel 10A*.)

Acute Herpetic Necrotizing Retinitis

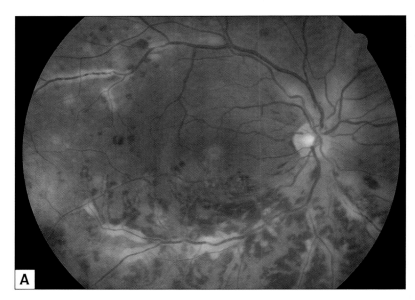

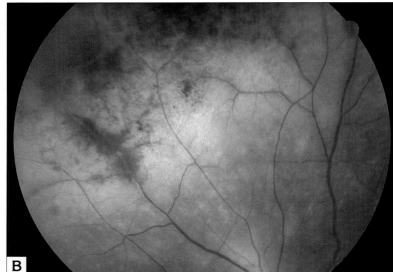

FIGURE 6-11 A, Acute herpetic necrotizing retinitis (acute retinal necrosis or progressive outer retinal necrosis), which developed 3 weeks after an aseptic meningitis presumed due to a herpes class virus. Such retinal infections are produced by herpes varicella zoster and herpes simplex. Small yellow-white patches of retinitis are seen in the posterior pole of the right eye, including one in the center of the macula. The retinal veins are sheathed with inflammatory cells and partially obstructed. Vision is 20/200. (Duker JS, Nielsen JC, Eagle RCJ, *et al.*: Rapidly progressive acute retinal necrosis secondary to herpes simplex virus, type 1. *Ophthalmology* 1990, 97:1638. Margolis TP, Lowder CY, Holland GN, et al.: Varicella-zoster virus retinitis in patients with the acquired immunodeficiency syndrome. *Am J Ophthalmol* 1991, 112:119–131.) **B,** Confluent, peripheral, herpetic necrotizing retinitis in the left eye of the patient in *panel 11A.* Older, total necrosis of the retina is seen at the top of the frame, confluent retinal whitening with venous obstruction in the middle of the frame, and fresh, large, indistinct lesions of retinitis at the bottom of the frame. For orientation, the peripheral edge of the retina (ora serrata) is superior to the frame and the optic nerve is inferior to the frame. The photograph demonstrates the orderly progression of the retinitis from peripheral to posterior retina in approximately 60° wedge; all 360° of the retinal periphery were similarly involved in both eyes. Treatment consisted of combination therapy with intravenous foscarnet and ganciclovir and retinal detachment repair with silicone oil. The patient retains ambulatory vision in the left eye 9 months after onset. The right eye is blind.

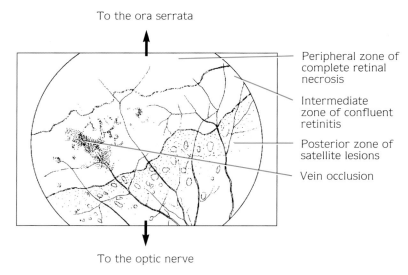

Fungal Endophthalmitis

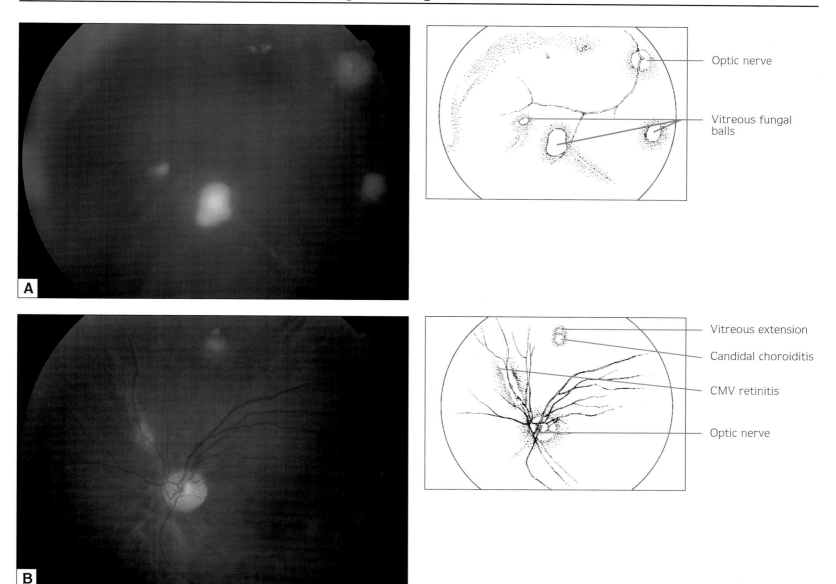

FIGURE 6-12 A, Candidal endophthalmitis that developed after fluconazole treatment was discontinued because of elevated liver enzymes. Large fungus balls float freely in the vitreous cavity and there is diffuse vitritis. (Heinemann MH, Bloom AF, Horowitz J: *Candida albicans* endophthalmitis in a patient with AIDS: Case report. *Arch Ophthalmol* 1987, 105:1172–1173.) **B,** A smaller choroidal lesion which is just beginning to bud into the vitreous cavity in the left eye of the same patient as *panel 12A.* A streak of CMV retinitis is adjacent to the optic nerve.

Resumption of fluconazole treatment for 6 weeks cured the choroidal lesion in this eye, but the vitreal fungal balls in the other eye continued to grow. The patient's physical condition precluded conventional therapy for candidal endophthalmitis, which is vitrectomy and injection of intravitreal amphotericin B, usually with adjunctive oral antifungal agents. (Brod RD, Flynn HJ, Clarkson JG, *et al.*: Endogenous Candida endophthalmitis: Management without intravenous amphotericin B. *Ophthalmology* 1990, 97:666–672.)

Toxoplasmic Chorioretinitis

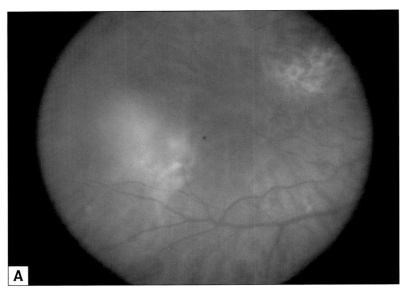

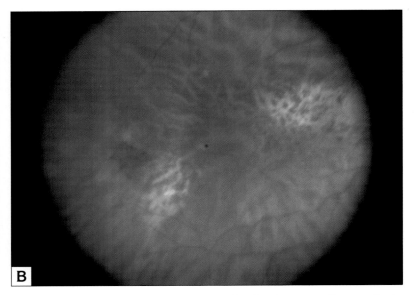

FIGURE 6-13 A, Toxoplasmic chorioretinitis. Full-thickness retinitis, usually without hemorrhage, and an overlying focal vitreous reaction is typical for toxoplasmosis. The depigmentation adjacent to the retinitis may be due to a preexisting toxoplasmosis scar from which the retinitis has reactivated or the patient's high myopia. A similar area of depigmentation adjacent to the optic nerve is seen to the right of the frame. Vision is 20/30. Toxoplasmic chorioretinitis is usually unilateral but may be bilateral in the AIDS population. Cerebral toxoplasmosis may coexist in 30% of cases. Initial response to medication is generally excellent. (Cochereau MI, LeHoang P, Lautier FM, *et al.*: Ocular toxoplasmosis in human immunodeficiency virus-infected patients. *Am J Ophthalmol* 1992, 114:130–135.) **B,** One month after treatment with pyrimethamine, 50 mg/d, and sulfadiazine, 4 g/d, the retinitis has resolved completely. Vision is 20/20. Remission was maintained by treatment with trimethoprim-sulfamethoxazole three times weekly.

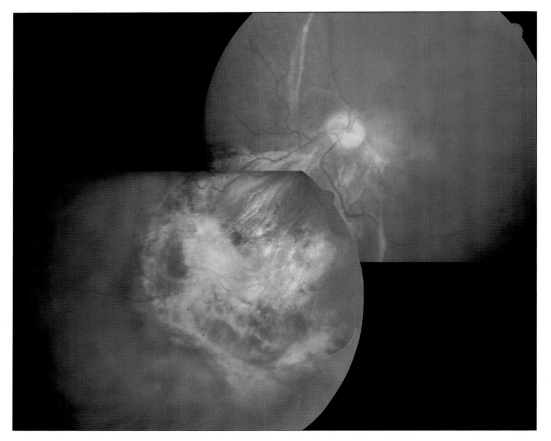

FIGURE 6-14 Toxoplasmic chorioretinitis. The very large healed lesion remains in remission after 1 year of treatment with trimethoprim-sulfamethoxazole three times weekly. Vision is poor because of an associated retinal detachment. Photographs of the acute lesion are not available because the intense inflammatory reaction precluded visualization of the fundus. Clindamycin and atovaquone are possible alternate treatments in patients who cannot tolerate sulfa medications. (Iannucci AA, Hart LL: Clindamycin in the treatment of toxoplasmosis in AIDS. *Ann Pharmacother* 1992, 26:645–647. Kovacs JA: Efficacy of atovaquone in treatment of toxoplasmosis in patients with AIDS: The NIAID-Clinical Center Intramural AIDS Program. *Lancet* 1992, 340:637–638.)

Pneumocystis Choroiditis

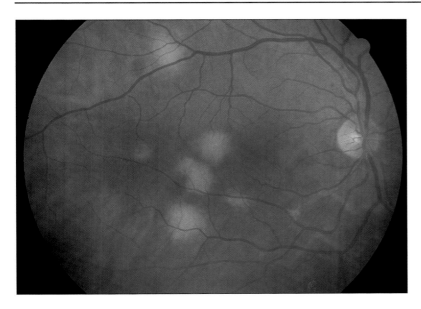

FIGURE 6-15 Pneumocystis choroiditis. A 41-year-old man recovered from pneumocystis pneumonia 3 months earlier and was being maintained on monthly inhalational pentamidine treatment. Despite the posterior location of the lesions, vision was 20/15. He was hospitalized at the same time with *Pneumocystis carinii* pneumonia. Treatment of *P. carinii* with systemic prophylactic agents rather than inhalational pentamidine may reduce the risk of disseminated disease including choroiditis. (Rao NA, Zimmerman PL, Boyer D, *et al.*: A clinical, histopathologic, and electron microscopic study of *Pneumocystis carinii* choroiditis. *Am J Ophthalmol* 1989, 107:218–228. Dugel PU, Rao NA, Forster DJ, *et al.*: *Pneumocystis carinii* choroiditis after long-term aerosolized pentamidine therapy. *Am J Ophthalmol* 1990, 110:113–117.)

Tuberculous Choroiditis

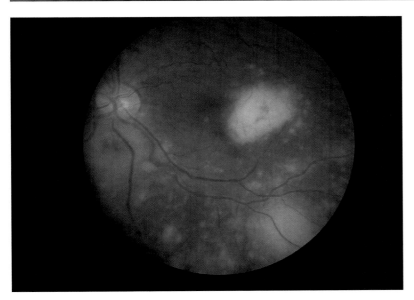

FIGURE 6-16 Presumed tuberculous choroiditis. A 30-year-old man with tuberculous myelitis on ethambutol, pyridoxine, pyrazinamide, and rifampin presented with pain and decreased vision in the right eye. The fundus in that eye could not be seen due to an intense inflammatory reaction; ultrasonography showed large choroidal nodules. The left eye had multiple choroidal lesions, as shown in the photograph. Death ensued rapidly. (Blodi BA, Johnson MW, McLeish WM, Gass JD: Presumed choroidal tuberculosis in a human immunodeficiency virus infected host. *Am J Ophthalmol* 1989, 108:605–607.) *Mycobacterium avium-intracellular* infection of the choroid also occurs, but most cases reported are autopsy specimens as the infection seems to produce few clinical symptoms. (Pepose JS, Holland GN, Nestor MS, *et al.*: Acquired immune deficiency syndrome: Pathogenic mechanisms of ocular disease. *Ophthalmology* 1985, 92:472–484.)

Endogenous Bacterial Retinitis

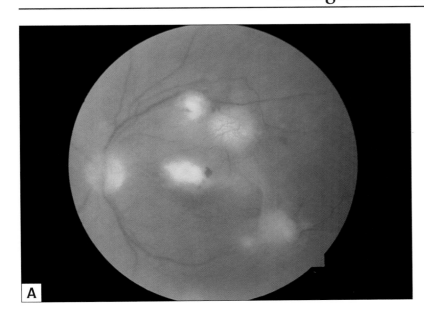

FIGURE 6-17 A, Bacterial retinitis. Bilateral multiple nodular lesions with serious detachment of the macula and small intraretinal hemorrhages developed slowly over several weeks. Enlargement of the most central lesion toward the fovea in the left eye was observed; vision was 20/200. Retinal biopsy was undertaken of the more severely affected right eye. (Davis JL, Nussenblatt RB, Bachman DM, *et al.*: Endogenous bacterial retinitis in AIDS. *Am J Ophthalmol* 1989, 107:613–623.) *(continued)*

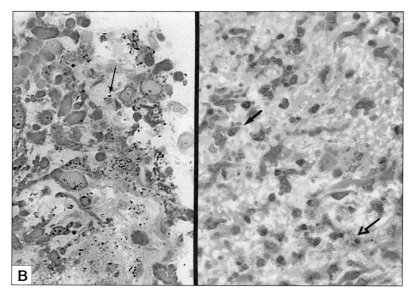
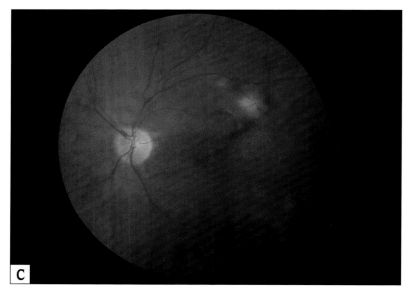

FIGURE 6-17 *(continued)* **B,** Retinal biopsy from the right eye of the patient in *panel 17A. Left,* Iodine-positive coccobacillary forms with surrounding clear zones *(arrow)* are identified both intracellularly and extracellularly (Brown's iodine stain, original magnification × 400). Some are diplococcoid *(arrow)*. *Right,* the bacteria are variably glycogen-positive *(open arrow)* (periodic acid-Schiff, original magnification × 400). Culture of the specimen failed to grow bacteria or other organisms. Viral inclusions were not present. (Published with permission from the American Journal of Ophthalmology; copyright by The Ophthalmic Publishing Co.) **C,** Because of the biopsy findings of an indolent, intracellular bacteria, doxycycline, 100 mg three times daily, was prescribed. After 6 weeks of treatment, the lesions regressed to scars. Vision improved to 20/40.

PANOPHTHALMITIS

Syphilis

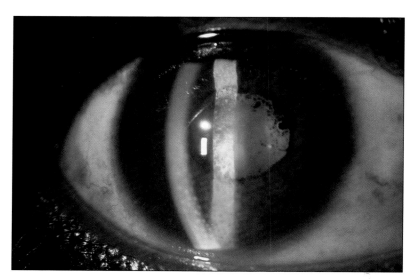
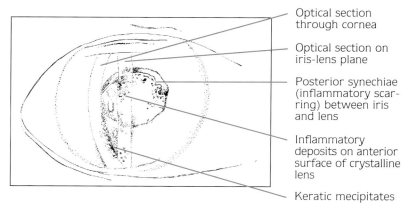

Optical section through cornea

Optical section on iris-lens plane

Posterior synechiae (inflammatory scarring) between iris and lens

Inflammatory deposits on anterior surface of crystalline lens

Keratic mecipitates

FIGURE 6-18 Syphilitic panuveitis. Inflammation involving the anterior and posterior segments obscured the view of intraocular structures and decreased the vision to 20/40 in this eye and to 20/400 in the other. A quantitative rapid plasma reagin test was 1:128. Cerebrospinal fluid VDRL test was nonreactive. Treatment with intravenous aqueous penicillin G, 24 million units/d for 10 days, led to rapid visual improvement in the left eye to 20/60 after 6 days of treatment. (McLeish WM, Pulido JS, Holland S, *et al.*: The ocular manifestations of syphilis in the human immunodeficiency virus type 1-infected host. *Ophthalmology* 1990, 97:196–203.)

Exogenous Endophthalmitis

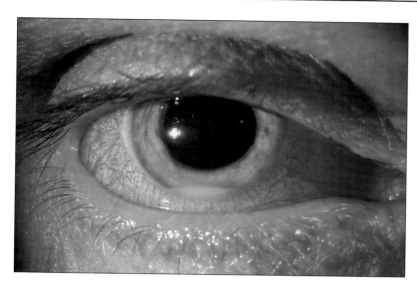

FIGURE 6-19 Coagulase-negative staphylococcal endophthalmitis following intravitreal injection of ganciclovir for the treatment of CMV retinitis. A hypopyon is present in the anterior segment. The view of the fundus was poor due to dense vitritis. Treatment with intravitreal injection of antibiotics and vitrectomy controlled the infection, but vision was lost due to retinal detachment. A similar presentation with hypopyon could occur in acute endogenous endophthalmitis or in drug-induced uveitis. (Young SH, Morlet N, Heery S, *et al.*: High-dose intravitreal ganciclovir in the treatment of cytomegalovirus retinitis. *Med J Aust* 1992, 157:370–373. Alvarez R, Adan A, Martinez JA, *et al.*: Haematogenous *Serratia marcescens* endophthalmitis in an HIV-infected intravenous drug addict. *Infection* 1990, 18:29–30. Shafran SD, Deschenes J, Miller M, *et al.*: Uveitis and pseudojaundice during a regimen of clarithromycin, rifabutin, and ethambutol: MAC Study Group of the Canadian HIV Trials Network [letter]. *N Engl J Med* 1994, 330:438–439.)

ACKNOWLEDGMENT

Dr. Stephen Pflugfelder, Dr. Barry Fishbourne, Dr. Barbara Blodi, Dr. Elaine Chuang, and the residents of the Bascom Palmer Eye Institute provided clinical care for some of the patients presented here. Their help is appreciated. The photographic department of the Bascom Palmer provided valuable technical assistance.

SELECTED BIBLIOGRAPHY

Gross JG, Bozzette SA, Matthews WC, *et al.*: Longitudinal study of cytomegalovirus retinitis in acquired immune deficiency syndrome. *Ophthalmology* 1990, 97:681–686.

Jabs DA, Green WR, Fox R, *et al.*: Ocular manifestations of acquired immune deficiency syndrome. *Ophthalmology* 1989, 96:1092–1099.

Shuler JD, Engstrom RJ, Holland GN: External ocular disease and anterior segment disorders associated with AIDS. *Int Ophthalmol Clin* 1989, 29:98–104.

CHAPTER 7

Oral Cavity Manifestations

Deborah Greenspan
John S. Greenspan

NEOPLASTIC DISEASE

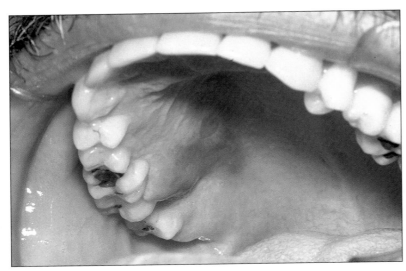

FIGURE 7-1 Kaposi's sarcoma of the palate. The oral mucosa is one of the commonest sites for Kaposi's sarcoma and is often the first or presenting location, with the palate being the most common intraoral site. A nodular purple lesion is seen in this patient, but larger lesions may ulcerate and can become secondarily infected. These lesions can be treated with intralesional chemotherapy, *eg*, vinblastine. Very extensive lesions may warrant radiation therapy. (Ficarra G, Person AM, *et al.*: Kaposi's sarcoma of the oral cavity: A study of 134 patients with a review of the pathogenesis, epidemiology, clinical aspects, and treatment. *Oral Surg Oral Med Oral Pathol* 1988, 66:543–550. Epstein JB, Scully C: Intralesional vinblastine for oral Kaposi's sarcoma in HIV infection. *Lancet* 1989, 2:1100–1101.)

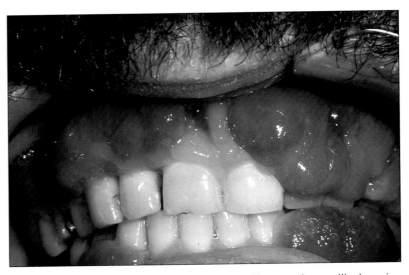

FIGURE 7-2 Kaposi's sarcoma of the maxillary and mandibular gingiva. Multiple and extensive nodular purple lesions are apparent on the gingiva in this patient. The gingiva is the second commonest intraoral site, and these lesions often become infected with dental plaque microorganisms, causing severe pain. Careful debridement, scaling, and curettage result in reduction of inflammation, making surgical excision or radiotherapy more effective.

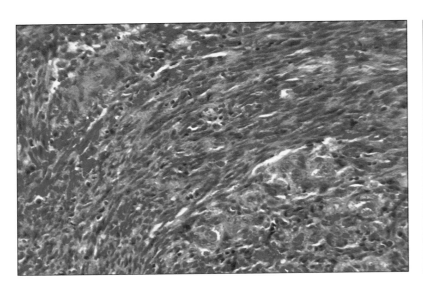

FIGURE 7-3 Kaposi's sarcoma, histopathology. Histopathologic examination of nodular lesion shows spindle cells and extravasated erythrocytes (hematoxylin-eosin stain, × 40). Their histopathologic appearance is identical to that of Kaposi's sarcoma at other sites. (Regezi JALAM, Daniels TE, DeSouza YG, *et al.*: Human immunodeficiency virus-associated oral Kaposi's sarcoma: A heterogeneous cell population dominated by spindle-shaped endothelial cells. *Am J Pathol* 1993, 143:240–249.)

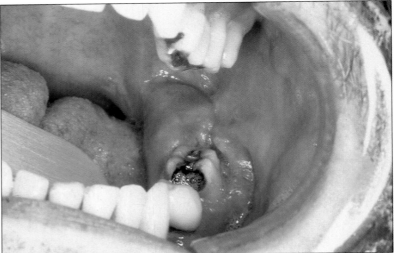

FIGURE 7-4 Non-Hodgkin's lymphoma. Most oral AIDS lymphomas are B-cell lymphoblastoid type, often Epstein-Barr virus–positive. Oral non-Hodgkin's lymphoma may present as ulcers or firm nodules, as seen on the posterior mandible of this patient. The oral lesions may be the first or only lesions of non-Hodgkin's lymphoma. (Dodd CL, Greenspan D, *et al.*: Multifocal oral non-Hodgkin's lymphoma in an AIDS patient. *Br Dent J* 1994, in press.)

FUNGAL AND VIRAL INFECTIONS

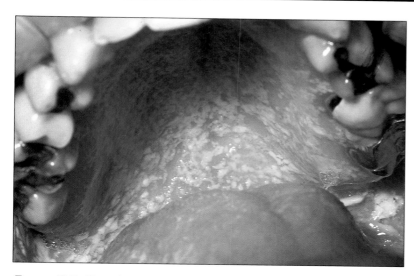

FIGURE 7-5 Pseudomembranous candidiasis of the palate. A creamy-white plaque consisting of fungal hyphae, desquamated epithelial cells, and polymorphonuclear cells can be easily removed, leaving a red surface. These lesions can appear at any location in the mouth and oropharynx. There may be symptoms of burning or changes in taste. (Greenspan D, Greenspan JS, *et al.: AIDS and the Mouth.* Copenhagen, Munksgaard, 1990.)

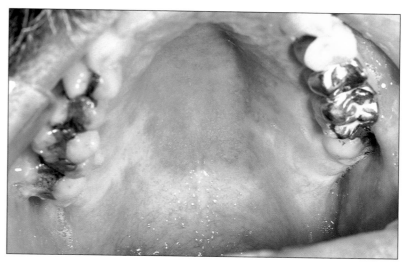

FIGURE 7-6 Erythematous candidiasis. Subtle red patches on the palate reveal *Candida* hyphae in a KOH preparation. This lesion is just as significant a predictor of progression to AIDS in HIV-positive individuals as the more obvious pseudomembranous form. (Dodd CL, Greenspan D, Katz MH, *et al.*: Oral candidiasis in HIV infection: Pseudomembraneous and erythematous candidiasis show similar rates of progression to AIDS. *AIDS* 1991, 5:1339–1343.)

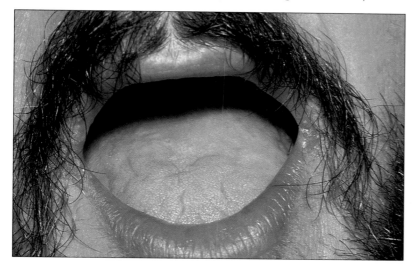

FIGURE 7-7 Angular cheilitis. Cracking, redness, and fissures at the corners of the mouth may be seen alone or in association with intraoral candidiasis. Antifungal creams applied to the lesions are a useful adjunct to other antifungal therapy.

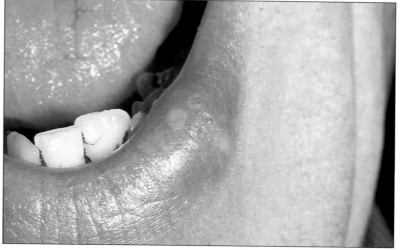

FIGURE 7-8 Herpes labialis of the lower lip. Recurrent herpes simplex virus lesions start as small vesicles, which ulcerate and coalesce. They are usually self-limiting. Treatment with oral acyclovir capsules is effective if administered early.

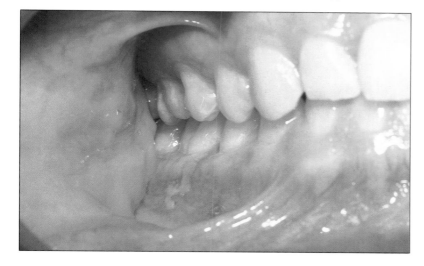

FIGURE 7-9 Recurrent intraoral herpes simplex. Crops of recurring vesicles that ulcerate can appear in HIV-infected persons. In immunocompetent individuals, this condition is seen only on the keratinized mucosa of the gingiva and palate, where the lesions are usually self-limiting. However, in those with HIV infection, the lesions may be seen also on other oropharyngeal surfaces, such as the dorsal tongue, and they may be persistent. Oral acyclovir may be indicated for early or persistent lesions. Rare cases of acyclovir-resistance occur. (MacPhail LA, Greenspan D, *et al.*: Acyclovir-resistant, foscarnet-sensitive oral herpes simplex type 2 lesion in a patient with AIDS. *Oral Surg Oral Med Oral Pathol* 1989, 67:427–432.)

HAIRY LEUKOPLAKIA

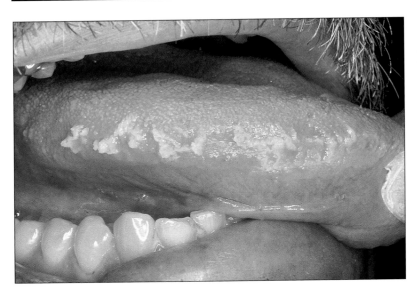

FIGURE 7-10 Hairy leukoplakia of the tongue. The lesion, consisting of corrugations on the lateral margin continuous with flat areas on the ventral surface, is seen most commonly on the lateral tongue. Originally described in HIV-positive individuals, in whom it is common, hairy leukoplakia has now been seen in a number of other immunodeficient groups, including transplant recipients and those on long-term steroid therapy. Like oral candidiasis, hairy leukoplakia is predictive of progression to AIDS in HIV-infected individuals. (Greenspan D, Greenspan JS, *et al.*: Oral "hairy" leucoplakia in male homosexuals: Evidence of association with both papillomavirus and a herpes-group virus. *Lancet* 1984, 2:831–834. Feigal DW, Katz MH, *et al.*: The prevalence of oral lesions in HIV-infected homosexual and bisexual men: Three San Francisco epidemiological cohorts. *AIDS* 1991, 5:519–525. Greenspan D, Greenspan JS: The significance of oral hairy leukoplakia. *Oral Surg Oral Med Oral Pathol* 1992, 73:151–154. Katz MH, Greenspan D, *et al.*: Progression to AIDS in HIV-infected homosexual and bisexual men with hairy leukoplakia and oral candidiasis. *AIDS* 1992, 6:95–100.)

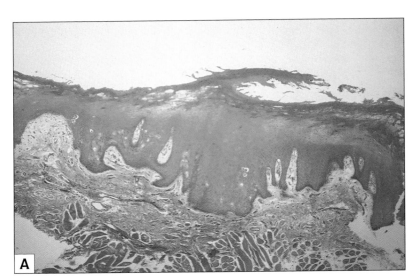

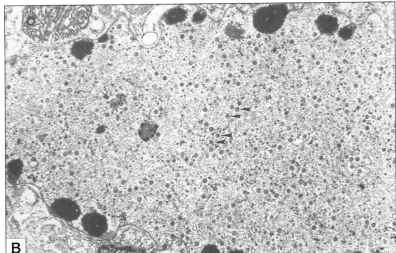

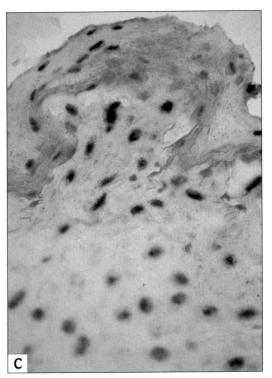

FIGURE 7-11 Hairy leukoplakia of the tongue. **A,** Histopathologic examination discloses epithelial thickening with surface projections, acanthosis, vacuolation of groups of cells in the stratum granulosum, and little or no inflammatory cell infiltration (hematoxylin-eosin stain, × 10). **B,** Electron microscopy shows large numbers of Epstein-Barr virus (EBV) particles. (Greenspan JS, Greenspan D, *et al.*: Replication of Epstein-Barr virus within the epithelial cells of "hairy" leukoplakia, an AIDS-associated lesion. *N Engl J Med* 1985, 313:1564–1571.) **C,** On *in-situ* hybridization for EBV-DNA, infected nuclei show a purple signal. (DeSouza YG, Freese UK, *et al.*: Diagnosis of Epstein-Barr virus infection in hairy leukoplakia by using nucleic acid hybridization and noninvasive techniques. *J Clin Microbiol* 1990, 28:2775–2778.)

WARTS, PERIODONTAL DISEASE, AND APHTHOUS ULCERS

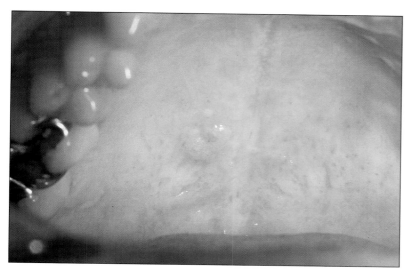

FIGURE 7-12 Wart, palate. Lesions due to human papillomavirus (HPV) infection are seen in all regions of the oral mucosa. Many are associated with HPV-7, a papillomavirus type associated previously with warts on the hands of butchers and not seen in the mouths of HIV-negative individuals. (Greenspan D, de Villiers EM, *et al.*: Unusual HPV types in the oral warts in association with HIV infection. *J Oral Pathol* 1988, 17:482–487.)

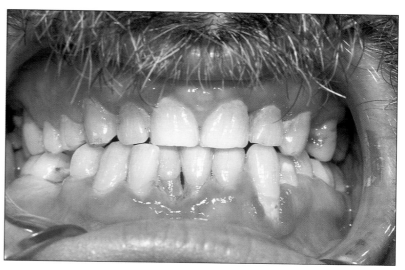

FIGURE 7-13 Necrotizing periodontitis ("HIV periodontitis"). This rapidly destructive inflammation, seen here on the anterior mandible, is associated with the same wide range of anaerobic bacteria as is found in conventional periodontal disease in immunocompetent individuals. The lesions respond to thorough local debridement (scaling and root planing) plus local antibacterial irrigation supplemented with systemic antibiotics. (Zambon JJ, Reynolds H, *et al.*: Are unique bacterial pathogens involved in HIV-associated periodontal diseases? In *Oral Manifestations of HIV Infection: Proceedings of the Second International Workshop*. Chicago, Quintessence Publishing Co., 1994. Palmer GD: Periodontal therapy for patients with HIV infection. In *Oral Manifestations of HIV Infection: Proceedings of the Second International Workshop*. Chicago, Quintessence Publishing Co., 1994.)

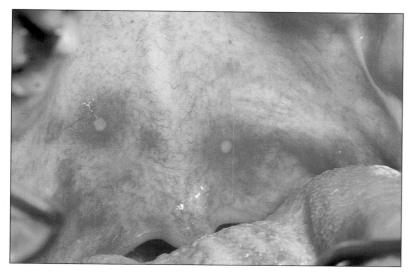

FIGURE 7-14 Minor recurrent aphthous ulcers on the buccal mucosa. Recurrent aphthous ulcers are only slightly more common in the HIV-infected population, but there they tend to be more frequent, severe, and prolonged. The cause is unknown, but autoimmunity may play a role. (MacPhail LA, Greenspan D, *et al.*: Recurrent aphthous ulcers in association with HIV infection: Description of ulcer types and analysis of T-cell subsets. *Oral Surg Oral Med Oral Pathol* 1991, 71:678–683.)

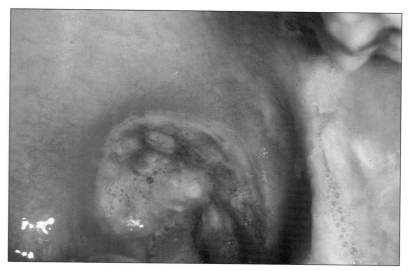

FIGURE 7-15 Severe major recurrent aphthous ulcers. Such lesions, as seen on the right soft palate in this patient, can be the cause of significant pain and difficulty with speech, mastication, and swallowing. Biopsy is usually indicated to rule out lymphoma and other chronic ulcerative lesions.

SIGNIFICANCE OF ORAL LESIONS

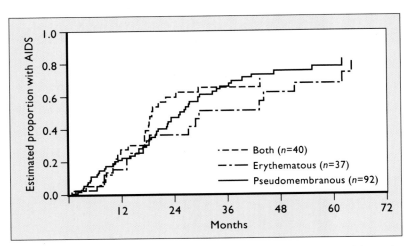

FIGURE 7-16 Time to development of AIDS for patients with oral candidiasis. As studied in a clinic population in San Francisco, erythematous candidiasis is as predictive as pseudomembranous candidiasis for indicating the time to development of AIDS. In this study, a rapid progression to AIDS (median, 25 months) and to death (median, 43.8 months) was seen for all three groups. (*From* Dodd CL, Greenspan D, Katz MH, *et al.*: Oral candidiasis in HIV infection: Pseudomembranous and erythematous candidiasis show similar rates of progression to AIDS. *AIDS* 1991, 5:1339–1343; with permission.)

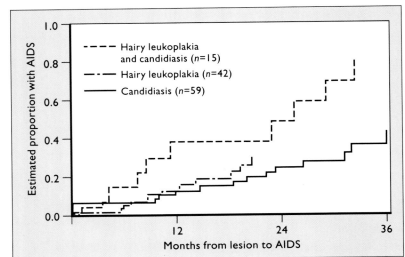

FIGURE 7-17 Progression to AIDS, according to the presence of oral manifestations. In three San Francisco cohorts, both oral candidiasis and hairy leukoplakia proved to be indicators of progression of HIV disease. After CD4 counts were adjusted for, men with hairy leukoplakia and candidiasis on baseline examinations had a significantly higher rate of progression to AIDS than men with normal oral findings. (*From* Katz MH, Greenspan D, Westenhouse J, *et al.*: Progression to AIDS in HIV-infected homosexual and bisexual men with hairy leukoplakia and oral candidiasis. *AIDS* 1992, 6:95–100; with permission.)

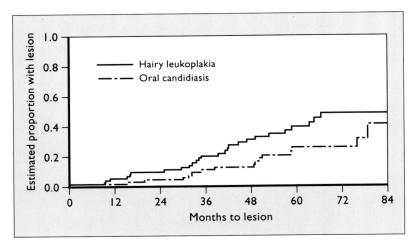

FIGURE 7-18 Estimated progression rates from seroconversion to oral lesions. In three cohorts of homosexual and bisexual men in San Francisco, men who acquired HIV infection during the course of the investigation were followed prospectively, and time to development of oral candidiasis or hairy leukoplakia was assessed. These lesions appeared frequently and relatively soon after HIV seroconversion, with oral candidiasis developing in 4% of patients by 1 year, 8% by 2 years, and 26% by 5 years, and hairy leukoplakia developing in 9% by 1 year, 16% by 2 years, and 42% by 5 years. (*From* Lifson AR, Hilton JF, Westenhouse JL, *et al.*: Time from HIV seroconversion to oral candidiasis or hairy leukoplakia among homosexual men and bisexual men enrolled in three prospective cohorts. *AIDS* 1994, 8:73–79; with permission.)

ACKNOWLEDGMENT

This paper was supported by PO1-DE-07946.

SELECTED BIBLIOGRAPHY

Dodd CL, Greenspan D, Katz MH, *et al.*: Oral candidiasis in HIV infection: Pseudomembraneous and erythematous candidiasis show similar rates of progression to AIDS. *AIDS* 1991, 5:1339–1343.

Feigal DW, Katz MH, *et al.*: The prevalence of oral lesions in HIV-infected homosexual and bisexual men: Three San Francisco epidemiological cohorts. *AIDS* 1991, 5:519–525.

Greenspan D, Greenspan JS, *et al.*: *AIDS and the Mouth.* Copenhagen, Munksgaard, 1990.

Katz MH, Greenspan D, *et al.*: Progression to AIDS in HIV-infected homosexual and bisexual men with hairy leukoplakia and oral candidiasis. *AIDS* 1992, 6:95–100.

Lifson AR, Hilton JF, Westenhouse JL, *et al.*: Time from HIV seroconversion to oral candidiasis or hairy leukoplakia among homosexual and bisexual men enrolled in three prospective cohorts. *AIDS* 1994, 8:73–79.

CHAPTER 8

Pulmonary Complications

Mark J. Rosen

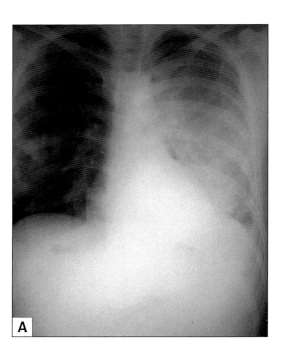

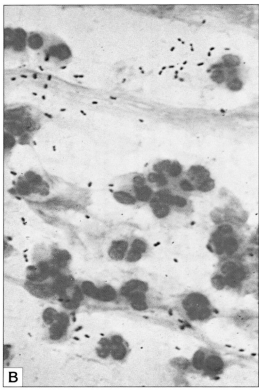

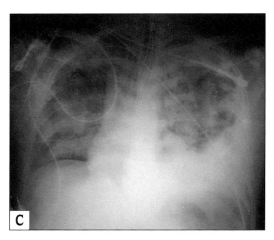

FIGURE 8-1 A, Chest radiograph of a 32-year-old man who presented with fever, chills, and shortness of breath. There is bilateral pulmonary consolidation, worse on the left. **B,** Gram stain of sputum showed numerous polymorphonuclear leukocytes and gram-positive diplococci. Blood cultures were positive for pneumococcus, type III. (Pesola GR, Charles A: Pneumococcal bacteremia with pneumonia. Mortality in acquired immunodeficien-cy syndrome. *Chest* 1992, 101:150–155.) **C,** Chest radiograph taken 4 days later shows bilateral diffuse areas of consolidation and a large left pleural effusion. The patient was intubated and on mechanical ventilation. His course was complicated by empyema, renal failure, and prolonged mechanical ventilation. He eventually recovered, only to develop Kaposi's sarcoma 6 months later.

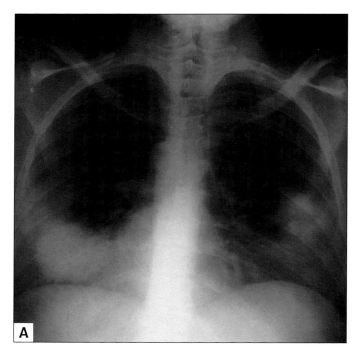

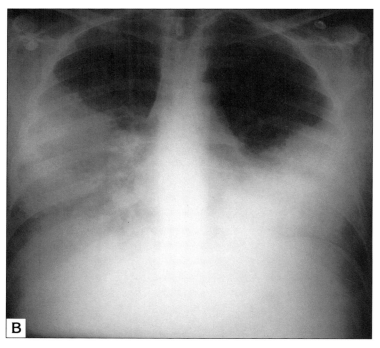

FIGURE 8-2 A, Haemophilus influenzae. Bilateral lower lobe dense consolidations. The blood cultures were positive for *H. influenzae*. **B,** Chest radiograph taken 12 hours later. The patient had a rapidly fulminating course and died.

PNEUMOCYSTIS CARINII PNEUMONIA

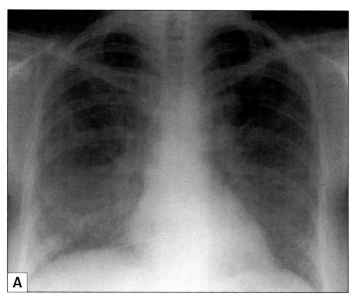

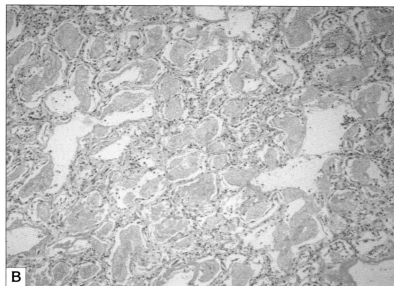

FIGURE 8-3 **A**, *Pneumocystis carinii* pneumonia. Chest radiograph showing typical changes of *P. carcinii* pneumonia. There are bilateral diffuse pulmonary infiltrates. (Masur H: Prevention and treatment of pneumocystis pneumonia. *N Engl J Med* 1992, 326:1853–1860.) **B**, An open lung biopsy (hematoxylin-eosin stain) shows most alveoli are filled with foamy pink material, typi- cal of *P. carinii* pneumonia. Profound ventilation-perfusion mis- matching causes severe hypoxemia. (Maxfield RA, Sorkin B, Fazzini EP, *et al.*: Respiratory failure in patients with acquired immunodeficiency syndrome and *Pneumocystis carinii* pneumonia. *Crit Care Med* 1986, 14:443–449.)

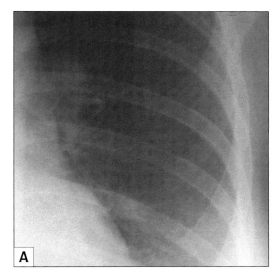

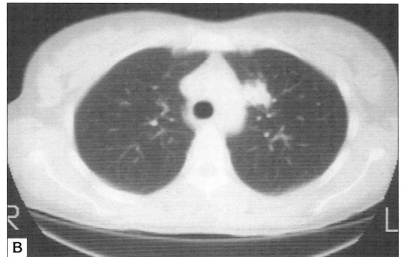

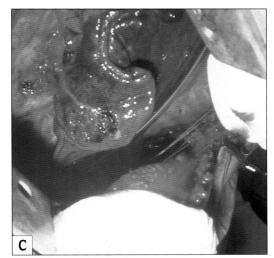

FIGURE 8-4 **A**, Atypical presentation of *Pneumocystis carinii* pneumonia. Detail of a chest radiograph shows a mass in the para-aortic area. **B**, Computed tomography (CT) of the chest con- firms this nodule. **C**, A nodule as seen during surgery. On histo- logic section, this nodule contained granulomas and *P. carinii* organisms.

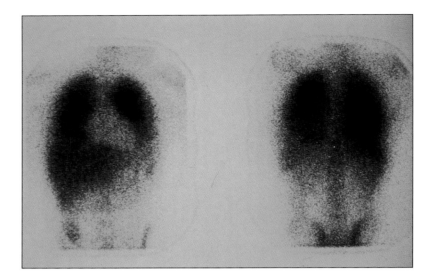

FIGURE 8-5 A gallium scan is 4+ positive in a patient with *Pneumocystis carinii* pneumonia and a normal chest radiograph. There is almost always intense uptake of gallium in the lung in cases of *P. carinii* pneumonia. (Golden JA, Sollitto RA: The radiology of pulmonary disease: Chest roentgenography, computed tomography and gallium scanning. *Clin Chest Med* 1988, 9:481–495.)

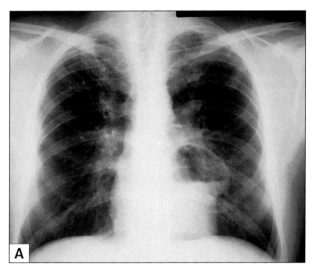

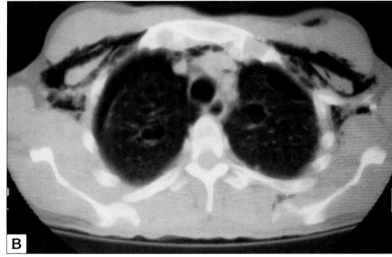

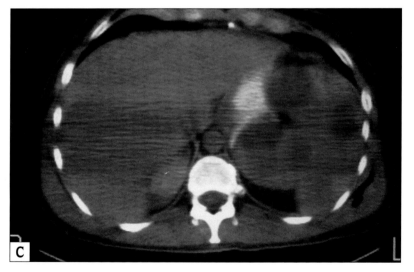

FIGURE 8-6 **A**, Chest radiograph of a patient using aerosolized pentamidine prophylaxis for *Pneumocystis carinii* pneumonia. There is a large cystic space with an air-fluid level and bilateral upper lobe linear densities. Bronchoscopic washings confirmed the presence of *P. carinii* pneumonia. **B**, Computed tomography (CT) scan of the chest in the same patient shows cystic changes in both upper lung fields, small bilateral pneumothoraces, and subcutaneous emphysema. Upper lobe cystic changes and pneumothoraces are common complications of *P. carinii* pneumonia in patients taking aerosolized pentamidine prophylaxis. (Masur H: Prevention and treatment of pneumocystis pneumonia. *N Engl J Med* 1992, 326: 1853–1860. **C**, CT scan of the abdomen in the same patient shows the presence of mass lesions in the spleen. These are presumed to be due to *P. carinii*, because they later resolved following anti-*Pneumocystis* treatment. Extrapulmonary *P. carinii* infection occurs more frequently in the setting of aerosolized pentamidine prophylaxis, presumably because the drug is distributed only to the lung.

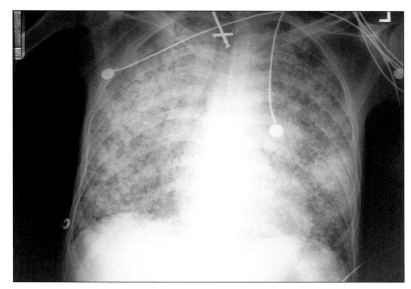

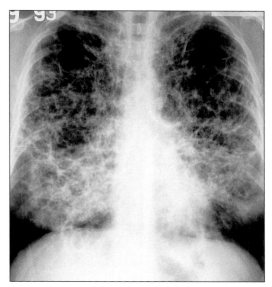

FIGURE 8-8 Numerous cystic lesions in a patient with confirmed *Pneumocystis carinii* pneumonia. This patient received no prior prophylaxis.

FIGURE 8-7 Miliary pattern in a patient with *Pneumocystis carinii* pneumonia.

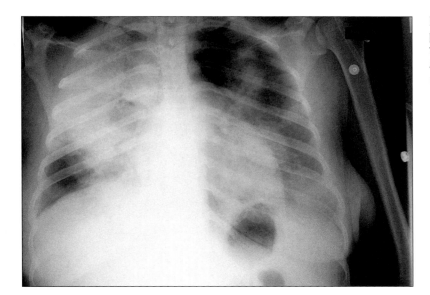

FIGURE 8-9 Patients may be infected with more than one pathogen. This chest radiograph discloses bilateral dense, but focal, consolidations. Blood and sputum cultures were positive for *Streptoccus pneumoniae*, but bronchoalveolar lavage also revealed *Pneumocystis carinii*.

TUBERCULOSIS

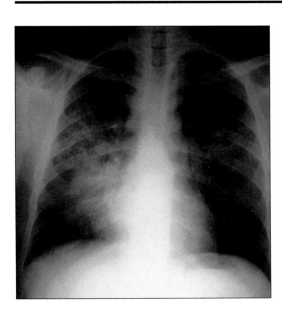

FIGURE 8-10 A chest radiograph in a patient with HIV infection and a low CD4 lymphocyte count (150×10^6/L) shows right lower lobe consolidation and paratracheal lymphadenopathy. (Pitchenik AE, Rubinson HA: The radiologic appearance of tuberculosis in patients with the acquired immune deficiency syndrome (AIDS) and pre-AIDS. *Am Rev Respir Dis* 1985, 131:393–396.)

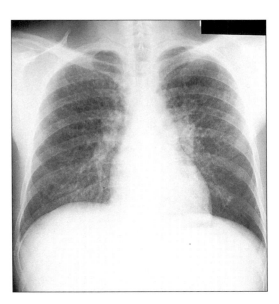

FIGURE 8-11 Miliary tuberculosis in a patient with HIV infection.

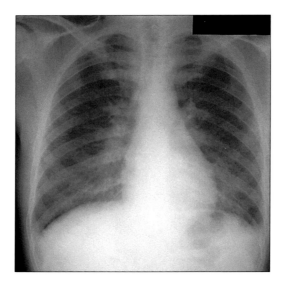

FIGURE 8-12 Chest radiograph of a patient with pulmonary tuberculosis and HIV infection. Note bilateral interstitial and cavitary changes, worse on the right than the left. (Chaisson RE, Schecter GF, Theuer CP, *et al.*: Tuberculosis in patients with acquired immunodeficiency syndrome: Clinical features, response to therapy, and survival. *Am Rev Respir Dis* 1987, 136:570.)

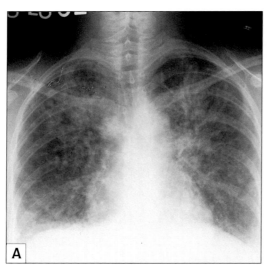

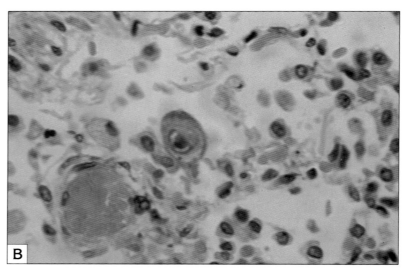

FIGURE 8-13 A, Cytomegalovirus pneumonitis. Chest radiograph of a patient with cytomegalovirus (CMV) pneumonitis. Although, CMV causes devastating infection in patients with HIV infection, clinically significant pneumonitis is rare. CMV is commonly cultured from bronchoalveolar lavage fluid in patients with HIV infection, but the diagnosis of CMV pneumonia depends on histologic demonstration of infection. (Drew WL: Cytomegalovirus infection in patients with AIDS. *Clin Infect Dis* 1992, 14:608.) **B,** Hematoxylin-eosin stain of an open lung biopsy sample shows a typical inclusion body of CMV.

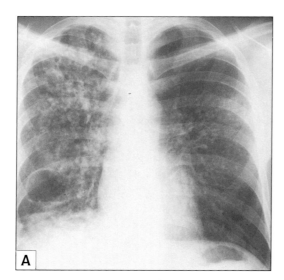

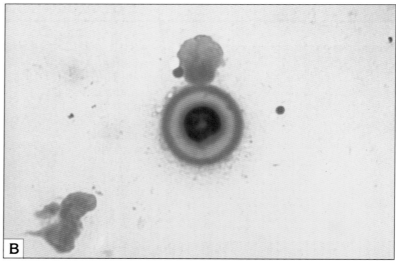

FIGURE 8-14 A, *Cryptococcus* infection. Chest radiograph of a patient with disseminated infection with *Cryptococcus neoformans*. These bilateral diffuse infiltrates are similar to those of *Pneumocystis carinii* pneumonia, but right paratracheal lymphadenopathy suggests another diagnosis. (Chechani V, Kamholz SL: Pulmonary manifestations of disseminated cryptococcosis in patients with AIDS. *Chest* 1990, 98:1060–1066.) *(continued)*

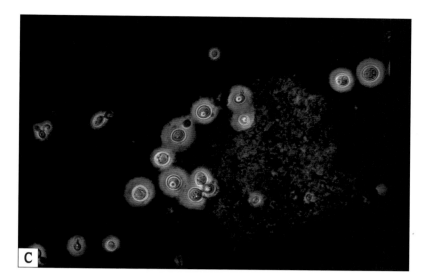

FIGURE 8-14 *(continued)* **B,** Periodic acid-Schiff stain of bronchoalveolar lavage fluid shows encapsulated organism typical of *C. neoformans*. **C,** India ink stain of bronchoalveolar lavage fluid confirms the presence of encapsulated organisms.

KAPOSI'S SARCOMA

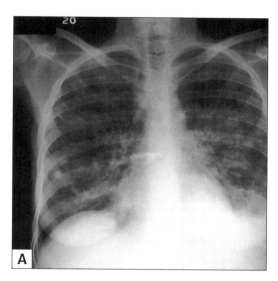

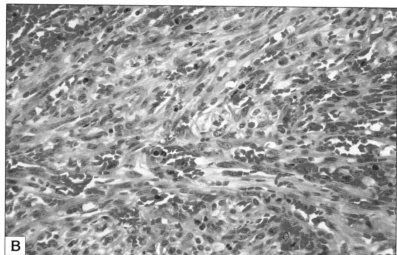

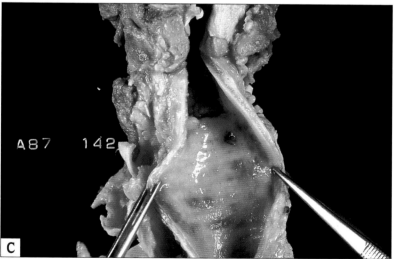

FIGURE 8-15 A, Chest radiograph showing bilateral diffuse linear and nodular infiltrates. This patient was a 32-year-old African-American woman who was an injection drug user. **B,** Fiberoptic bronchoscopy, including transbronchial biopsy and bronchoalveolar lavage, were nondiagnostic. An open lung biopsy specimen (hematoxylin-eosin stain) shows spindle cells and vascular clefts, typical of Kaposi's sarcoma. This malignancy usually involves the skin, but may disseminate to internal organs. For unknown reasons, it is much more common in gay men than in other risk groups. The patient died of respiratory failure. (Ognibene FP, Steis RG, Macher AM, *et al.*: Kaposi's sarcoma causing pulmonary infiltrates and respiratory failure in the acquired immunodeficiency syndrome. *Ann Intern Med* 1985, 102:471–475. **C,** Airway appearance of Kaposi's sarcoma. This autopsy specimen shows purple submucosal lesions within the trachea. When seen with the bronchoscope, these lesions should be considered diagnostic of Kaposi's sarcoma.

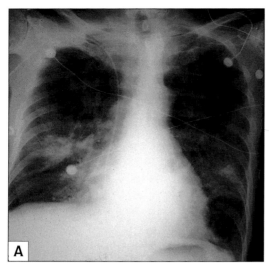

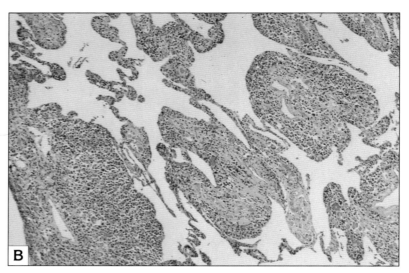

FIGURE 8-16 A, B-cell lymphoma. Chest radiograph of a 42-year-old man with hemophilia and HIV infection showing a right lower lobe pulmonary infiltrate. **B,** Autopsy specimen (hematoxylin-eosin stain) disclos- ing infiltration of the pulmonary parenchyma with B-cell lymphoma. (Polish LB, Cohn DL, Ryder JW, *et al.*: Pulmonary non-Hodgkin's lymphoma in AIDS. *Chest* 1989, 96:1321–1326.

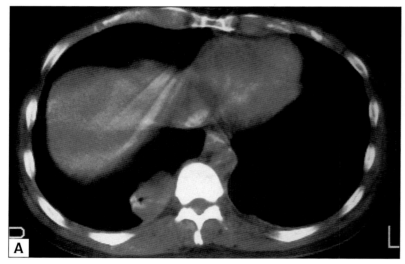

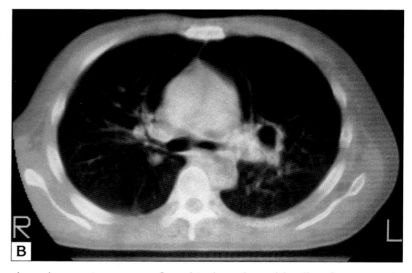

FIGURE 8-17 A, Chest computed tomography (CT) scan in a 40-year-old homosexual man showing a right lower lobe posterior mass. **B,** A later CT scan in the same patient shows another mass in the left midlung field. The patient developed massive hemopty- sis and, on autopsy, was found to have been bleeding from a cavi-tary mass of B-cell lymphoma.

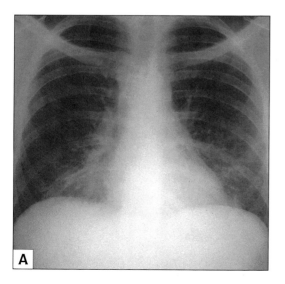

FIGURE 8-18 A, Lymphocytic interstitial pneumonitis. Chest radiograph of a 30-year-old African-American homosexual man with bilateral interstitial infiltrates, predominantly involving the lower lobes. Fiberoptic bronchoscopy with transbronchial biopsy and bron-choalveolar lavage were nondiagnostic. *(continued)*

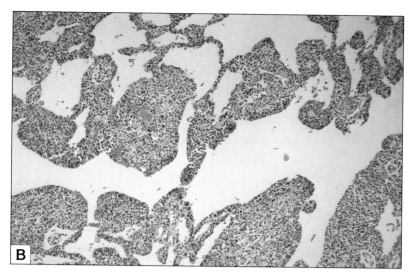

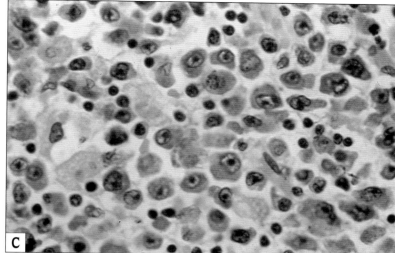

FIGURE **8-18** *(continued)* **B,** Hematoxylin-eosin stain of an open lung biopsy shows histiocytic and plasma cell infiltrates, diagnostic of lymphocytic interstitial pneumonitis. **C,** High-power view.

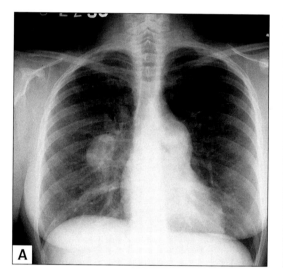

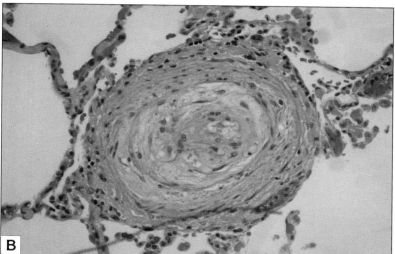

FIGURE **8-19 A,** Primary pulmonary hypertension. A 32-year-old injection drug user presented with progressive shortness of breath. There is marked dilatation of both pulmonary arteries. **B,** Open lung biopsy discloses arterial medial hypertrophy and intimal hyperplasia, typical of primary pulmonary hypertension. For unknown reasons, the incidence of primary pulmonary hypertension is increased in patients with HIV infection.

SELECTED BIBLIOGRAPHY

Murray JF, Felton CP, Garay SM, *et al.*: Pulmonary complications of the acquired immunodeficiency syndrome: Report of National Heart, Lung and Blood Institute Workshop. *N Engl J Med* 1984, 310:1682.

Murray JF, Mills J: Pulmonary infectious complications of human immunodeficiency virus infection. *Am Rev Respir Dis* 1990, 141:1356–1372, 1582–1598.

White DA, Matthay RA: Noninfectious complications of infection with the human immunodeficiency virus. *Am Rev Respir Dis* 1989, 140:1763–1787.

Janoff EN, Breiman RE, Daley CL, *et al.*: Pneumococcal disease during HIV infection. Epidemiologic, clinical and immunologic perspectives. *Ann Intern Med* 1992, 117:314.

Barnes PF, Bloch AB, Davidson PT, *et al.*: Tuberculosis in patients with human immunodeficiency virus infection. *N Engl J Med* 1991, 324:1644.

CHAPTER 9

Gastrointestinal Manifestations

Christine A. Wanke

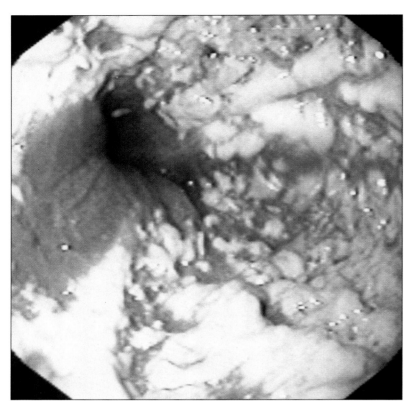

FIGURE 9-1 Manifestations of HIV infection extend throughout the gastrointestinal tract. Candidal infection of the oral cavity or thrush may be one of the first manifestations of immune compromise in an HIV-infected patient. Apthous ulcers of unclear etiology also occur. Some of these can be persistent, painful, and refractory to therapy, although some response to thalidomide has been seen. Esophagitis caused by *Candida albicans* is a frequent complication in AIDS patients and may develop as an extension of untreated oral thrush. The use of the effective oral prophylactic antifungal agent, fluconazole, has decreased the incidence of this opportunistic infection. Severe disease may also be treated by a short course of intravenous amphotericin B. The appearance of severe candidal esophagitis is distinctive as seen in this figure, but confirmation of the diagnosis depends on scrapings demonstrating the classic gram-positive candidal forms. (Laine L, Dretler RH, Conteas CN, *et al.*: Fluconazole compared with ketoconazole for the treatment of candidal esophagitis in AIDS: A randomized trial. *Ann Intern Med* 1992, 117:655–660.)

CYTOMEGALOVIRUS

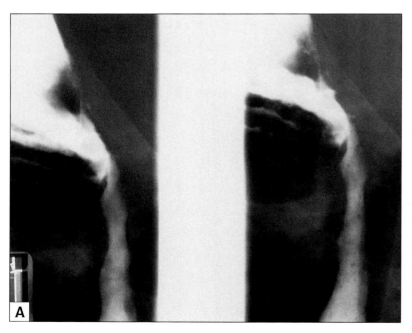

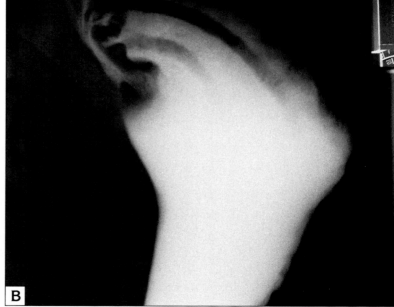

FIGURE 9-2 A, Additional causes of esophagitis in the HIV-infected population include herpes virus and cytomegalovirus (CMV), which is shown in the radiograph. The secure diagnosis of these agents rests on endoscopic evaluation and biopsy demonstrating typical inclusion bodies. (Wilcox CM, Diehl DL, Cello JP, *et al.*: Cytomegalovirus esophagitis in patients with AIDS: A clinical, endoscopic, and pathologic correlation. *Ann Intern Med* 1990, 113:589–593. Sacks SL, Wanklin RJ, Reece DE, *et al.*: Progressive esophagitis from acyclovir-resistant herpes simplex: Clinical roles for DNA polymerase mutants and viral heterogeneity? *Ann Intern Med* 1989, 111:893–899.) **B,** CMV also may cause disease throughout the gastrointestinal tract. This radiograph demonstrates a gastric mass lesion that biopsy proved to be an inflammatory mass caused by CMV. It resolved on therapy with ganciclovir. (Rich JD, Crawford JM, Kazanijian SN, Kazanijian PH: Discrete gastrointestinal mass lesions caused by cytomegalovirus in patients with AIDS: Report of three cases and review. *Clin Infect Dis* 1992, 15:609–614.)

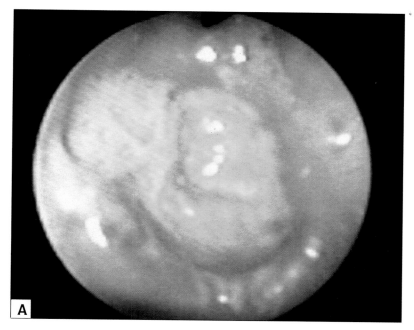

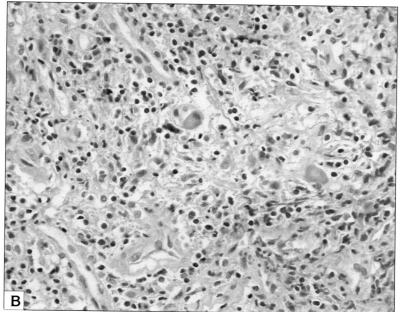

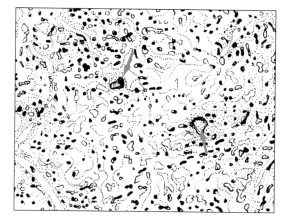

FIGURE 9-3 CMV must also be considered as a potential pathogen in an AIDS patient presenting with a gastric or duodenal ulcer or with acalculous cholecystitis. **A**, A deep gastric CMV ulcer. **B**, Typical CMV inclusion bodies (*arrows*) in the gall bladder mucosa. (Kavin H, *et al.*: Acalculous cholecystitis and CMV infection in AIDS. *Ann Intern Med* 1986, 104:53–54. Schneiderman DJ, *et al.*: Papillary stenosis and sclerosing cholangitis in AIDS. *Ann Intern Med* 1987, 106:546.)

HIV ENTEROPATHY

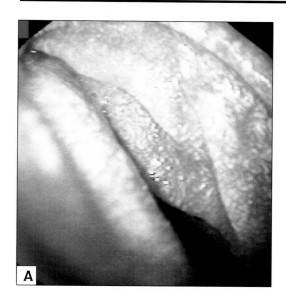

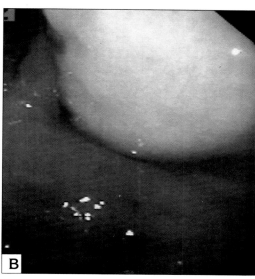

FIGURE 9-4 Small bowel illness in HIV-infected individuals may be caused by opportunistic pathogens, but HIV infection of the intestinal mucosa may also play a role. HIV has been demonstrated in the lamina propria, macrophages, and, on occasion, enterocytes by immunohistochemical staining and *in situ* hybridization. HIV may also cause an intestinal autonomic neuropathy, induce cytokines or inflammatory cells to migrate to the intestine, or induce enteric immune dysfunction to produce the pathogen-negative enteropathy known as HIV enteropathy. In this syndrome, villi are flattened and crypts are hypertrophied. **A** and **B**, This is visible grossly as can be seen in the endoscopic view in (*panel 4A*), compared with normal intestinal mucosa (*panel 4B*) as well as histologically. *(continued)*

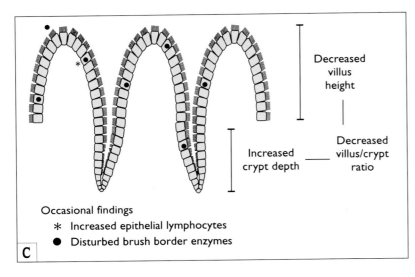

C

Occasional findings
* * Increased epithelial lymphocytes
* ● Disturbed brush border enzymes

Decreased villus height

Increased crypt depth ___ Decreased villus/crypt ratio

FIGURE 9-4 *(continued)* **C.** The expected histologic findings in HIV enteropathy are shown schematically. (Greenson JK, Belitsos PC, Yardley JH, Bartlett JG: AIDS enteropathy: Occult enteric infections and duodenal mucosal alterations in chronic diarrhea. *Ann Intern Med* 1991, 114:366–372. Ullrich R, Zeitz M, Heise W, *et al.*: Small intestinal structure and function in patients infected with human immunodeficiency virus (HIV): Evidence for HIV-induced enteropathy. *Ann Intern Med* 1989, 111:15–21.) It remains unclear what role viral pathogens play in this syndrome; Norwalk virus, rotavirus, and picobirnavirus have all been described as contributing to diarrhea in this population but are not routinely sought in clinical or study evaluations. (Grohmann GS, Glass RI, Pereira HG, *et al.*: Enteric viruses and diarrhea in HIV-infected patients. *N Engl J Med* 1993, 329:14–20. Kaljot KT, Ling JP, Gold JWM, *et al.*: Prevalence of acute enteric viral pathogens in acquired immunodeficiency syndrome patients with diarrhea. *Gastroenterology* 1989, 97:1031–1032.)

MYCOBACTERIUM AVIUM COMPLEX

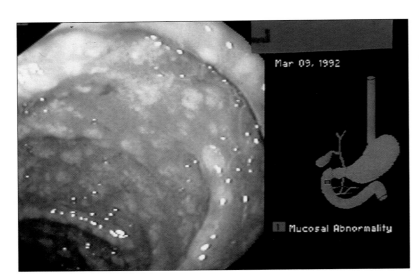

FIGURE 9-5 *Mycobacterium avium* complex may infiltrate the small bowel of AIDS patients with low CD4 counts. In addition to systemic symptoms such as fever, it may result in severe malabsorption with weight loss and diarrhea. Such malabsorption also complicates therapy, as the oral drugs routinely used to treat *M. avium* complex would be poorly absorbed in this situation. When biopsy and culture-proven infiltration of the small bowel occurs, therapy may need to include intravenous modalities as well, such as amikacin and one of the intravenous quinolones (Gillin JS, Urmacher C, West R, Shike M: Disseminated *Mycobacterium avium-intracellulare* infection in acquired immunodeficiency syndrome mimicking Whipple's disease. *Gastroenterology* 1983, 85:1187–1191. Kemper CA, Meng TC, Nussbaum J, *et al.*: Treatment of *Mycobacterium avium* complex bacteremia in AIDS with a four-drug oral regimen: Rifampin, ethambutol, clofazimine, and ciprofloxacin. *Ann Intern Med* 1992, 116:466–472.) (*Courtesy of* Dr. Douglas Pleskow, Division of Gastroenterology, New England Deaconess Hospital, Boston, MA.)

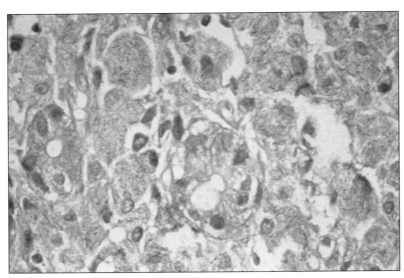

FIGURE 9-6 *M. avium* complex is visible on histologic sections stained with an acid-fast stain. As shown in this micrograph, these acid-fast organisms may be present extensively in foamy macrophages and often do not form granulomas. *M. avium* complex organisms cannot be distinguished from other mycobacterium on histologic grounds alone. Although severe small bowel infiltrative disease in this population is most commonly caused by *M. avium* complex, *M. tuberculosis* can produce an identical syndrome. *M. kansasii* and *M. genavense* have also been reported to cause severe infiltrative intestinal disease as well as severe systemic disease in the HIV population. (Bottger EC, Teske A, Kirschner P, *et al.*: Disseminated *Mycobacterium genavense* infection in patients with AIDS. *Lancet* 1992, 340:76–80.)

MYCOBACTERIUM TUBERCULOSIS

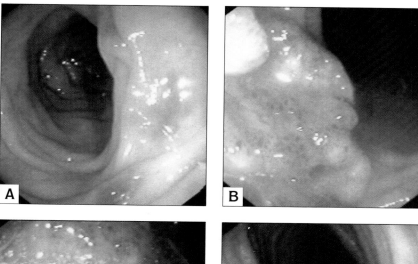

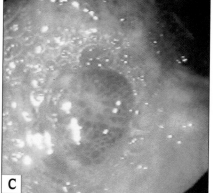

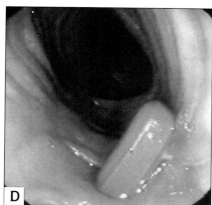

FIGURE 9-7 *M. tuberculosis* infection of the small bowel may be localized to the ileum in HIV-infected individuals, as it is in uncompromised hosts. It is likely that the gastrointestinal tract is the portal of entry for these infiltrative enteric illnesses. The gastrointestinal tract may be the portal of entry for disseminated *M. avium* complex disease as well. **A**, **B**, and **C**, The gross appearance of *M. tuberculosis* infiltrating the terminal ileum. **D**, An intact tablet in the terminal ileum, suggesting bowel dysfunction and malabsorption. (Chaisson RE, Schecter GF, Theuer CP, *et al.*: TB in patients with immunodeficiency syndrome: Clinical features, response to therapy and survival. *Am Rev Respir Dis* 1987, 136:570–574.)

CRYPTOSPORIDOSIS

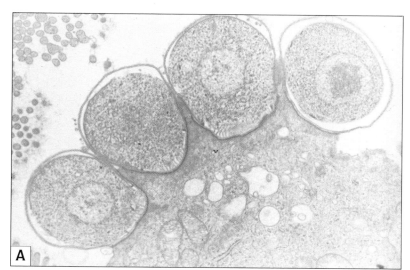

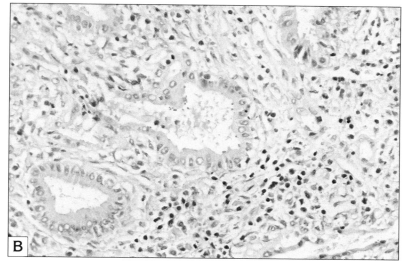

FIGURE 9-8 The protozoan parasite, *Cryptosporidium parvum*, causes a severe watery diarrhea in AIDS patients with advanced disease and low CD4 lymphocyte counts by closely adhering to the intestinal mucosa and invading the host cell membrane. The organism may produce a self-limited syndrome in HIV-infected individuals with a CD4 count above 200, but the disease is refractory to therapy in individuals with a suppressed CD4 count. Dehydration and malnutrition, as well as acalculous cholecystitis are frequent complications of small bowel cryptosporidial infections. Therapy may be attempted, but there is no clearly effective agent recognized at present. **A**, The organisms on small bowel mucosa as seen by electron microscopy. **B**, The organisms on the gall bladder mucosa. (Ungar BLP, Ward DJ, Fayer R, Quinn CA: Cessation of *Cryptosporidium*-associated diarrhea in an acquired immunodeficiency syndrome patient after treatment with hyperimmune bovine colostrum. *Gastroenterology* 1990, 98:486–489. McGowan I, Hawkins AS, Weller IVD: The natural history of cryptosporidial diarrhea in HIV-infected patients. *AIDS* 1993, 7:349–354.)

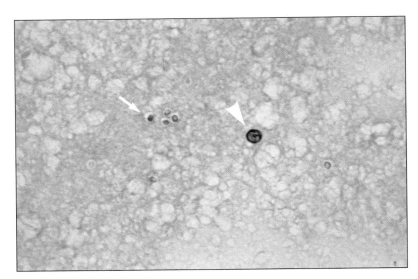

FIGURE 9-9 Cryptosporidial organisms (*arrow*) may be identified in stool by modified acid-fast stain or fluorescent antibody stains. *Cyclospora cayatenensis* (*arrowhead*) is a recently recognized parasite, which may also be detected by modified acid-fast stain. This organism has been described in travelers and in sporadic cases in noncompromised hosts, but is similar to cryptosporidium in the prolonged nature of the diarrheal illness in immunocompromised hosts. Other protozoan parasites, such as *Isospora belli, Giardia lamblia,* or the controversial *Blastocystis hominis,* may also be identified in stool by the modified acid-fast (Isospora) or trichrome stain. (*Courtesy of* Dr. J Fishman, Division of Infectious Diseases, Massachusetts General Hospital, Boston, MA). (Weber R, Bryan RT, Juranek DD: Improved stool concentration procedure for detection of *Crytosporidium* oocysts in fecal specimens. *J Clin Microbiol* 1992, 30:2869–2873. Wurtz RM, Kocka FE, Peters CS, *et al.*: Clinical characteristics of seven cases of diarrhea associated with a novel acid-fast organism in the stool. *Clin Infect Dis* 1993, 16:136–138.)

MICROSPORIDIOSIS

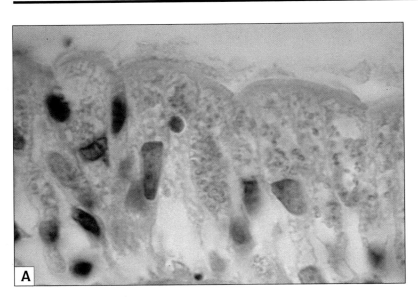

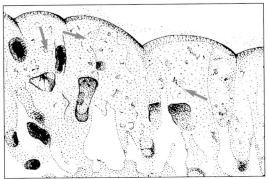

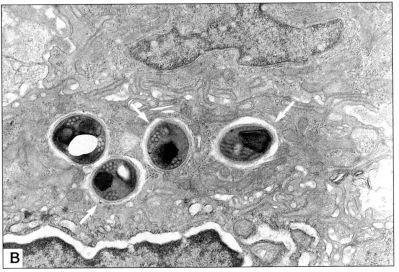

FIGURE 9-10 A, Microsporidial species have been recently recognized as potentially associated with up to 40% to 50% of the persistent diarrhea seen in patients with advanced AIDS. Although several microsporidial species are able to infect humans, to date only two species are known to infect the intestine. These organisms primarily infect the small bowel. Microsporidial organisms may be missed on routine histopathologic examination, although to an experienced observer they are readily visible, (as in this hematoxylin-eosin–stained biopsy section) where they may be expected to occur supranuclearly (*arrows*). Speciation of microsporidia cannot be done at a light microscopic level. (Simon D, Weiss LM, Tanowitz HB, *et al.*: Light microscopic diagnosis of human microsporidiosis and variable response to octreotide. *Gastroenterology* 1991, 100:271–273.) **B,** Electron microscopic examination of intestinal biopsy specimens allows speciation of microsporidial organisms as either *Enterocytozoon bineusi* or *Septada intestinalis.* The typical electron micrographic appearance of *E. bineusi* is shown (*arrows*). *(continued)*

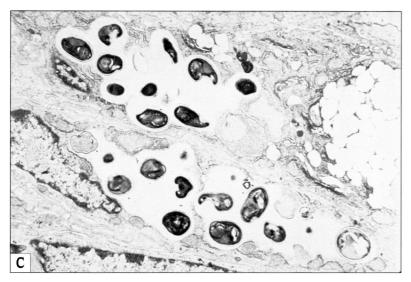

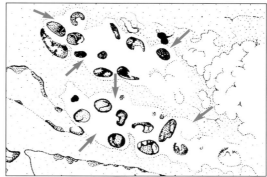

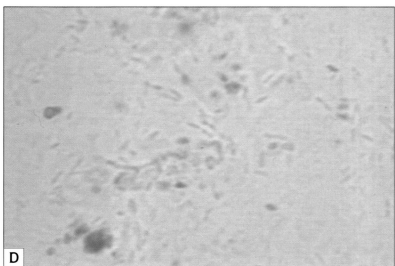

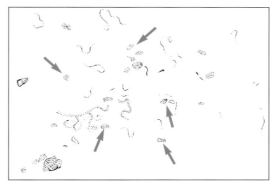

FIGURE 9-10 *(continued)* *E. bineusi* infection is generally limited to the small bowel, although direct extension into the gall bladder presenting as acalculous cholecystitis has been reported. Infected patients often develop malabsorption and diarrhea and suffer weight loss; they may not appear to respond well to any known therapy. The course of illness is relapsing and remitting, so responses are difficult to judge. (Molina JM, Sarfati C, Beauvais B, *et al.*: Intestinal microsporidiosis in human immunodeficiency virus-infected patients with chronic unexplained diarrhea: Prevalence and clinical and biologic features. *J Infect Dis* 1993, 167:217–221. Dieterich DT, Lew EA, Kotler DP, *et al.*: Treatment with albendazole for intestinal disease due to *Enterocytozoon bineusi* in patients with AIDS. *J Infect Dis* 1994, 169:178–183.) **C**, The microsporidial species *S. intestinalis*, seen in this electron micrograph (*arrows*), is the second microsporidal species that frequently infects the small bowel. It may also disseminate and organisms have been documented in the colon, renal epithelium, urine, and bronchial washings. Patients with *S. intestinalis* present with the same symptom complex as patients with *E. bineusi*, but symptoms in these patients appear to respond to therapy with albendazole. Patients may be infected with *S. intestinalis* without dissemination of the organisms beyond the bowel mucosa. (Cali A, Kotler DP, Orenstein JM: *Septata intestinalis* n. g., n. sp., an intestinal microsporidian associated with chronic diarrhea and dissemination in AIDS patients. *J Eur Microbiol* 1993, 40:101–112. Asmuth DM, DeGirolami PC, Federman M, *et al.*: Clinical features of microsporidiosis in patients with acquired immunodeficiency syndrome. *Clin Infect Dis* 1994, 18:819–825. **D**, Both microsporidial organisms that infect the small bowel may be visible in stool, when stained with a modified trichrome stain (*arrows*). Attempts to develop more specific stains are underway. When patients with *S. intestinalis* are treated with albendazole, they can clear the organisms from their stool, whereas patients with *E. bineusi* seem to remain stool smear positive while on therapy. (Weber R, Bryan RT, Owen RL, *et al.*: Improved light-microscopical detection of microsporidia spores in stool and duodenal aspirates. *N Engl J Med* 1992, 326:161–166.)

KAPOSI'S SARCOMA

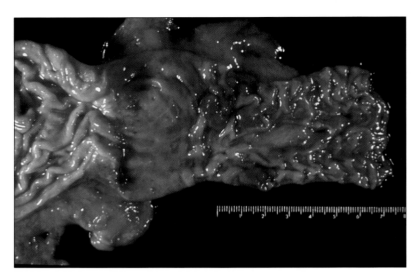

FIGURE 9-11 Kaposi's sarcoma may invade the gastrointestinal tract in patients with AIDS. These patients may present with diarrhea, gastrointestinal bleeding, or, on rare occasions, bowel obstruction. This figure grossly demonstrates Kaposi's sarcoma lesions in the small bowel. (Krigel RL, Friedman-Lien AE: Epidemic Kaposi's sarcoma. *Semin Oncol* 1990, 17:350–360.) (*Courtesy of* the Department of Pathology, New England Deaconess Hospital, Boston, MA.)

COLITIS

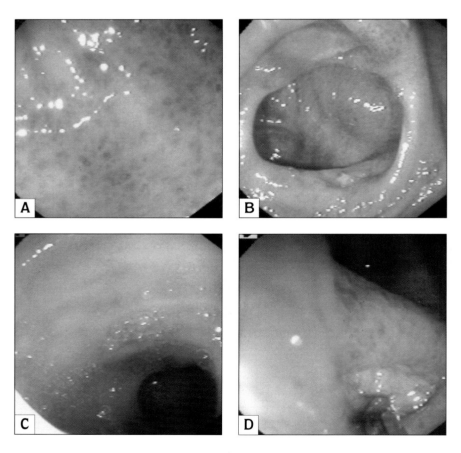

FIGURE 9-12 Colitis in HIV-infected individuals may be caused by a variety of organisms: usual bacterial pathogens such as salmonella, shigella, campylobacter, yersinia, and *Clostridium difficile*. Often these bacterial pathogens cause a more complicated or relapsing diarrheal illness than in the noncompromised host. **A, B, C,** and **D,** The pancolitis seen in the endoscopic view (*panels 4A, 4B, and 4D* compared with the normal mucosa seen in *panel 4C*) was produced by *Campylobacter jejuni* and was refractory to usual antibiotic therapy including erythromycin, azithromycin, and ciprofloxacin, but responded to long-term oral gentamicin therapy. Potential complications also include a higher than usual rate of bacteremias with these organisms, as well as a more protracted course. The complication rate may be higher in those patients who have a lower CD4 count. Spirochetes have also been considered as a potential cause of colitis in the HIV population. (Nelson MR, Shanson DC, Hawkins DA, Gazzard BG: Salmonella, campylobacter and shigella in HIV-seropositive patients. *AIDS* 1992, 6:1495–1498. Perlman DM, Ampel NM, Schifman RB, *et al.*: Persistent *Campylobacter jejuni* in patients infected with human immunodeficiency virus. *Ann Intern Med* 1988, 108:540–546. Cozart JC, Kalangi SS, Clench MH, *et al.*: *Clostridium difficile* diarrhea in patients with AIDS versus non-AIDS controls: Methods of treatment and clinical response to treatment. *J Clin Gastroenterol* 1993, 16:192–194.)

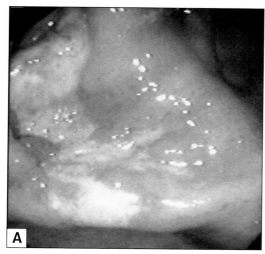
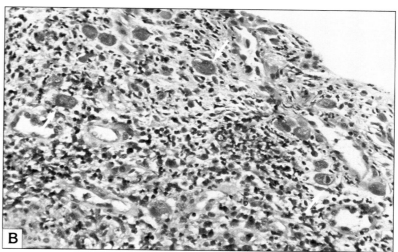

FIGURE 9-13 Colitis in AIDS patients may also be caused by viral pathogens such as cytomegalovirus (CMV). CMV colitis is often, but not invariably, seen in patients who have other end-organ evidence of CMV disease. Diagnosis requires biopsy with identification of the typical inclusion bodies and inflammation. The true efficacy of therapy for CMV colitis with either ganciclovir or foscarnet remains unclear. **A,** CMV may produce a full spectrum of disease in the colon, from mild ulcerations to deeply inflamed ulcerations. **B,** Typical CMV inclusion bodies (*arrows*) with inflammation on a colonic biopsy. Diarrheal disease may be either fulminant and watery or scant and bloody. Diarrheal disease caused by CMV is often accompanied by fever. Other viral causes of colitis in this population, such as adenovirus, must also be diagnosed by biopsy and demonstration of organisms by electron microscopy. (Goodgame RW: Gastrointestinal cytomegalovirus disease. *Ann Intern Med* 1993, 119:924–935. Janoff EN, Orenstein JM, Manischewitz JF, Smith PD: Adenovirus colitis in the acquired immunodeficiency syndrome. *Gastroenterology* 1991, 100:976–979.)

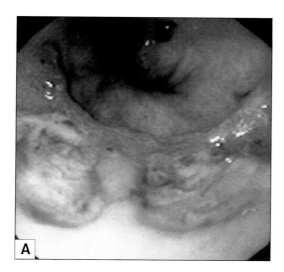
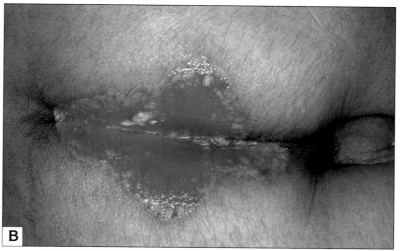

FIGURE 9-14 A, More distal colonic lesions or proctitis may be caused by a variety of organisms including herpes simplex virus, as seen on this endoscopic view. **B,** These patients may also have perianal disease with severe pain as well as diarrhea. Patients who have been repeatedly exposed to acyclovir may develop refractory disease with resistant viral strains. Proctitis may also be caused by chlamydial organisms, and spirochetes. (*Panel B from* Seigel FP, Lopez C, Hammer GS, *et al.*: Severe acquired immunodeficiency in male homosexuals manifest by chronic perianal ulcerative herpes simplex lesions. *N Engl J Med* 1981, 305:1439–1444; with permission. Safrin S, Crumpacker C, Chatis P, *et al.*: A controlled trial comparing foscarnet with vidarabine for acyclovir-resistant mucocutaneous herpes simplex in the acquired immunodeficiency syndrome. *N Engl J Med* 1991, 325:551–555.)

SELECTED BIBLIOGRAPHY

Wanke CA, Mattia AR: A 36-year-old man with AIDS, increasing chronic diarrhea, and intermittent fever and chills. *N Engl J Med* 1993, 329:1946-1955.

CHAPTER 10

Neurologic Manifestations

David M. Simpson
Susan Morgello
Michele Tagliati

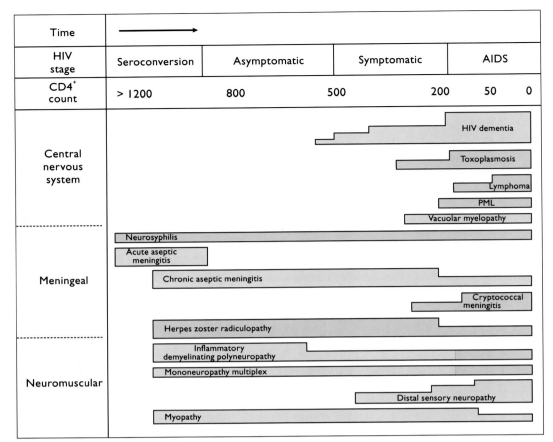

Time	→			
HIV stage	Seroconversion	Asymptomatic	Symptomatic	AIDS
CD4⁺ count	> 1200 800	500	200	50 0

Central nervous system
- HIV dementia
- Toxoplasmosis
- Lymphoma
- PML
- Vacuolar myelopathy

Meningeal
- Neurosyphilis
- Acute aseptic meningitis
- Chronic aseptic meningitis
- Cryptococcal meningitis

Neuromuscular
- Herpes zoster radiculopathy
- Inflammatory demyelinating polyneuropathy
- Mononeuropathy multiplex
- Distal sensory neuropathy
- Myopathy

FIGURE 10-1 Time line of primary (*blue*) and secondary (*red*) neurologic complications of HIV infection. As patients progress from seroconversion to progressive HIV disease, a constellation of central and peripheral neurologic complications may occur, in isolation or together. The CD4 cell count is the best predictor of the likelihood of a specific disorder and thus provides guidance for empiric and prophylactic therapy. (*Adapted from* Johnson RD, McArthur JC, Narayano O: The neurobiology of human immunodeficiency virus infections. *FASEB J* 1988, 2:2970–2981.)

PRIMARY HIV NEUROLOGIC DISEASE

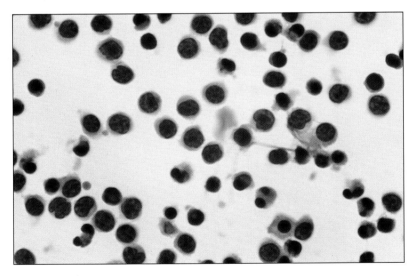

FIGURE 10-2 Aseptic leptomeningitis. Cerebrospinal fluid (CSF) cytospin displays an increased number of mononuclear cells, typical of HIV infection. CSF abnormalities including pleocytosis and anti-HIV antibodies are common throughout the course of HIV infection in both neurologically symptomatic and asymptomatic individuals. This likely reflects early entry of HIV into the central nervous system (CNS). (McArthur JC, Cohen BA, Farzedegan H, *et al.*: Cerebrospinal fluid abnormalities in homosexual men with and without neuropsychiatric findings. *Ann Neurol* 1988, 23(suppl):534–537.)

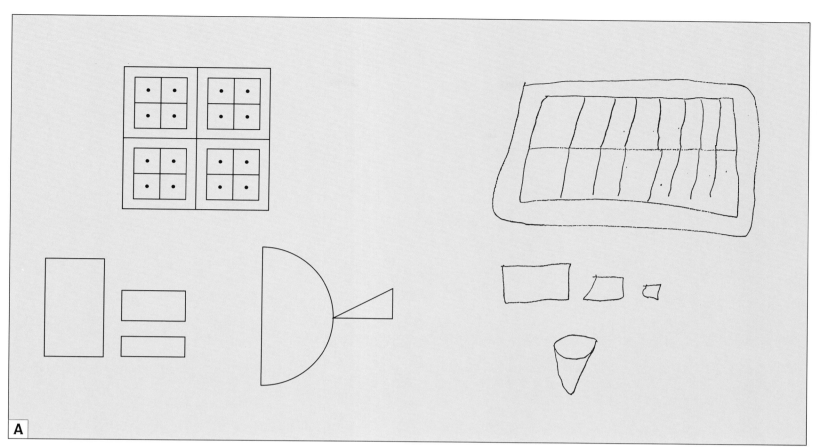

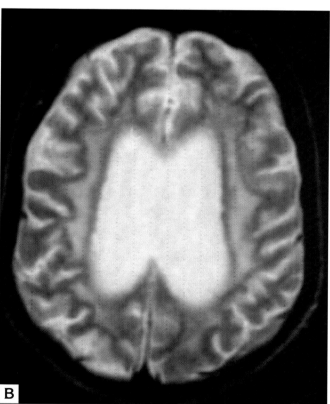

FIGURE 10-3 A, Visual memory test (Wechsler Memory Scale—Revised) in a 40-year-old man with HIV dementia. The patient was asked to observe the figures (*left*) for 10 seconds and then to reproduce them (*right*). Neuropsychological tests are the best quantitative markers of progression of AIDS dementia and of the efficacy of therapy. High-dose zidovudine therapy resulted in significant improvement in neuropsychologic performance in a placebo-controlled study of HIV dementia. (*Figure courtesy of* David Dorfman, PhD.) (Sidtis JJ, Gatsonis C, Price RW, *et al.*: Zidovudine treatment of the AIDS dementia complex: Results of a placebo-controlled trial. *Ann Neurol* 1993, 33:343–349.) **B,** Brain magnetic resonance imaging (MRI) scan (T2-weighted image) of a 34-year-old man with HIV dementia demonstrates ventricular enlargement, white matter hyperintensity, and cortical atrophy. Radiologic studies have shown a significant correlation between cerebral atrophy and degree of HIV dementia. The greatest degree of brain atrophy appears in the subcortical regions, in parallel with neuropathologic findings. (Dal Pan PJ, McArthur JH, Aylward E, *et al.*: Patterns of cerebral atrophy in HIV-1 infected individuals: Results of a quantitative MRI analysis. *Neurology* 1992, 42:2125–2130.)

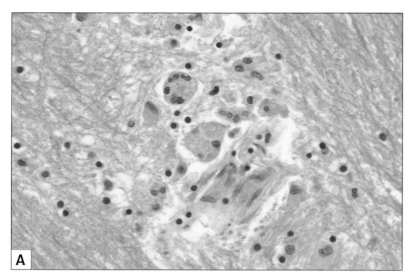

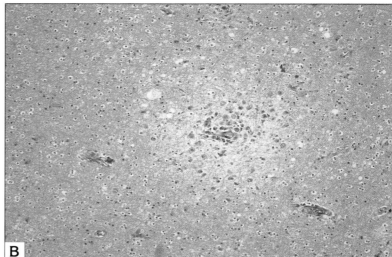

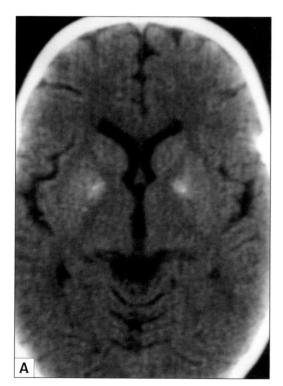

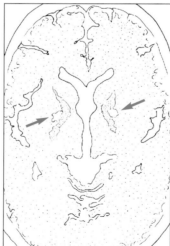

FIGURE 10-4 HIV encephalitis. **A,** Primary CNS infection with HIV is characterized by a microglial nodule encephalitis with multinucleated cells (*arrow*) (hematoxylin and eosin). **B,** Virus is located within these nodules, which are present in subcortical structures and are often accompanied by white matter pallor (Luxol fast blue stain for myelin). Although all patients with HIV encephalitis are demented, not all individuals with dementia have HIV encephalitis. The histopathologic substrate of dementia in this latter group is unclear. (Navia BA, Cho ES, Petito CK, Price RW: The AIDS dementia complex: II. Neuropathology. *Ann Neurol* 1986, 19:525–535.)

FIGURE 10-5 A, Pediatric AIDS encephalopathy. Brain computed tomography (CT) scan of a child with AIDS encephalopathy reveals bilateral mineralization of the basal ganglia (*arrows*). There is a different spectrum of neuropathology in pediatric patients with AIDS when compared with adults. For example, a far lower incidence of opportunistic infections is seen in children. Characteristic neurologic findings in children include developmental delay, progressive encephalopathy, lethargy, and spasticity. (Belman A, Lantos G, Horoupian D, *et al.*: Calcification of the basal ganglia in infants and children. *Neurology* 1986, 36:1192–1199.) (*continued*)

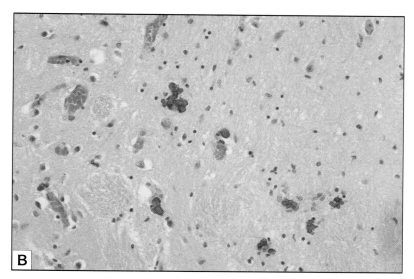

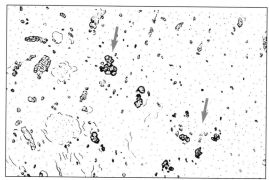

FIGURE 10-5 *(continued)* **B,** The most common histopathologic finding in pediatric AIDS encephalopathy is dystrophic mineralization of cerebral blood vessels and parenchyma (*arrows*, mineralizations appear purple) (hematoxylin and eosin). Microcephaly, white matter pallor, and microglial nodule encephalitis may also be seen. (Sharer LR, Epstein LG, Cho ES, *et al.*: Pathologic features of AIDS encephalopathy in children: Evidence for LAV/HTLV-III infection of brain. *Hum Pathol* 1986, 17:271–284.)

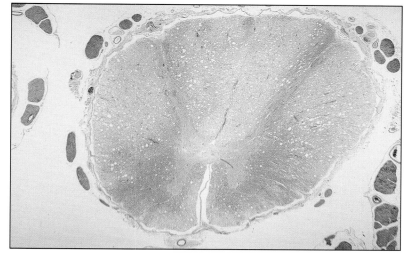

FIGURE 10-6 Vacuolar myelopathy. Vacuolization and sparse macrophage infiltrates are present predominantly in posterior and lateral columns at thoracic levels of the spinal cord, as displayed in this Luxol fast blue stain for myelin (abnormal areas appear pink). Vacuolar myelopathy is the most common cause of spinal cord pathology in AIDS, although its pathogenesis is unknown. Presenting symptoms include lower extremity weakness, sensory loss, spasticity, and sphincter impairment. Other treatable causes of myelopathy, including lymphoma, tuberculosis, and toxoplasmosis, should be excluded in these patients by radiologic and CSF studies. (Petito CK, Navia BA, Cho ES, *et al.*: Vacuolar myelopathy pathologically resembling subacute combined degeneration in patients with the acquired immunodeficiency syndrome. *N Engl J Med* 1985, 312:874–879.)

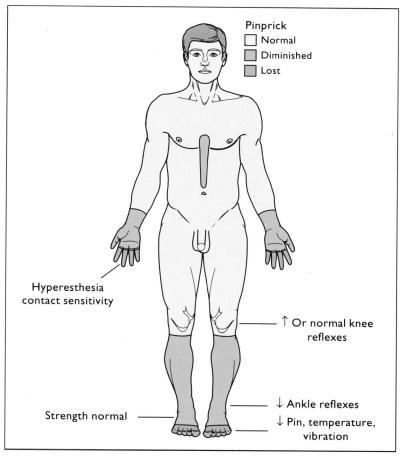

FIGURE 10-7 Typical "stocking-glove" pattern of sensory impairment in distal symmetrical polyneuropathy. This condition is a primary manifestation of HIV infection or may result from metabolic or nutritional abnormalities (*ie*, vitamin B12 deficiency). Neurotoxins such as vincristine, didanosine (ddI), zalcitabine (ddC), and stavudine (d4T) may initiate or exacerbate neuropathic symptoms, particularly in patients with preexisting HIV neuropathy. (*Adapted from* Schaumburg HH, Spencer PS, Thomas PK (eds): Anatomical classification of PNS disorder. In *Disorders of Peripheral Nerves.* Philadelphia: FA Davis, Co; 1983, with permission.)

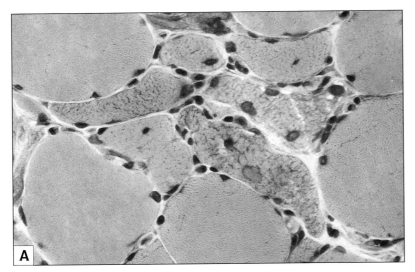

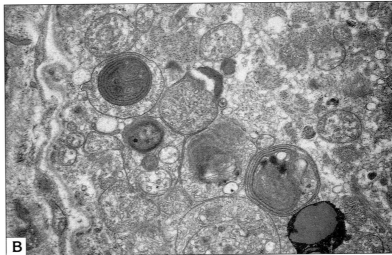

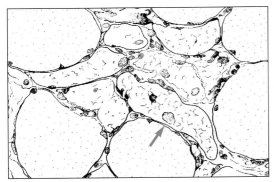

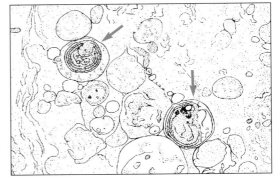

FIGURE 10-8 HIV-associated myopathy. Patients with myopathy present with progressive proximal weakness, often associated with myalgia. Elevated serum creatine phosphokinase and electromyography are supportive laboratory features. **A**, Muscle biopsy specimens often display basophilic, degenerating fibers with cytoplasmic bodies. The *arrow* indicates a cytoplasmic body (hematoxylin and eosin). **B**, Abnormalities in mitochondrial structure, with loss of crystal architecture and occasional paracrys-

talline inclusions. *Arrows* indicate representative mitochondria with abnormal cristae, seen in this electron micrograph. Although zidovudine may contribute to myopathy in some patients, the frequency of this association and the clinical significance of pathologic alterations of muscle mitochondria are not established. (Simpson D, Citak K, Godfrey E, *et al.*: Myopathies associated with human immunodeficiency virus and zidovudine: Can their effects be distinguished? *Neurology* 1993, 43:971–976.)

OPPORTUNISTIC NERVOUS SYSTEM INFECTIONS

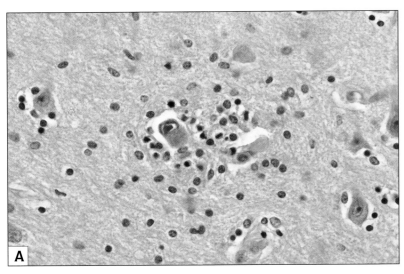

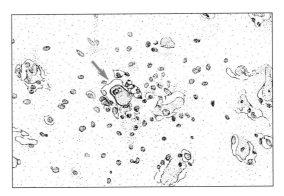

FIGURE 10-9 Cytomegalovirus encephalitis. The clinical manifestations of CNS infection with cytomegalovirus (CMV) are diverse and include dementia, brainstem syndromes, and myelitis. CNS involvement often occurs in the setting of systemic CMV infection. **A**, The

most common finding in the brain is a microglial nodule encephalitis with rare CMV inclusions. The *arrow* indicates inclusion in the nodule seen (hematoxylin and eosin). Most patients with CMV-related encephalitis are not detected antemortem. *(continued)*

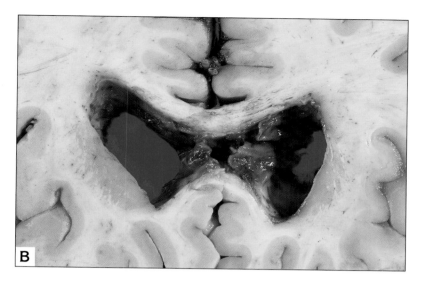

B

FIGURE 10-9 *(continued)* **B**, In approximately 10% of patients, necrotizing ventriculoencephalitis may occur, where the ventricular system is rimmed by hemorrhagic necrosis. These patients may manifest more obvious and rapidly progressive neurologic abnormalities. (Morgello S, Cho ES, Nielsen S, *et al*.: Cytomegalovirus encephalitis in patients with acquired immunodeficiency syndrome: An autopsy study of 30 cases and a review of the literature. *Hum Pathol* 1987, 18:289–297.)

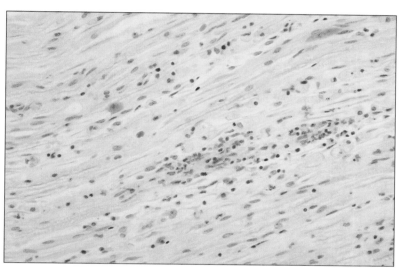

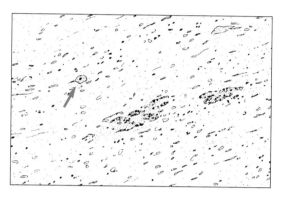

FIGURE 10-10 CMV neuropathy. CMV has been demonstrated as a primary pathogen in at least two forms of peripheral neuropathy in AIDS. *Progressive polyradiculopathy* presents with lower extremity weakness, sensory loss, areflexia, and sphincter dysfunction and is associated with a CSF polymorphonuclear pleocytosis. *Mononeuropathy multiplex* is characterized by multifocal cranial or peripheral nerve lesions. Histopathologically, endoneurial inflammation and CMV inclusions (*arrow*) are seen in peripheral nerve (hematoxylin and eosin). The neuropathy may display both axonal and demyelinating features. Empirical ganciclovir or foscarnet therapy is warranted in these disorders, even before CSF culture results are available. (Miller R, Storey J, Greco C: Ganciclovir in the treatment of progressive AIDS-related polyradiculopathy. *Neurology* 1990, 40:569–574.)

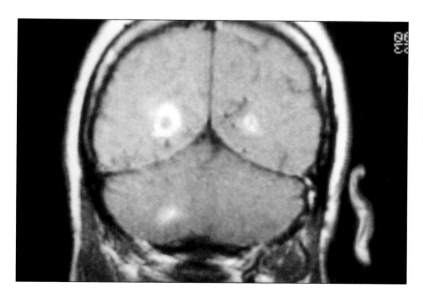

FIGURE 10-11 Cerebral toxoplasmosis. Coronal brain MRI reveals multiple subtentorial and supratentorial contrast-enhancing toxoplasma lesions. CNS toxoplasmosis is the most common brain mass lesion in AIDS and generally represent the reactivation of latent infection. Empirical therapy with sulfadiazine, pyrimethamine, or clindamycin generally results in rapid clinical and radiologic improvement. (Luft B, Hafner R, Korzun A, *et al*.: Toxoplasmic encephalitis in patients with acquired immunodeficiency syndrome. *N Engl J Med* 1993, 329:995–1000.)

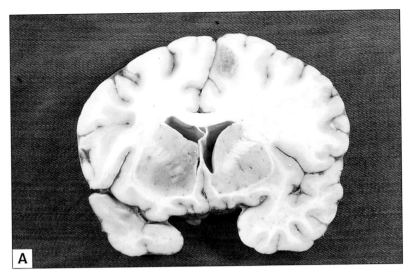

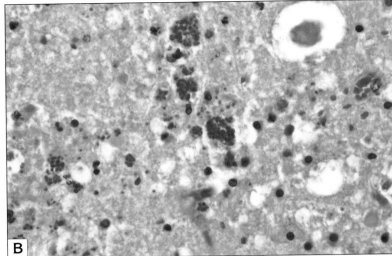

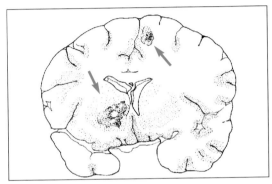

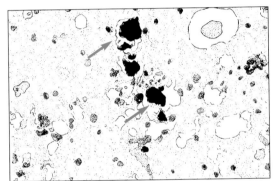

FIGURE 10-12 A, Cerebral toxoplasmosis typically produces multifocal abscesses with central yellow necrosis and hyperemic borders; *arrows* indicate two macroscopic lesions. There is sometimes a predilection for a subpial location, as seen in the right medial cerebral hemisphere of this coronal brain section. (*Specimen courtesy of* H. Laufer, MD). **B**, Microscopically, both encysted and individual organisms may be seen in zones of necrosis; *arrows* show represen- tative pseudocysts (hematoxylin and eosin). Individual tachyzoites may be difficult to distinguish from necrotic debris in tissue sections, and their identification is aided by immunohistochemistry with antitoxoplasma antisera. (Navia BA, Petito CK, Gold JWM, *et al.*: Cerebral toxoplasmosis complicating the acquired immunodeficiency syndrome: Clinical and neuropathological findings in 27 patients. *Ann Neurol* 1986, 19:224–238.)

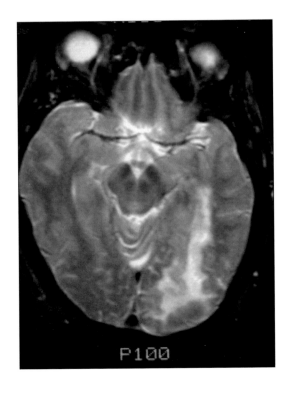

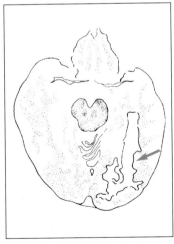

FIGURE 10-13 Progressive multifocal leukoencephalopathy (PML). Brain MRI reveals a large confluent hyperintense lesion in left parietal white matter (*arrow*), biopsy proven as PML. Approximately 4% of patients with AIDS develop PML, with a higher incidence found in autopsy series. Uncontrolled case series have reported favorable therapeutic responses to high-dose antiretroviral therapy and intravenous or intrathecal cytarabine, although some patients have had spontaneous prolonged remissions. These agents are under investigation in controlled studies. (Berger J, Kaszovitz B, Post J, Dickinson G: Progressive multifocal leukoencephalopathy associated with human immunodeficiency virus infection. *Ann Intern Med* 1987, 107:78–87.)

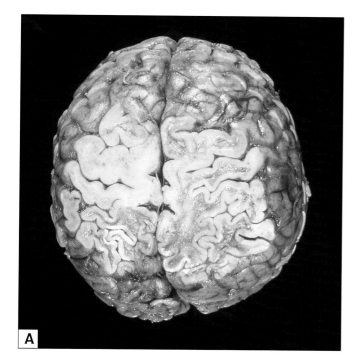

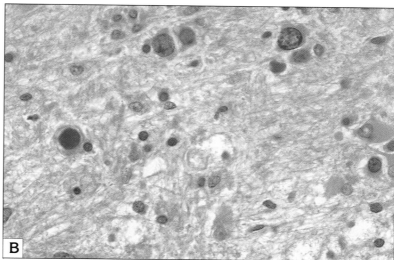

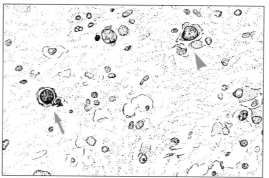

FIGURE 10-14 A, Demyelinated PML foci may involve large regions of cerebral white matter in patients with AIDS, as demonstrated in a semihorizontal section, where the entire right and posterior portions of the left hemispheric white matter are replaced by brown-gray lesions (horizontal section throughout the superior portions of the cerebral hemisphere). (*Courtesy of* H. Laufer, MD.) **B**, Microscopically, demyelinated foci contain atypical astrocytes (*arrowheads*) and oligodendroglia (*arrow*) with intranuclear inclusions characteristic of JC virus, the etiologic agent of PML. There is a suggestion that in patients with prolonged clinical course, marked inflammatory infiltrates may accompany the demyelinated foci. (Hair LS, Nuovo G, Powers JM, *et al.*: Progressive multifocal leukoencephalopathy in patients with human immunodeficiency virus. *Hum Pathol* 1992, 23:663–667.)

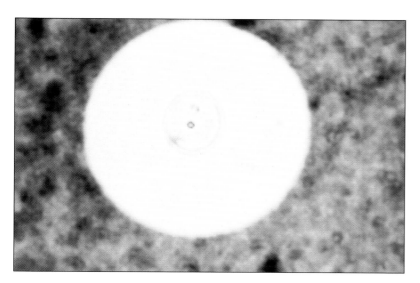

FIGURE 10-15 *Cryptococcus neoformans* suspended in india ink, with its distinctive thick capsule. Although patients with cryptococcal meningitis may present with headache, fever, and meningeal signs, these classic findings are often absent in patients with AIDS. Antifungal therapy, including amphotericin B or fluconazole, should be continued as life-long suppressive therapy following the acute course of treatment in AIDS patients. (*Courtesy of* Edward Bottone, MD.) (Powderly W, Saag M, Gretcher G, *et al.*: A controlled trial of fluconazole or amphotericin-B to prevent relapse of cryptococcal meningitis in patients with the acquired immunodeficiency syndrome. *N Engl J Med* 1992, 326:793–798.)

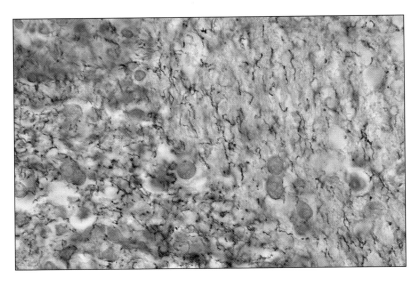

FIGURE 10-16 Neurosyphilis. Both neurosyphilis and HIV may result in chronic meningitis, dementia, cranial neuropathies, and myelopathies. Additionally, both are associated with similar CSF abnormalities, particularly a persistent pleocytosis. Although a positive CSF VDRL test is diagnostic of neurosyphilis, this assay has a sensitivity of only 30% to 70%. In an HIV-infected patient with symptoms consistent with neurosyphilis, even in the absence of a positive CSF VDRL, a reactive CSF profile justifies treatment with intravenous penicillin. HIV infection may alter the natural history of syphilis, with an increased incidence of neurologic disease and possibly a worsened clinical course. In the untreated autopsied case demonstrated here, a fulminant encephalitis with numerous treponemes was seen (modified Steiner's stain with tangles of black-appearing organisms). (Morgello S, Laufer H: Quaternary neurosyphilis in a Haitian man with human immunodeficiency virus infection. *Hum Pathol* 1989, 20:805–811.)

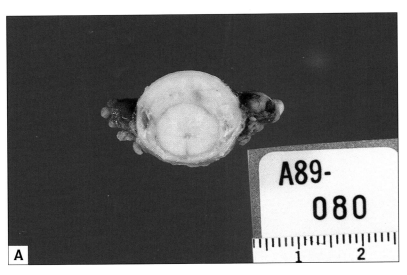

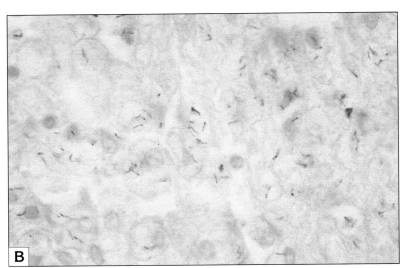

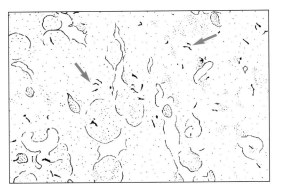

FIGURE 10-17 Tuberculous meningitis. Neurologic manifestations of *Mycobacterium tuberculosis* infection include cerebral mass lesions, chronic meningitis, and cranial neuropathies. The incidence of neurologic complications appears to be increased in HIV-infected patients. **A,** Thick leptomeningeal infiltrates surround this cross-section of low thoracic spinal cord (spinal roots are seen at *right* and *left*). **B,** Numerous acid-fast bacilli are present in regions of exudate and necrosis. (Berenguer J, Moreno S, Laguna F, *et al.*: Tuberculous meningitis in patients infected with the human immunodeficiency virus. *N Engl J Med* 1992, 26:668–672.)

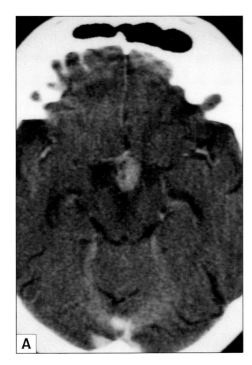
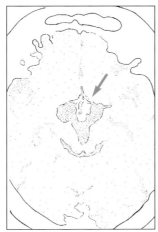
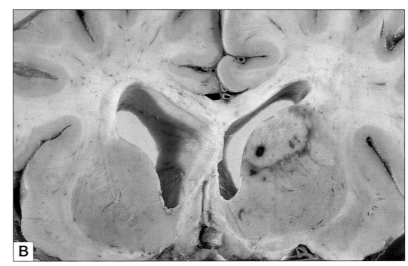
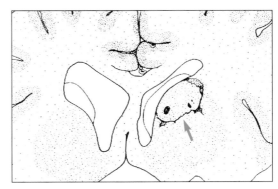

FIGURE 10-18 A, Primary CNS lymphoma. Brain MRI of lymphoma reveals a hyperintense lesion in the hypothalamic region (*arrow*). It may be difficult to differentiate between lymphoma and toxoplasmosis on clinical and radiologic grounds. Definitive diagnosis is achieved in most cases with stereotactic brain biopsy. Although the prognosis of AIDS-associated CNS lymphoma is poor, radiation therapy improves quality of life and survival. The addition of chemotherapy is under investigation in controlled trials. (Baumgarten J, Rachlin J, Beckstead J, *et al.*: Primary central nervous system lymphomas: Natural history and response to radiation therapy in 55 patients with acquired immunodeficiency syndrome. *J Neurosurg* 1990, 73:206–211.) **B**, Primary CNS lymphomas may have a wide variety of gross appearances but typically are white, firm expansile lesions with a predilection for deep gray matter structures (*arrow*). (Morgello S, Petito CK, Mouradian JA: Central nervous system lymphoma in the acquired immunodeficiency syndrome. *Clin Neuropathol* 1990, 9(4):205–215.)

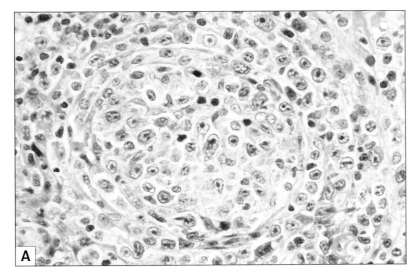
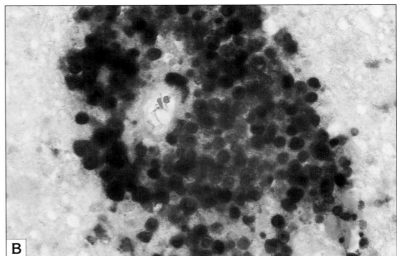

FIGURE 10-19 A, Many AIDS-related CNS lymphomas have large cell histology (hematoxylin and eosin). **B**, One hundred percent of AIDS-associated lymphomas contain Epstein-Barr virus nucleic acids, as demonstrated by RNA *in situ* hybridization for EBER-1 transcripts, with nitroblue tetrazolium reaction product. This extraordinary viral association is unlike CNS lymphoma arising in nonimmunocomprised individuals, in which only 30% of tumors contain the virus. (MacMahon EME, Glass JD, Haywards SD, *et al.*: Epstein-Barr virus in AIDS-related primary central nervous system lymphoma. *Lancet* 1991, 338:969–973.)

ACKNOWLEDGMENT

The authors thank Aryeh Stollman, MD, for radiographic images.
Arlene Rivera provided expert technical assistance.

SELECT BIBLIOGRAPHY

Snider WD, Simpson DM, Nielsen S, *et al.*: Neurological complications of acquired immunodeficiency syndrome: Analysis of 50 patients. *Ann Neurol* 1983, 14:403–418.

Price RW, Brew B, Sidtis JJ, *et al.*: The brain in AIDS: Central nervous system HIV-1 infection and the AIDS dementia complex. *Science* 1988, 239:586–592.

Simpson DM, Olney RK: Peripheral neuropathies associated with human immunodeficiency virus infection. *In Dyck PJ, ed: Peripheral Neuropathies: New Concepts and Treatments.* Philadelphia: WB Saunders; 1992:685–711.

Budka H, Wiley CA, Kleinves P, *et al.*: HIV-associated disease of the nervous system: Review of nomenclature and proposal for neuropathology-based terminology. *Brain Pathol* 1991, 1(3):143–152.

DeGirolami U, Smith TW, Henin D, Hauw JJ: Neuropathology of the acquired immunodeficiency syndrome. *Arch Pathol Lab Med* 1990, 114:643–655.

CHAPTER 11

Metabolic Manifestations

Carl Grunfeld
Peter Jensen

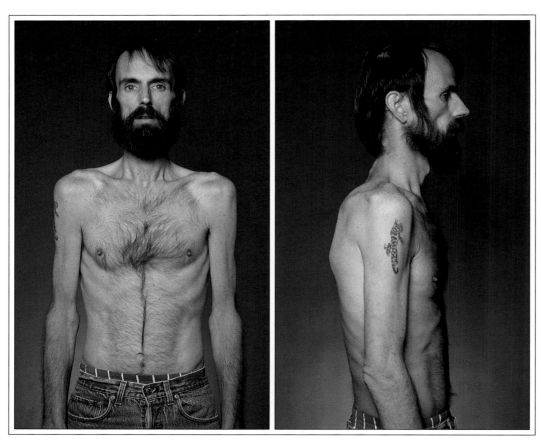

FIGURE 11-1 The wasting syndrome in AIDS is accompanied by marked muscle wasting with variable loss of body fat. Patients with the wasting syndrome show tissue loss in the extremities and viscera.

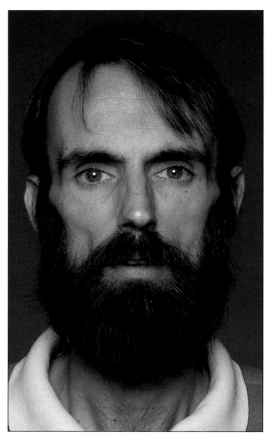

FIGURE 11-2 In the wasting syndrome, prominent loss of temporal muscle and cheek tissue can be seen.

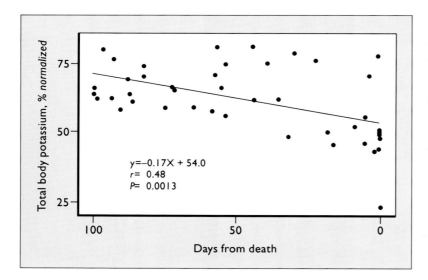

$y = -0.17X + 54.0$
$r = 0.48$
$P = 0.0013$

FIGURE 11-3 Body cell mass as measured by total body potassium in 43 patients with AIDS who died with the wasting syndrome. Total body potassium is plotted against the days before death on which the measurement was made. These values extrapolate to a body cell mass at the time of death at 54% of normal. Projected body weight at death was 66% of ideal body weight, a percentage that is similar to that seen during death from starvation. (*From* Kotler DP, Tierney AR, Wang J, Pierson RN Jr: Magnitude of body-cell-mass depletion and the timing of death from wasting in AIDS. *Am J Clin Nutr* 1989, 50:444–447.)

ABNORMALITIES IN LIPID METABOLISM

Plasma lipid and lipoprotein levels in HIV infection and aids

	Control	HIV+	AIDS
Triglycerides, *mg/dL*	102 ± 10.8	110 ±14.8	203 ± 24.9[†]
Cholesterol, *mg/dL*	183 ± 6.67	150 ± 7.86*	151 ± 11.4*
HDL Cholesterol, *mg/dL*	49.2 ± 2.55	31.3 ± 1.67[†]	31.1 ± 1.90[†]
LDL Cholesterol, *mg/dL*	121 ± 6.53	102 ± 7.34	84.4 ± 10.3*

*$P < 0.02$ vs controls.
[†]$P < 0.001$ vs controls.

FIGURE 11-4 Serum lipid and lipoprotein levels in HIV infection and AIDS. Compared with levels seen in age-matched men, serum cholesterol levels (in both the LDL and HDL fractions) decrease early in the course of HIV infection. Subsequently, serum triglyceride levels rise. It is estimated that 10% of patients with AIDS have severe hypertriglyceridemia (> 500 mg/dL), which puts them at risk for triglyceride-induced pancreatitis. This syndrome is of particular concern for patients on antiretroviral therapies (*eg*, didanosine, dalcitabine) that may induce pancreatitis. (Grunfeld C, Pang M, Doerrler W, *et al*.: Lipids, lipoproteins, triglyceride clearance, and cytokines in human immunodeficiency virus infection and the acquired immunodeficiency syndrome. *J Clin Endocrinol Metab* 1992, 74:1045–1052.)

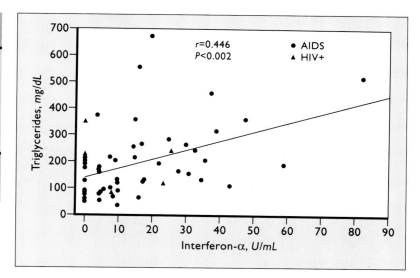

FIGURE 11-5 Serum triglyceride levels correlate with the increased levels of interferon-α seen in patients with AIDS. There is no correlation between serum triglyceride levels and other circulating cytokines, such as tumor necrosis factor or interleukin-1. Interferon-α has previously been shown to modulate triglyceride metabolism in cell culture, animal, and human studies. (*From* Grunfeld C, Kotler DP, Shigenaga JK, *et al*.: Circulating interferon-α levels and hypertriglyceridemia in the acquired immunodeficiency syndrome. *Am J Med* 1991, 90:154–162; with permission.)

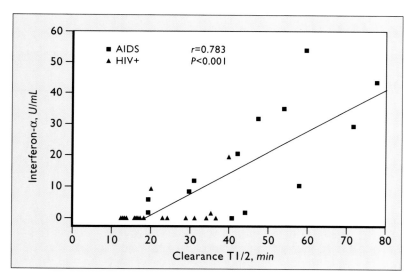

FIGURE 11-6 Triglyceride clearance is markedly slowed in AIDS and HIV infection. The decrease in triglyceride clearance strongly correlates with circulating levels of interferon-α. Decreased clearance is due, in part, to decreases in the enzyme lipoprotein lipase. (*Adapted from* Grunfeld C, Pang M, Doerrler W, *et al*.: Lipids, lipoproteins, triglyceride clearance, and cytokines in human immunodeficiency virus infection and the acquired immunodeficiency syndrome. *J Clin Endocrinol Metab* 1992; 74:1045–1052; with permission.)

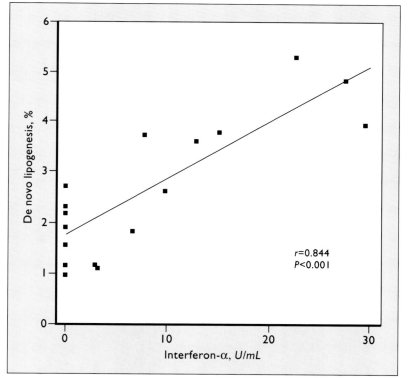

FIGURE 11-7 De novo lipogenesis (synthesis of fatty acids) by the liver is increased in AIDS. In the fasting state, this increase in lipogenesis (expressed as percentage of C-16 palmitic acid that is newly synthesized) correlates with circulating levels of interferon-α. (*Adapted from* Hellerstein MK, Grunfeld C, Wu K, *et al*.: Increased de novo hepatic lipogenesis in human immunodeficiency virus infection. *J Clin Endocrinol Metab* 1993, 76:559–565; with permission.)

Effect of zidovudine treatment on interferon-α and triglyceride levels in HIV infection and AIDS			
Serum level	**ZDV** $(n=9)$	**Placebo** $(n=9)$	**P value***
Interferon-α, *U/mL*			
Change from baseline	-143[†]	6.33	0.077
Slope with time	-9.22[‡]	4.50	0.017
Triglycerides, *mg/dL*			
Change from baseline	-61.2[§]	42	0.017
Slope with time	-15.1[¶]	19.1	0.027

*Wilcoxon 2-sample rank test.
P values vs zero in 1-sample signed rank test:
[†]0.022
[‡]0.052
[§]0.024
[¶]0.009.

FIGURE 11-8 The relationship between serum triglycerides and interferon-α levels was demonstrated in therapeutic studies. The administration of antiretroviral therapy (zidovudine [ZDV]) to previously untreated patients reduced both circulating triglyceride levels and circulating interferon-α levels compared with those patients treated with placebo. The decreases in triglyceride and interferon-α levels occurred within 1 month of initiating zidovudine therapy and were sustained for 5 months. Control patients showed a trend toward increases in these values. (Mildvan D, Machado SG, Wilets I, Grossberg SE: Endogenous interferon and triglyceride concentrations to assess response to zidovudine in AIDS and advanced AIDS-related complex. *Lancet* 1992, 339: 453–456.)

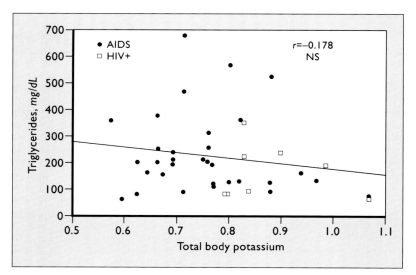

FIGURE 11-9 There is no correlation between the presence of hypertriglyceridemia and wasting as detected by measurement of body cell mass using total body potassium (normalized to 1.0). It had previously been speculated that certain metabolic disturbances, in particular those of triglyceride metabolism, directly caused weight loss. Studies in animal models and in patients with AIDS indicate that there is no direct relationship between hypertriglyceridemia and wasting. Patients with hypertriglyceridemia can have long periods of stable weight and body cell mass (total body potassium). (*Adapted from* Grunfeld C, Kotler DP, Hamadeh R, *et al.*: Hypertriglyceridemia in the acquired immunodeficiency syndrome. *Am J Med* 1989, 86:27–31; with permission.)

THYROID ABNORMALITIES

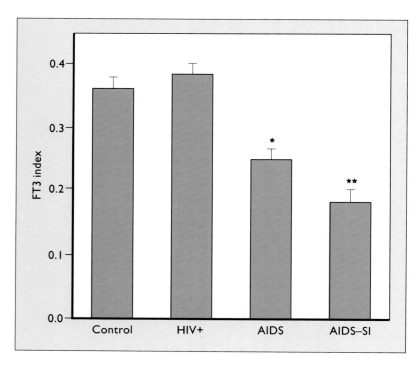

FIGURE 11-10 Free triiodothyronine (FT3) levels are reduced in AIDS. FT3 is known to be reduced in other severe illnesses, a phenomenon that is characteristic of the "euthyroid-sick syndrome." This reduction of FT3 is thought to lower resting energy expenditure, reduce protein loss, and help to conserve nitrogen balance. Although FT3 levels may be normal in stable patients with HIV infection or AIDS, FT3 levels decrease appropriately when illness or malnutrition is superimposed in such patients. (*$P < 0.0001$ vs control; **$P < 0.0001$ vs control, $P < 0.05$ vs HIV+.) (Grunfeld C, Pang M, Doerrler W, *et al.*: Indices of thyroid function and weight loss in human immunodeficiency virus infection and the acquired immunodeficiency syndrome. *Metabolism* 1993, 42:1270–1276.)

WEIGHT LOSS AND WASTING

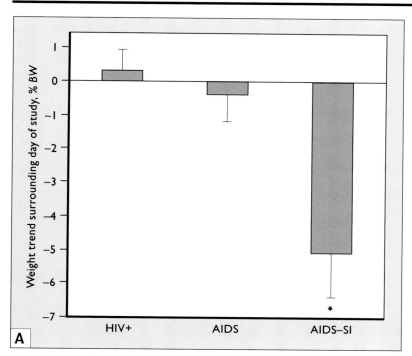

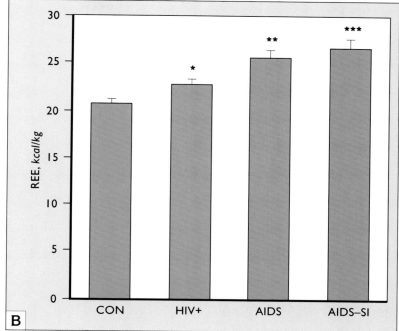

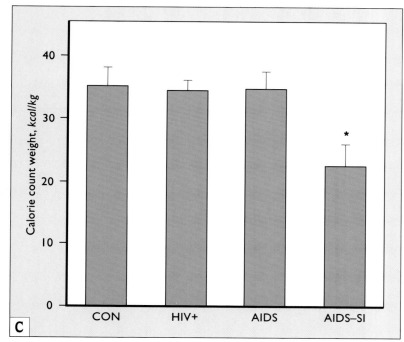

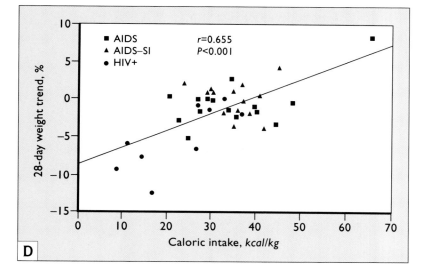

FIGURE 11-11 **A**, Average weight change in selected cohorts of patients with HIV infection and AIDS. Weight change during a 28-day period surrounding a metabolic study was determined for patients with early HIV infection (HIV+), patients with AIDS in the absence of opportunistic or secondary infection (AIDS), and patients with AIDS during the course of an acute opportunistic or secondary infection (AIDS-SI). Although some patients in the HIV+ and AIDS cohort gained weight and others lost weight, patients in the AIDS-SI cohort consistently showed a rapid weight loss, averaging 5% of body weight in 4 weeks (*$P < 0.002$ vs HIV+; $P = 0.02$ vs AIDS). Patients with significant diarrhea (> five bowel movements/day) were excluded from this study. **B**, Resting energy expenditure (REE) is significantly elevated in persons with HIV infection and AIDS. Previous theories had suggested that excess energy expenditure, particularly due to increased REE, was a major cause of weight loss. However, in AIDS (without known active secondary infection), REE is elevated nearly to the same extent as in AIDS-SI (with active secondary infection), yet only the latter group consistently shows weight loss. There was no correlation between REE and weight change (*$P < 0.025$ vs control (CON); **$P < 0.0001$ vs control, $P < 0.025$ vs HIV+; ***$P < 0.0001$ vs control, $P < 0.01$ vs HIV+). **C**, Caloric intake in HIV infection and AIDS. Caloric intake was normal in HIV+ and AIDS (without secondary infection), whereas caloric intake was markedly reduced in AIDS-SI (with active secondary infection) (*$P < 0.01$ vs control and HIV+, $P < 0.02$ vs AIDS). In fact, caloric intake in AIDS-SI was only 83% of REE, a level that would lead to weight loss even if these patients were bedridden. Caloric intake was measured during a metabolic ward admission at the time of studying REE. **D**, Weight change correlates with caloric intake in AIDS. Weight change over 28 days is significantly correlated with caloric intake studied on a metabolic ward. From the mechanistic studies illustrated in *panels A–D*, we proposed that rapid weight loss, particularly when accompanied by anorexia, is a harbinger of secondary infection. (*Adapted from* Grunfeld C, Pang M, Shimizu L, *et al.*: Resting energy expenditure, caloric intake, and short-term weight change in human immunodeficiency virus infection and the acquired immunodeficiency syndrome. *Am J Clin Nutr* 1992, 55:455–460; with permission.)

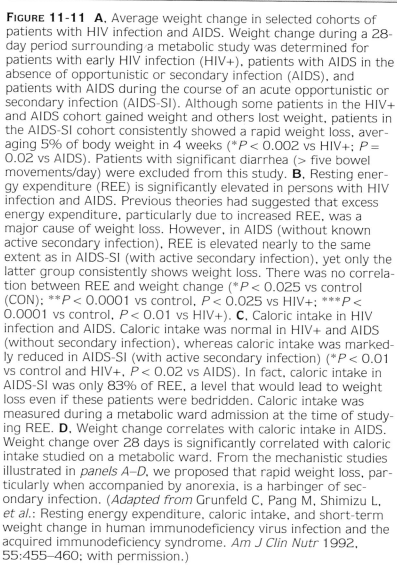

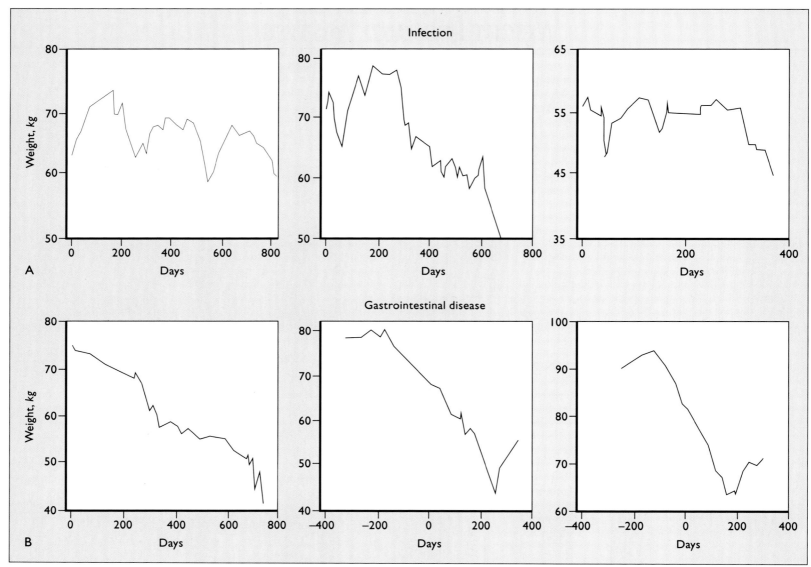

FIGURE 11-12 **A**, Acute weight loss pattern accompanying secondary infection in AIDS. In a prospective study of weight change in HIV infected patients, it was noted that episodes of rapid weight loss (> 4 kg in < 4 months) were frequently (82%) associated with acute infection. The patterns presented for these three patients are notable both for the periods of rapid weight loss and the fact that weight was often not fully regained after successful treatment of secondary infection. A wide variety of secondary infections have been associated with weight loss, including *Pneumocystis carinii* pneumonia, *Mycobacterium avium* complex infection, tuberculosis, sinusitis, urosepsis, bronchitis, cryptococcosis, salmonellosis, cytomegalovirus infection, and indwelling catheter infection. (*From* Macallan DC, Noble C, Baldwin C, *et al.*: Prospective analysis of weight changes in IV human immunodeficiency virus infection. *Am J Clin Nutr* 1993, 58:417–424; with permission.) **B**, Slow pattern of weight loss seen in HIV infection and AIDS. Compared with the patients in *panel 12A*, other patients showed a slower, more progressive period of weight loss. These patients frequently (65%) had gastrointestinal disorders often accompanied by diarrhea. Gastrointestinal disorders and infections associated with slow weight loss include severe refractory diarrhea, malabsorption, candidiasis, cryptosporidiosis, giardiasis, herpes simplex and other forms of esophagitis, and anogenital disease. Day 0 notes the day of diagnosis of stage-IV AIDS. (*From* Macallan DC, Noble C, Baldwin C, *et al.*: Prospective analysis of weight changes in IV human immunodeficiency virus infection. *Am J Clin Nutr* 1993, 58:417–424; with permission.)

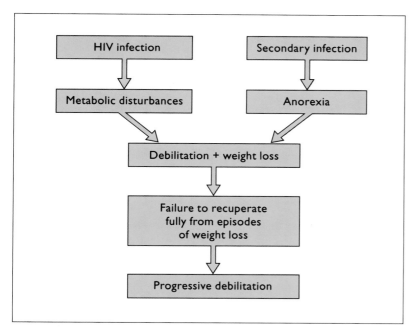

FIGURE 11-13 The mechanisms and consequences of weight loss in AIDS. HIV infection (and to a certain extent, secondary infection) leads to metabolic disturbances that contribute to debilitation. Secondary infection (and to a lesser extent primary HIV infection itself) leads to anorexia, which in the presence of the metabolic disturbances leads to rapid weight loss. Because the underlying metabolic disturbances cause debilitation, patients often fail to recuperate fully from episodes of weight loss. The net consequence is progressive debilitation and, in the extreme, death from inanition. (*From* Grunfeld C, Feingold KR: Metabolic disturbances and wasting in the acquired immunodeficiency syndrome. *N Engl J Med* 1992, 327:329–337; with permission.)

Effect of total parental nutrition on body cell mass

Underlying cause	Change in body cell mass (TBK)
Gastrointestinal disease	14.4% ± 6.8%
Systemic infection	-8.5% ± 5.1%

FIGURE 11-14 The effect of hyperalimentation with total parenteral nutrition (TPN) in HIV infection and AIDS. A cohort of patients with the wasting syndrome (averaging 78% of ideal body weight) was treated with hyperalimentation. Body cell mass was determined by measuring total body potassium (TBK) before and after TPN. In a retrospective analysis, patients with decreased intake due to gastrointestinal disease showed improvement in body cell mass with TPN. Patients with untreatable systemic infection lost body cell mass despite TPN. (Kotler DP, Tierney AR, Culpepper-Morgan JA, *et al.*: Effect of home total parenteral nutrition on body composition in patients with acquired immunodeficiency syndrome. *JPEN J Parenter Enteral Nutr* 1990, 14:454–458.)

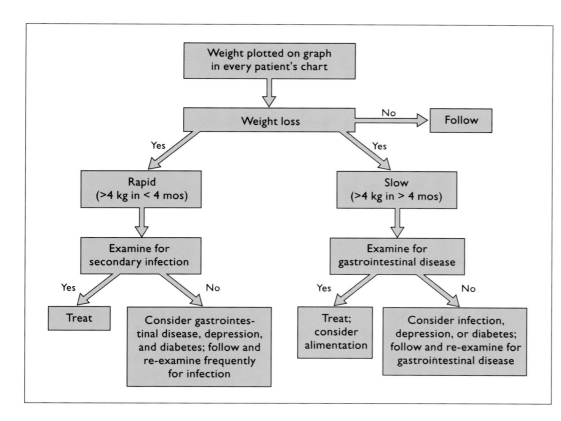

FIGURE 11-15 The use of weight loss as a clinical marker in HIV infection in AIDS. The weight of each patient with HIV infection for each visit should be plotted on a graph in the patient's chart. Rapid episodes of weight loss should first prompt investigation for secondary infection, whereas slower weight loss should first prompt investigation for gastrointestinal disease. However, infection, gastrointestinal disease, depression, and diabetes should be considered in all HIV-infected patients with weight loss.

Direct treatment of weight loss in HIV infection and AIDS

Approved therapies
  Dronabinol
  Megestrol acetate
Experimental approaches
  Growth hormone
  Insulin-like growth factor-1 (IGF-1)
  Anabolic steroids

FIGURE 11-16 Treatment of the wasting syndrome. Although it is most important to treat the underlying causes of weight loss, there is considerable morbidity and potential mortality from weight loss *per se*. Therefore, direct treatment of the wasting syndrome has been proposed. The approved agents, dranabinol and megestrol acetate, stimulate appetite and lead to weight gain that is primarily adipose tissue. Experimental agents are currently being tested in clinical trials, which may promote the formation of lean body mass and muscle.

SELECTED BIBLIOGRAPHY

Grunfeld C, Feingold KR: Metabolic disturbances and wasting in the acquired immunodeficiency syndrome. *N Engl J Med* 1992, 327:329–337.

Macallan DC, Noble C, Baldwin C, *et al.*: Prospective analysis of weight change in stage IV human immunodeficiency virus infection. *Am J Clin Nutr* 1993, 58:417–424.

Grunfeld C, Feingold KR: Body weight as essential data in the management of patients with human immunodeficiency virus infection and the acquired immunodeficiency Syndrome. *Am J Clin Nutr* 1993, 58:317–318.

Schambelan M, Grunfeld C: Endocrine abnormalities associated with human immunodeficiency virus infection and AIDS. *In* Broder S, Merigan T, Bolognesi DP (eds): *Textbook of AIDS Medicine.* Baltimore: Williams & Wilkins, 1994.

CHAPTER 12

Hematologic Manifestations

W. Christopher Ehmann
Christopher D. Gocke
M. Elaine Eyster

EFFECTS OF HIV INFECTION

Cytopenias

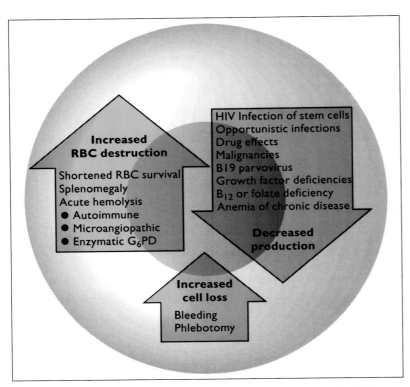

FIGURE 12-1 Anemia. Anemia has many possible causes in HIV-infected subjects, and these causes can be divided into those causing decreased production of red blood cells, increased destruction of red blood cells, and increased red cell loss. Most HIV-infected subjects develop anemia during the course of their illness, which is typically a hypoproliferative anemia (decreased production with a low reticulocyte count). Accelerated red blood cell destruction or loss can also contribute to the anemia. While acute hemolysis is rare, patients with congenital glucose-6-phosphate dehydrogenase (G_6PD) deficiency can develop acute hemolysis when given some medications, such as dapsone or trimethoprim/sulfamethoxazole.

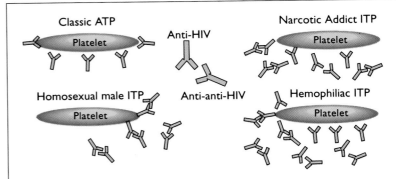

FIGURE 12-2 Thrombocytopenia. Three different types of immune-mediated thrombocytopenia (ITP) can occur in HIV-infected individuals shown here contrasted to classic autoimmune thrombocytopenia (ATP). In ATP, platelet-specific antibodies bind by their $F(ab')_2$ portions to platelet antigens and mediate clearance by reticuloendothelial system macrophages which attach to the Fc portion of the immunoglobulin molecules. Homosexual men with ITP have immune complexes both circulating and on their platelet surface. These complexes consist of one immunoglobulin molecule directed against HIV antigens, with the other molecule directed against a portion of the $F(ab')_2$ region of the first molecule. These complexes bind to the platelets via the platelet Fc receptor. Narcotic addicts with ITP have both platelet-specific antibodies and immune complexes. Hemophiliacs with ITP have both forms but with a preponderance of platelet-specific antibodies. (Karpatkin S: HIV-1 related thrombocytopenia. *Hematol/Oncol Clin North Am* 1990, 4(1):193-218.)

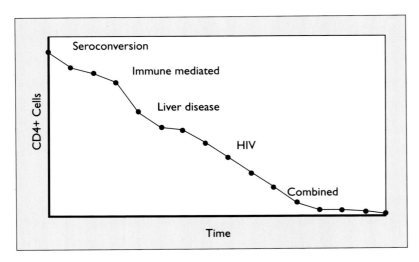

FIGURE 12-3 Possible causes of thrombocytopenia during the course of HIV infection. Some patients become thrombocytopenic during the acute viral illness which results in seroconversion. As CD4 counts decline, B-cell derangement may produce one of the forms of immune-mediated thrombocytopenia. In hemophiliacs with chronic liver disease caused by hepatitis C virus infection, thrombocytopenia may be caused either by the liver disease or the subsequent portal hypertension and splenomegaly. Later in the course of HIV infection, megakaryocytes may become infected with HIV, leading to a hypoproliferative thrombocytopenia. It is this form of thrombocytopenia that may respond to treatment with zidovudine. As patients develop severe immune deficiency, opportunistic infections and the drugs used to treat them impair platelet production.

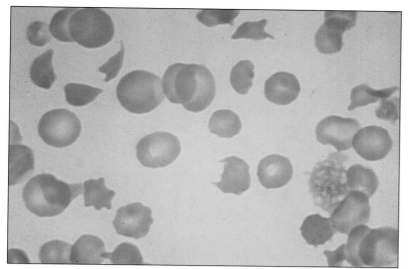

FIGURE 12-4 Thrombotic thrombocytopenia purpura (TTP). In this peripheral blood smear, note the fragmented red blood cells and thrombocytopenia. The incidence of TTP is increased in HIV-infected subjects and is characterized by a pentad of findings: thrombocytopenia, microangiopathic hemolytic anemia, renal insufficiency, neurologic symptoms, and fever. This entity has been described in all HIV risk groups and at all stages of disease. (Rarick MU, Espina B, Mocharnuk R, *et al.*: Thrombotic thrombocytopenia purpura in patients with human immunodeficiency virus infection: A report of three cases and review of the literature. *Am J Hematol* 1992, 40:103-109.)

BONE MARROW ABNORMALITIES

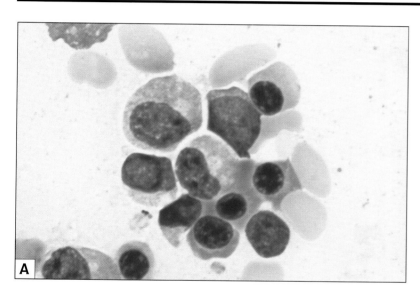

A

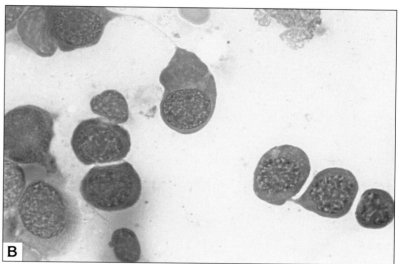

B

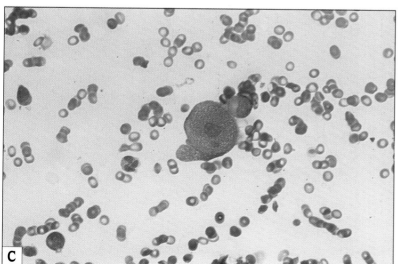

C

FIGURE 12-5 Bone Marrow Aspirates. There is no one abnormality that is pathognomonic for HIV infection in bone marrow aspirates of persons infected with HIV. Hypercellularity, hyperplasia of one or more lineage, myelodysplasia (including dyserythropoiesis), and increased iron stores either alone or in combination are the most common findings in the bone marrows of HIV-infected individuals. (Karcher DS, Frost AR: The bone marrow in human immunodeficiency virus (HIV)-related disease. *Am J Clin Pathol* 1991, 95:63-71.) **A**, Normal bone marrow erythroid activity (shown for comparison). (H+E; original magnification × 1000.) **B**, Megaloblastic maturation seen in patients treated with zidovudine. Almost all patients who take zidovudine develop megaloblastic maturation, and many develop anemia. The increased mean corpuscular volume (MCV) seen with zidovudine therapy can be an aid to monitoring compliance with this medication. Although didanosine (ddI) and zalcitabine (ddC) are nucleoside analogs with similar mechanisms of action, they do not produce the same megaloblastic changes in the red blood cell precursors. (H+E; original magnification × 1000.) **C**, A giant pronormoblast from an HIV-infected subject who was also infected with B19 parvovirus (*Courtesy of* N. Young, MD). *(continued)*

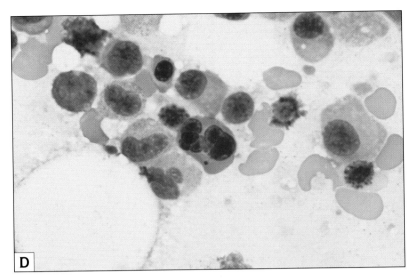

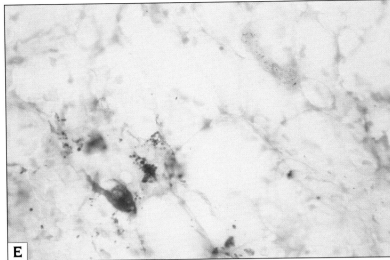

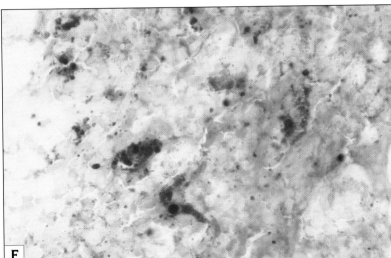

FIGURE 12-5 *(continued)* Such patients are characterized by severe anemia, low reticulocyte counts, and a response to intravenous immunoglobulins. (Frickhofen N, Abkowicz JL, Safford M, *et al.*: Persistent B19 parvovirus infection in patients infected with human immunodeficiency virus type I (HIV-1): A treatable cause of anemia in AIDS. *Ann Intern Med* 1990, 113:926.) (H+E; original magnification × 1000.) **D**, Dyserythropoiesis, characterized by bizarre red blood cell precursors, especially multinucleated cells. (H+E; original magnification × 1000.) **E** and **F**, *Panel 5E* shows a low-power view of a normal bone marrow aspirate stained for iron, which appears blue-green. *Panel 5F* shows an aspirate from an HIV-infected subject. The increased iron evident on such preparations is probably due to a metabolic block of iron utilization seen in anemias of chronic disease. (Potassium ferrocyanide, × 400.)

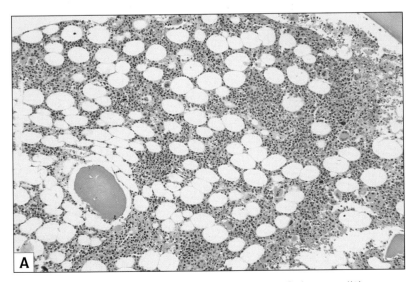

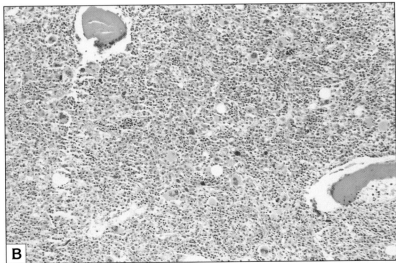

FIGURE 12-6 Bone marrow biopsies. A range of abnormalities are seen on bone marrow biopsy specimens of HIV-infected subjects. **A**, A normal bone marrow biopsy specimen, shown for comparison. About 50% of bone marrow is fat, which is dissolved during preparation and appears as acellular spaces on hematoxylin-eosin staining. **B**, A biopsy specimen from an HIV-infected subject demonstrates the increased cellularity frequently seen in HIV infection. *(continued)*

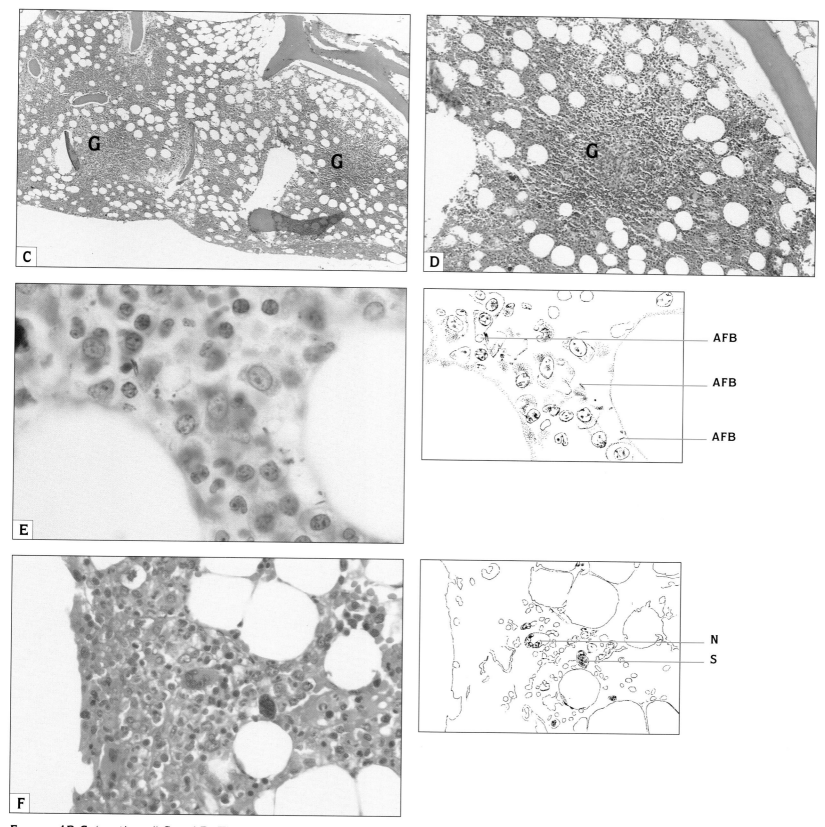

FIGURES 12-6 *(continued)* **C** and **D**, The granulomas (*G*) seen in HIV-infected subjects, shown at low (*panel 6C*) and higher power (*panel 6D*), are less compact with fewer histiocytes and more lymphoid cells than granulomas in immunocompetent hosts. Although it is uncommon to see acid-fast organisms if granulomas are not present, many HIV-infected subjects have bone marrow granulomas and no evidence of infection. (Nichols L, Florentine B, Lewis W, *et al.*: Bone marrow examination for the diagnosis of mycobacterial and fungal infections in the acquired immunodeficiency syndrome. *Arch Pathol Lab Med* 1991, 115:1125–1132.) **E**, A biopsy specimen stained with a Ziehl-Neelsen stain for acid-fast bacilli, which stain red on a blue background (*AFB*). Subsequent culture identified these as *Mycobacterium avium* complex. When patients are infected with *M. avium* complex, numerous organisms are typically seen, usually in granulomas. This patient was distinct, both for the low number of organisms and the lack of granuloma formation. **F**, Two megakaryocytes, one normal (*N*) and the other a stripped (*S*) or "naked" megakaryocyte, a characteristic finding in HIV infection. *(continued)*

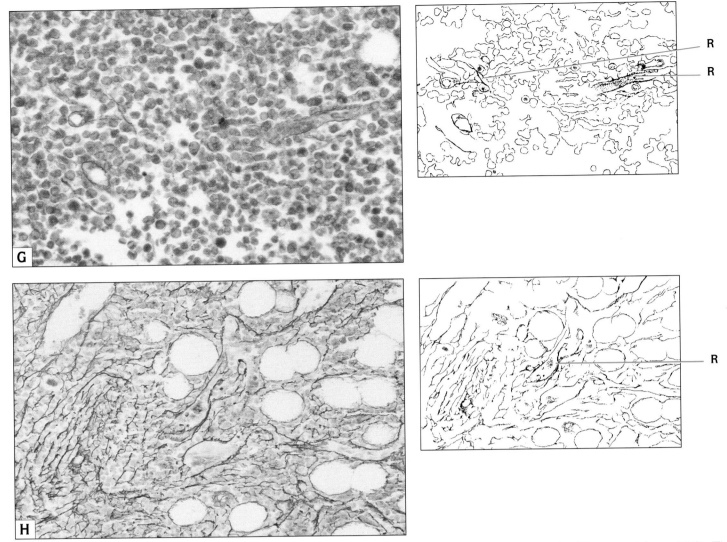

FIGURE **12-6** *(continued)* **G.** Biopsy specimens stained with a modified Gomori's stain for reticulum demonstrate the increase in black-staining reticulum fibers (*R*) seen in HIV-infected subjects *(panel 6H)* as compared with normal *(panel 6G)*. The increase in reticulum is probably responsible for the fact that bone marrow cannot be aspirated from many HIV-infected subjects.

Cellular Depletion of Lymph Nodes

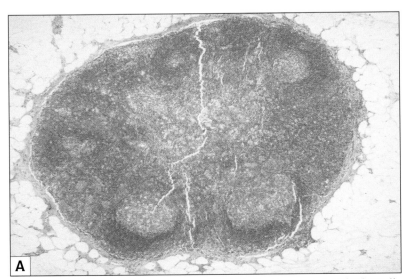

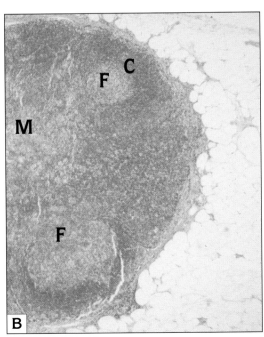

FIGURE **12-7** During the course of HIV infection, acute viral replication occurs in the lymph nodes, leading to progressive depletion of cells in the lymph node. **A** and **B,** A normal lymph node (at low and higher power, respectively). Note the presence of distinct medulla (*M*) and cortex (*C*), the latter containing small follicles (*F*). *(continued)*

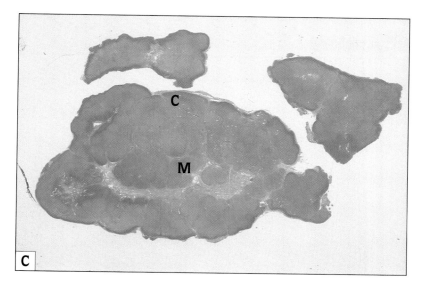

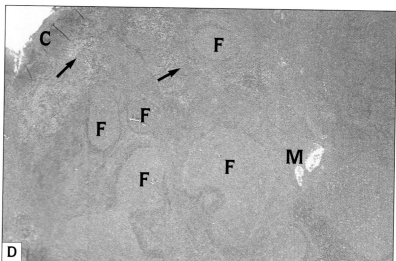

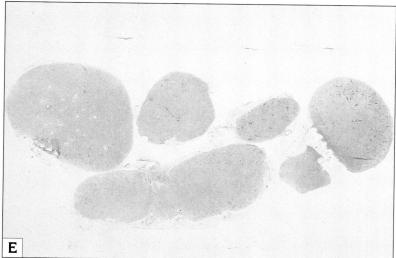

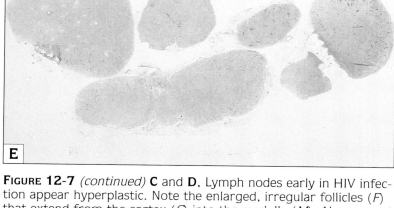

FIGURE 12-7 *(continued)* **C** and **D**, Lymph nodes early in HIV infection appear hyperplastic. Note the enlarged, irregular follicles (*F*) that extend from the cortex (*C*) into the medulla (*M*). Also present are characteristic clusters of pale monocytoid B cells (*arrows*). **E** and **F**, During late-stage infection, there is decreased cellularity of lymph nodes with follicles depleted of dendritic and lymphoid cells. This progressive depletion of cells in the lymph nodes during the course of HIV infection creates the pale appearance of the lymph node, despite adequate staining. Active viral replication is known to occur in the lymph nodes during the period after the seroconversion illness, even though the titer of HIV is low in the circulating blood. The dendritic cells in the lymph nodes may initially function as a filter, decreasing the amount of circulating free virus. Loss of these cells may increase the viral burden in the infected individual. Finally, all cell types are decreased, leading to the "burnt out" appearance of the end-stage lymph nodes. (*All*, hematoxylin-eosin.)

IMMUNOLOGIC ABNORMALITIES

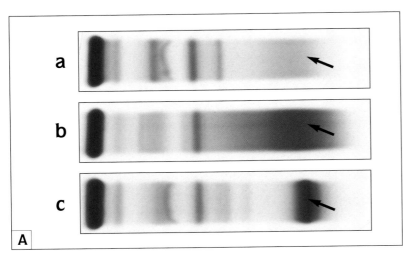

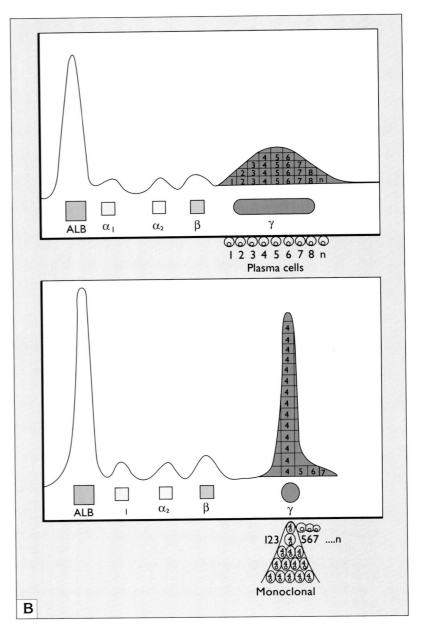

FIGURE 12-8 A, Serum electrophoresis demonstrates a normal pattern (*lane a*, for comparison), a polyclonal gammopathy (*lane b*), and a monoclonal gammopathy (*lane c*). Immunoglobulins (*arrows*) migrate toward the negatively charged electrode (to the right of the gel) and demonstrate a light staining diffuse pattern in normals, a heavy broad band in those with a polyclonal gammopathy, and a discrete heavy staining band in those with a monoclonal gammopathy. HIV-infected subjects often have a polyclonal gammopathy, which may be a manifestation of B-cell dysregulation occurring early in HIV infection. Polyclonal gammopathies may be responsible for some of the autoimmune phenomena that accompany HIV infection, such as a positive antinuclear antibody test or a positive direct Coombs' test. **B,** A polyclonal gammopathy is the result of immunoglobulin secretion from many different plasma cells (*upper panel*). In contrast, a monoclonal gammopathy is the result of immunoglobulin secretion from a single clone of plasma cells, all secreting the same immunoglobulin with the same electrophoretic mobility, resulting in a narrow band on the gel (*lower panel*). (*Modified from* Paraskevas F, Foerster J: Immunodiagnostics. Lee GR, Bithell TC, Foerster J, eds: In *Wintrobe's Clinical Hematology*, 9th ed. Philadelphia: Lea & Febiger; 1993:488; with permission.)

Coagulation Abnormalities

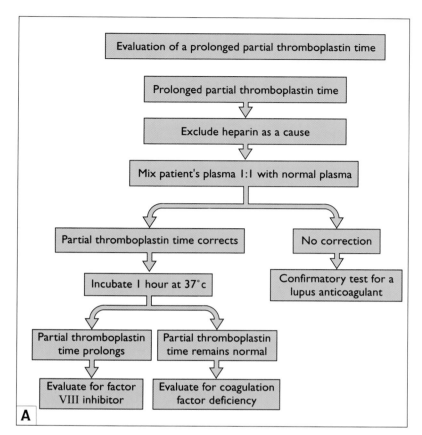

A

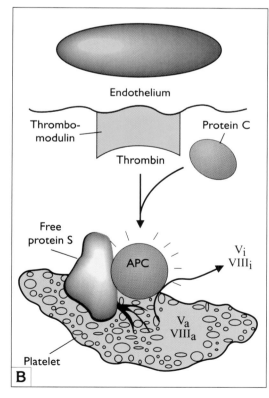

B

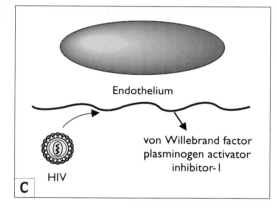

C

FIGURE 12-9 **A,** Evaluation of a prolonged partial thromboplastin time (PTT). Many HIV-infected subjects have lupus anticoagulants, which appear as patients become more acutely ill and disappear as they recover. These antibodies react with the phospholipid used in the PTT test. Although they prolong the PTT, they probably have no clinical significance. (Cohen AJ, Philips TM, Kessler CM: Circulating coagulation inhibitors in the acquired immunodeficiency syndrome. *Ann Intern Med* 1986, 104:175-180.) **B,** The function of protein S. The free form of this vitamin-K-dependent protein acts as a cofactor for activated protein C. The complex of proteins S and C assembles on the platelet surface and cleaves activated factors V and VIII, counteracting activation of the coagulation cascade. Protein S deficiency is associated with an increased risk of venous thrombosis. An acquired form of protein S deficiency is quite common in HIV-infected individuals, some of whom may be predisposed to developing thrombosis. (*Modified from* Rapaport SI: *Introduction to Hematology*, 2nd ed. Philadelphia: J.B. Lippincott; 1987:462; with permission. Stahl CP, Wideman CS, Spira TJ, *et al.*: Protein S in men with long term human immunodeficiency virus infection. *Blood* 1993, 81:1801-1807.) **C,** HIV infection affects endothelial cells by stimulating the release of a variety of factors, including von Willebrand's factor (VWF) and plasminogen activator inhibitor (PAI-1), into the circulating blood. The clinical consequences of these phenomena are unknown. (Lafeuillade A, Alessi MC, Poizot-Martin I, *et al.*: Endothelial cell dysfunction in HIV infection. *J Acq Immune Defic Syndr* 1992, 5:127-131.)

TOXICITY OF NUCLEOSIDE ANALOGS

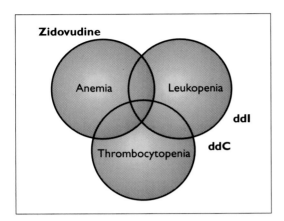

FIGURE 12-10 The hematologic toxicities of the nucleoside analogs presently approved for use. The principal toxicity of zidovudine is anemia, which is usually manifested within the first 12 weeks of therapy and is less common in subjects with high CD4 counts. Zidovudine also frequently produces leukopenia, especially in those with more advanced HIV disease. Thrombocytopenia is rare with zidovudine treatment; platelet counts often increase during therapy with this drug. Didanosine (ddI) and zalcitabine (ddC) are more frequently associated with leukopenia and thrombocytopenia than with anemia. Leukopenia is a fairly frequent dose-limiting toxicity of all of these drugs.

ROLE OF HEMATOPOIETIC GROWTH FACTORS

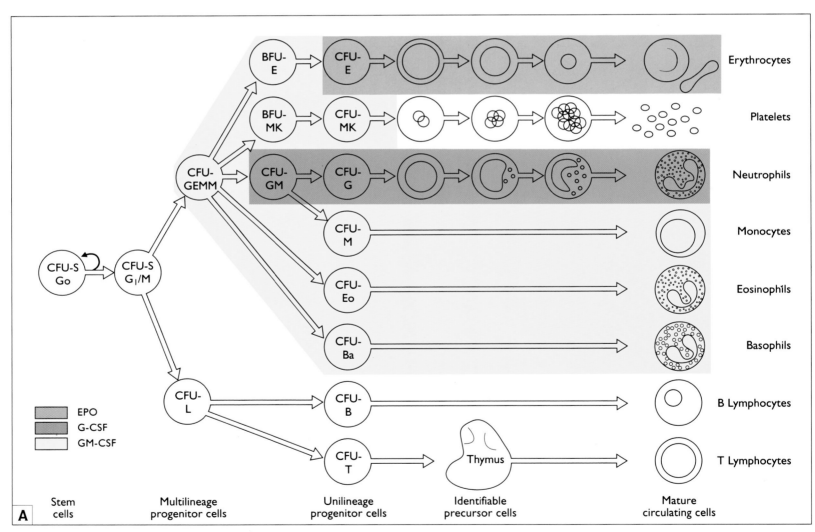

FIGURE 12-11 A, The hematopoietic effects of granulocyte–colony-stimulating factor (G-CSF), granulocyte-macrophage–colony-stimulating factor (GM-CSF), and epotin-alfa. *(continued)*

B. Use of growth factors

Compound	Trade names	Abbreviation	Current indications	Initial dose	Possible uses
Epotin alfa	Epogen (Amgen) Procrit (Ortho)	EPO	Anemia of chronic renal failure Zidovudine-induced anemia	50–100 U/kg 3 × weekly 100 U/kg 3 × weekly, increase by 100 U/kg every 4-8 wks to max 300 U/kg	Anemia of HIV
Filgrastim	Neupogen (Amgen)	G-CSF	Chemotherapy-induced neutropenia in non-myeloid malignancies	5µg/kg/d until neutrophils >10,000/mm^3	Other drug-induced neutropenia including ZDV* HIV-associated neutropenia Combined with epotin alfa for neutropenia and anemia* Extremely low doses may suffice (even 50 µg/mo) Combined with interferon-α as antiretroviral or for Kaposi's sarcoma
Sargramostim	Leukine (Immunex)	GM-CSF	Reconstitution after autogenous bone marrow transplantation For delayed engraftment after auto/allogenous transplantation	250 µg/m^2/d for 21 days as a 2-hr infusion	May potentiate intracellular effect of zidovudine May potentiate epotin-alfa May increase viral replication Intralesional therapy for Kaposi's sarcoma

*GM-CSF also useful.

FIGURE 12-11 *(continued)* **B**, The names, manufacturers, and current FDA-approved indications for the three growth factors that are presently available. In addition, the last column suggests other possible uses for these growth factors. (Figure 12A *modified from* Hoffman R, Benz EJ Jr, Shattil SJ, *et al.*, eds: *Hematology: Principles and Practice.* New York: Churchill-Livingstone; 1991:74; with permission. Mitsuyasu RT: Hematopoietic growth factors in the treatment of patients with HIV infection. *Biotherapy* 1990, 2:173-181.)

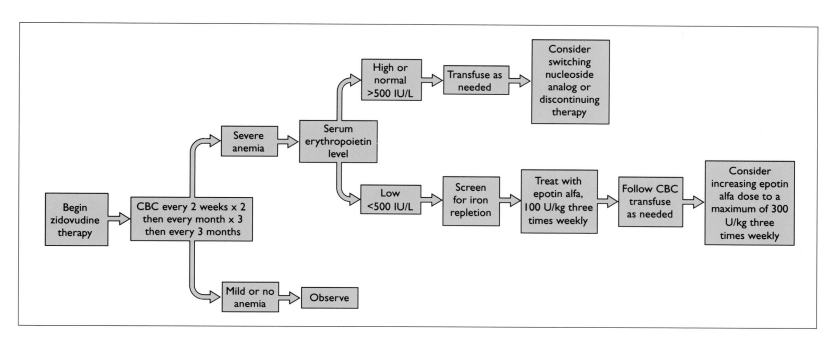

FIGURE 12-12 Evaluation of anemia in patients treated with zidovudine. Those with symptomatic anemia and a serum erythropoietin level of < 500 IU/L have been shown to require fewer transfusions when given epotin alfa, 100-200 U/kg subcutaneously or intravenously three times weekly. (CBC—complete blood count.)

HIV INFECTION IN HEMOPHILIACS

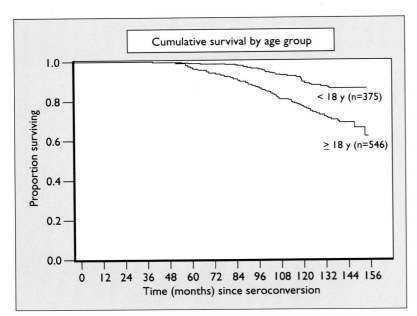

FIGURE 12-13 A Kaplan-Meier survival curve from a large multicenter cohort of hemophiliacs shows the effect of age on survival for those who HIV seroconverted at age < 18 years vs ≥ 18 years of age. It was initially thought that hemophiliacs were a distinct group who survived longer than other groups after they were infected with HIV. However, many hemophiliacs were infected as children, and survival data for hemophiliacs approximates that of homosexual men when corrected for the differences in age at seroconversion. (Ehmann WC, Eyster ME, Wilson SE, *et al.:* Relationship of CD4 lymphocyte counts to survival in a cohort of hemophiliacs infected with human immunodeficiency virus. *J Acquir Immune Defic Syndr,* in press.)

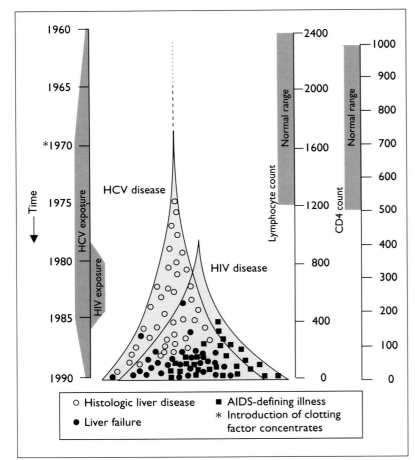

FIGURE 12-14 The hypothetical progression of HIV and liver disease in hemophiliacs infected with both HIV and hepatitis C virus (HCV). Almost all heavily treated hemophiliacs were infected with HCV, with exposures occurring from the 1970s when clotting factor concentrates were introduced (*asterisk*) or earlier (*far left*). HIV exposure occurred between 1978 and 1986, also shown on the left side. Over the ensuing years, the total lymphocyte and CD4-positive lymphocyte counts have decreased for these patients (*right*). In the center of the figure, the increasing incidence of histologic liver disease is depicted by *open circles*, and liver failure (still an important cause of death in hemophiliacs) by *closed circles*. AIDS-defining illnesses are depicted by the *closed squares*, with an increasing incidence since HIV infection. Many of the medications used to treat either HIV or opportunistic infections may accelerate the progression to liver failure in these patients. In a hemophilia cohort study, HIV has been shown to accelerate the course of HCV infection, with faster progression to liver failure for those who are both HCV and HIV infected. (*From* Eyster ME, Diamondstone LS, Lien JM, *et al.:* Natural history of hepatitis C virus infection in multitransfused hemophiliacs: Effect of coinfection with human immunodeficiency virus. *J Acq Immune Defic Syndr* 1993, 6:602-610; with permission.)

SELECTED BIBLIOGRAPHY

Mitsuyasu RT, Golde DW, eds: Hematologic and Oncologic Aspects of HIV Disease. *Hematol Clin North Am* 1991, 5(2):195-373.

Scadden DT, Zon LI, Groopman JE: Pathophysiology and Management of HIV Associated Hematologic Disorders. *Blood* 1989, 74:1455.

CHAPTER 13

Microbiology of Opportunistic Infections

Edward J. Bottone

BACTERIA

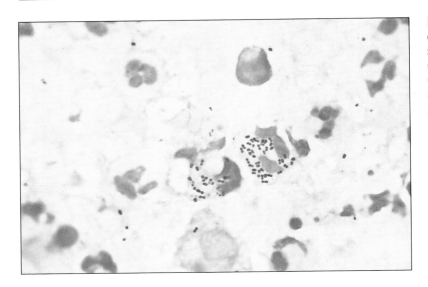

FIGURE 13-1 *Streptococcus pyogenes*. A smear of exudate from a cutaneous ulcer on a foot shows gram-positive cocci in pairs and short chains, some within polymorphonuclear leukocytes. Cultures of the lesion material on 5% sheep blood agar produced small compact colonies surrounded by a zone of complete (β) hemolysis. Serologic testing identified the isolate as *Streptococcus pyogenes*. (Gram stain, × 1000.)

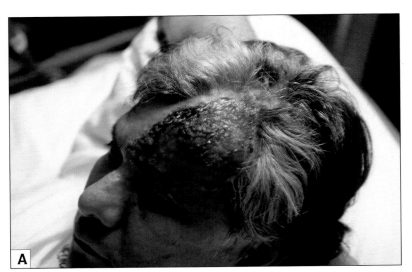

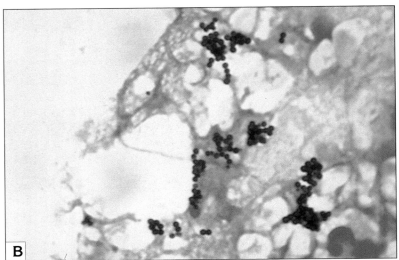

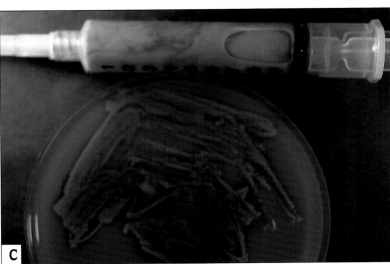

FIGURE 13-2 **A**, *Staphyloccocus aureus*. Large pulsatile scalp abscess in a patient with AIDS. The lesion was surgically drained of 300 mL of purulent material. Underlying bone was not involved. **B**, A smear of pus from the scalp abscess aspirated prior to surgical debridement shows gram-positive cocci singly, in pairs, and in clusters of varying coccal units. The morphologic presentation and staining characteristics of the coccus were consistent with a staphylococcal species. (Gram stain, × 1000.) **C**, A syringe containing purulent material from the scalp abscess. Culture of the purulence to sheep blood agar resulted in pure growth of yellow-pigmented colonies surrounded by a small zone of β hemolysis. The isolate was coagulase and catalase positive, leading to its identification as *Staphylococcus aureus*.

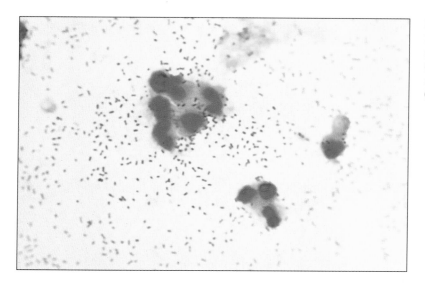

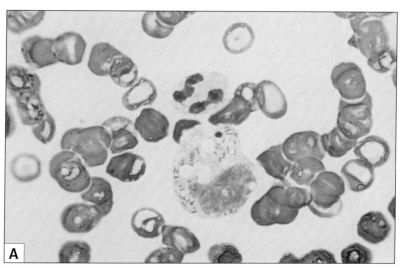

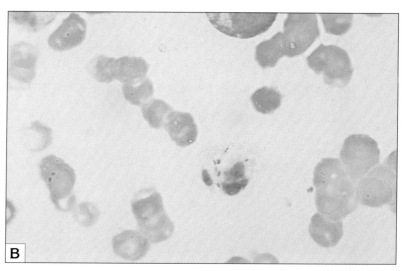

FIGURE 13-4 A, *Salmonella* sp. A bone marrow aspirate shows macrophages containing numerous intracellular bacilli, which on culture proved to be *Salmonella enteritidis* serovar *tymphimurium.* **B,** Gram stain of a bone marrow aspirate preparation shows gram-negative bacilli within polymorphonuclear leukocytes. Gram stain characteristics enabled the initial differentiation from *Listeria monocytogenes,* a gram-positive bacteria, which is also an intracellular pathogen and produces bacteremia and meningitis in the setting of immunosuppression. (Gram stain, × 1000.)

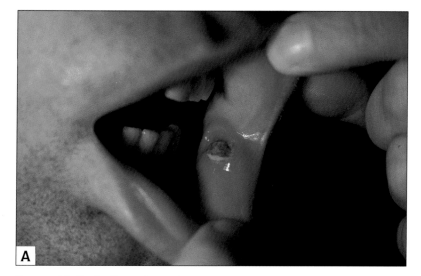

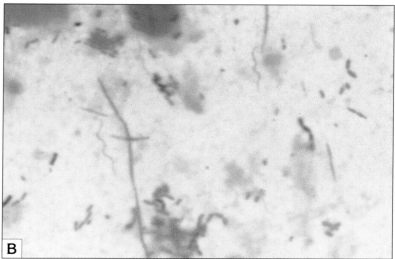

FIGURE 13-5 A, *Borrelia* sp. An erythematous and painful ulcer on the inner aspect of the cheek is encircled by an adherent membrane with a necrotic center. This developed from an initial ulcer of herpetic origin, which became secondarily infected with fusiforms and spirochetes (*Borrelia* species). The necrotic, painful aspect of the ulcer resolved after 24 hours of penicillin therapy. **B,** Gram stain of teased necrotic membrane from the cheek ulcer shows gram-negative slender fusiform bacilli with tapered ends admixed with gram-negative spiral forms. Other areas of smear showed massive entanglement of fusiforms and spirochetes forming membranous patches.

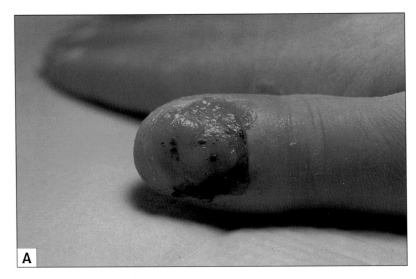

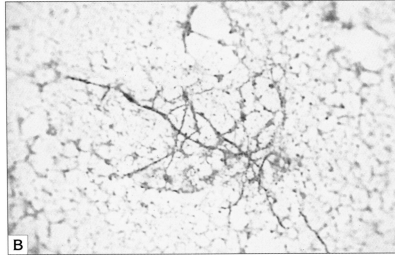

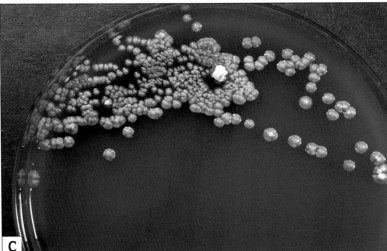

FIGURE 13-6 A, *Nocardia asteroides* infection of the nailbed of a finger. The nail was removed, exposing a painful underlying ulcer with a necrotic border. The patient had not sustained trauma to the finger. **B,** A smear from a scraping of the nailbed shows gram-positive branching filaments of *N. asteroides.* (Gram stain, × 1000.) Initial identification as a *Nocardia* species was achieved by showing that microorganism was acid-fast when subjected to a modified Kinyoun acid-fast stain. **C,** Blood agar culture of finger scraping shows dry, chalk-white colonies of *N. asteroides* after 72 hours' incubation at 37° C. The isolate was identified as *N. asteroides* on the basis of its growth in lysozyme broth, urease production, and failure to hydrolyze casein, xanthine, or tyrosine.

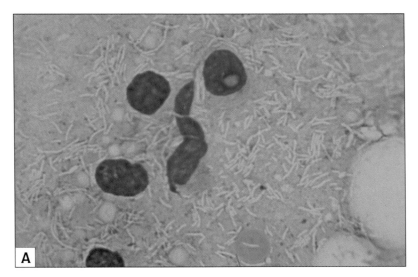

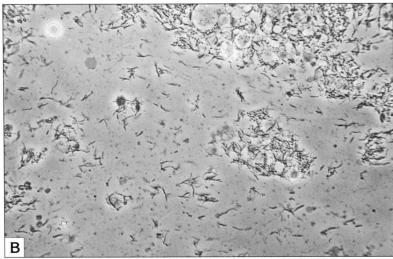

FIGURE 13-7 A, *Myocbacterium avium-intracellulare.* A touch preparation of lymph node biopsy shows innumerable unstained bacillary forms of *Myocbacterium avium-intracellulare.* These were subsequently confirmed by Kinyoun acid-fast stain of companion smears and by culture. (Giemsa stain, × 1000). **B,** Phase contrast microscopy of lymph node macerate shows numerous, slightly curved bacillary forms of *M. avium-intracellulare* singly and in small clumps of adherent bacilli. Adherence of mycobacterial cells to one another is a function of glycolipid (trehalose-6,6'-dimycolate) "cord factor" in the outer cell wall surface of mycobacteria. (× 400.) *(continued)*

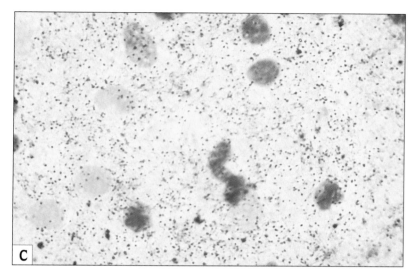

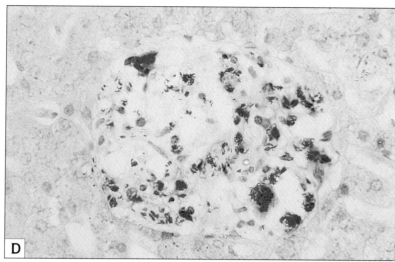

FIGURE 13-7 *(continued)* **C,** A touch imprint of lymph node biopsy shows innumerable, slightly curved, beaded, acid-fast bacilli subsequently identified as *M. avium-intracellulare*. Note the almost total absence of cellular component of lymph node. (Kinyoun stain, × 1000). **D,** Histologic section of liver from a patient with disseminated *M. avium-intracellulare* infection shows dense clumps of acid-fast bacilli. (Kinyoun stain, × 1000).

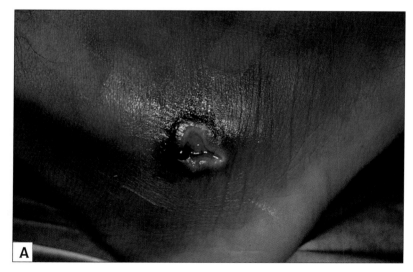

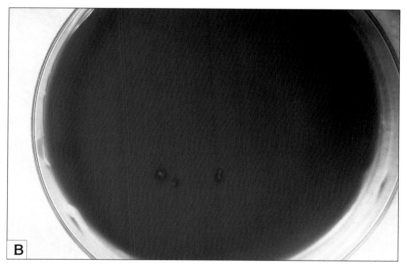

FIGURE 13-8 A, *Mycobacterium haemophilum*. An ulcerated lesion on an ankle caused by *Mycobacterium haemophilum*, a fastidious, slow-growing species requiring iron (hemin) supplementation of culture medium and reduced incubation temperatures (32° C) for growth. *M. haemophilum* produces mainly cutaneous infections in immunocompromised individuals and cervical and perihilar lymphadenitis in immunocompetent children. Its natural reservoir and mode of transmission are still unknown. (*Courtesy of* Marsha Gordon, MD.) **B,** Culture of ankle lesion material on chocolate agar shows growth of several colonies of *M. haemophilum*. This species may be differentiated from rapidly growing mycobacterial species such as *M. fortuitum*, which also grows on routine bacteriologic media, mainly by its requirement for iron (hemin) for growth.

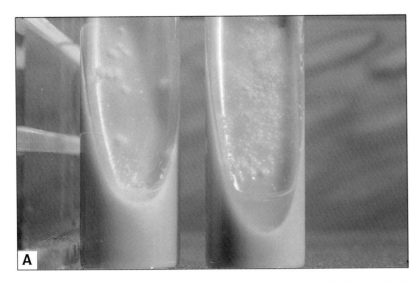

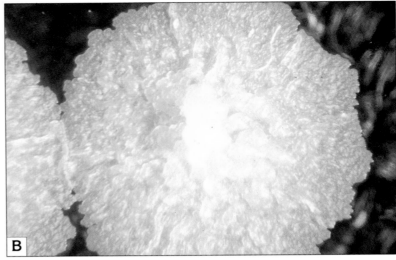

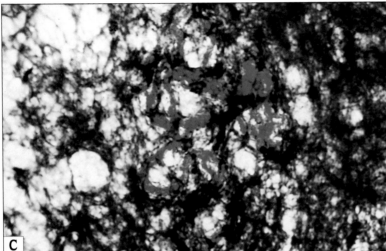

FIGURE 13-9 A, *Mycobacterium tuberculosis* cultured on Löwenstein-Jensen medium. Colonies are buff-colored, dry, and crumbly. In contrast, colonies of *M. avium-intracellulare* are usually smooth, although a mixture of smooth and rough colonies may be encountered as well as orange-pigmented colonies. **B,** Characteristic "cauliflower" morphology of a colony of *M. tuberculosis* growing on Middlebrook 7H10 agar medium. The roughened striated texture of the colony reflects hydrophobicity of the mycobacterial cell surface imparted by complex cellular lipids. **C,** Smear of the *M. tuberculosis* colony shows characteristic "serpentine" cords comprised of innumerable adherent bacilli arranged in parallel rows. This morphologic aspect can also be observed in smears prepared from tuberculosis lesions and directly in colonies of *M. tuberculosis*. Cording may also be observed in nontuberculous mycobacteria, but to a lesser intensity.

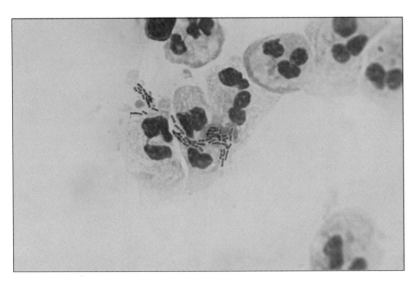

FIGURE 13-10 *Haemophilus ducreyi*. A touch imprint of a genital lesion shows parallel rows ("school of fish") of gram-negative, slightly curved bacilli characteristic of *Haemophilus ducreyi*. Organisms may also be found intracellularly. Note the coursing of bacilli between clusters of polymorphonuclear leukocytes. Banding of *H. ducreyi* cells through intercellular adhesion may also account for the compactness of *H. ducreyi* colonies on agar media, which allows them to be moved across the agar surface with an inoculation loop. (Gram stain, × 1000.)

FUNGI

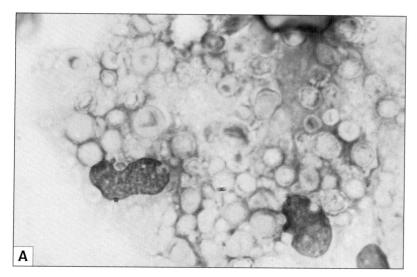

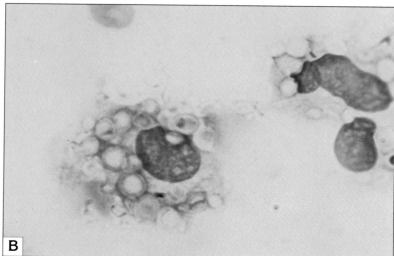

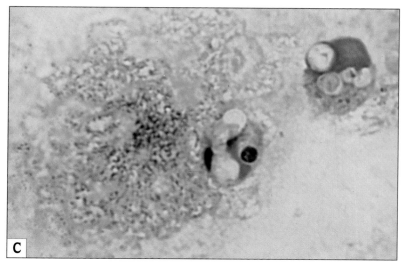

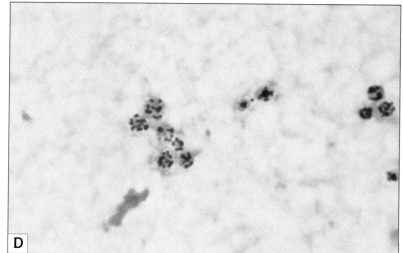

FIGURE 13-11 A, *Cryptococcus neoformans.* Bronchoalveolar lavage (BAL) fluid shows dense clusters of encapsulated yeast cells of *Cryptococcus neoformans.* (Giemsa stain, × 1000.) The diagnosis of pulmonary cryptococcosis may be advanced by assaying for cryptococcal capsular polysaccharide antigen in BAL fluid, in which fluid is reacted to an endpoint titration with latex particles coated with anticryptococcal antibody. Confirmation of *C. neoformans* infection rests on isolation of the mycotic agent. **B,** Bronchoalveolar lavage fluid shows encapsulated yeast cells of *C. neoformans* within a pulmonary macrophage. This microscopic presentation may mimic that seen with *Histoplasma capsulatum.* However, *C. neoformans* is larger and more spherical than the ovoid yeast cells of *H. capsulatum,* and budding is less frequently observed. (Giemsa stain, × 1000.) **C,** Bronchoalveolar lavage fluid shows irregularly stained, sparsely encapsulated yeast cells of *C. neoformans* within pulmonary macrophages. (Gram stain, × 1000.) **D,** Gram-stained smear of a blood culture positive for *C. neoformans* showing markedly stippled, oval yeast cells. In the Gram staining technique, the capsule of *C. neoformans* may prevent the entry of crystal violet to the interior part of the yeast cell, thereby reducing complete gram-positive staining. Irregular staining and absence of a clearly stained yeast cell wall give the appearance of discrete clusters of gram-positive cocci. Assessment of blood culture medium for cryptococcal antigen and isolation of mycotic agent will confirm the diagnosis. (Gram stain, × 1000.) *(continued)*

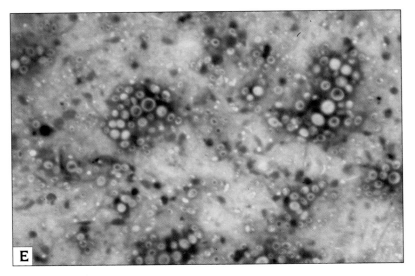

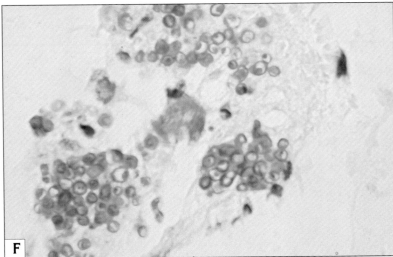

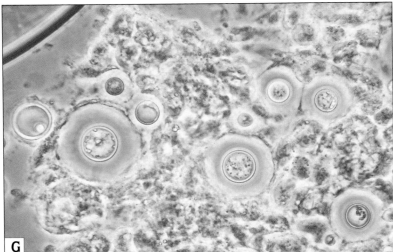

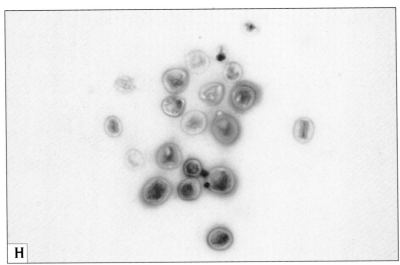

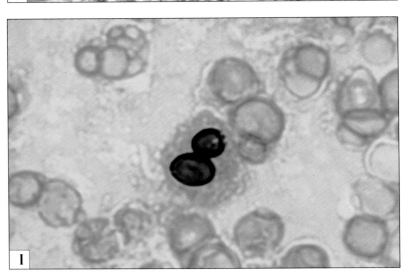

FIGURE 13-11 *continued* **E,** Scraping of gelatinous perisplenic exudate shows innumerable encapsulated yeast cells of *C. neoformans.* Note the presence of oval yeast cells of varying sizes, including sparsely encapsulated, infrequently budding cells. (Papanicolaou stain, × 1000.) Many *C. neoformans* cells were enmeshed in a viscous, glistening exudate covering the spleen. *C. neoformans* was also observed in lungs, brain, liver, and cerebrospinal fluid. **F,** Histologic section of lung shows dense clusters of oval yeast cells of *C. neoformans.* The cellular component of tissue has been almost completely supplanted by cryptococcal yeast cells. (Mucicarmine stain, × 1000.) **G,** A bronchoalveolar lavage (BAL) specimen shows yeast cells with capsules delineated by cellular constituents in the specimen. (Phase contrast microscopy, × 1000.) India ink preparation of BAL fluid confirmed the presence of encapsulated yeast cells. **H,** In cerebrospinal fluid, *C. neoformans* is distinguished by a rim of deep pink-staining capsular material surrounding the yeast cells. The internal aspect of the yeast cells may show linear invaginations, which distinguish cryptococcal yeast cells from those of *Candida* species. Single, more densely stained bodies near the periphery of the cell may also be discerned. (Giemsa stain, × 1000.) **I,** Methenamine silver staining of a lung biopsy specimen shows yeast cells of *C. neoformans* within a pulmonary macrophage. Rounded yeast cells with a suggestion of central folding and deep-staining oval bodies aid distinction from *Histoplasma capsulatum.* (Methenamine silver stain, × 1000.)

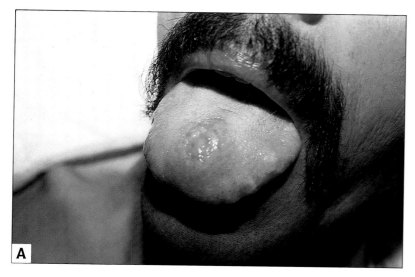

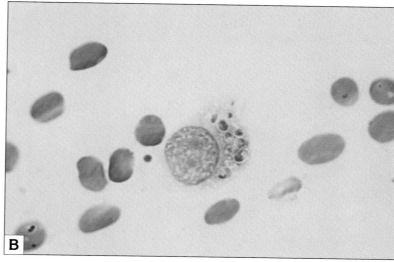

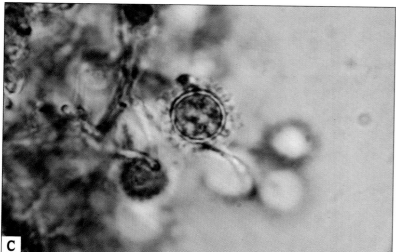

FIGURE 13-12 A, *Histoplasma capsulatum*. An ulcer on the tongue is a representative mucosal manifestation of disseminated *Histoplasma capsulatum* infection. The ulcer is well-circumscribed and firm, with a raised border suggestive of a chancre. Darkfield examination for *Treponema pallidum* and serologic tests for syphilis were negative, as were smears and cultures for mycobacteria. B, A scraping of the tongue ulcer shows oval yeast forms of *H. capsulatum* within a macrophage. Note the pseudohalo surrounding individual yeast cells. (Giemsa stain, × 1000.) C, Moldlike growth of *H. capsulatum* at 25° C is teased apart to demonstrate characteristic oval macroconidium with spiny projections (tuberculate macroconidium). Small oval microconidia are also visible, which are the infectious unit inhaled by air pertubations of the moldlike growth in soil. (Lactophenol cotton blue preparation, × 1000.)

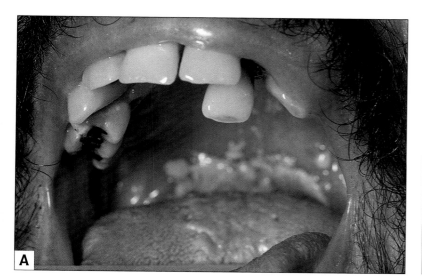

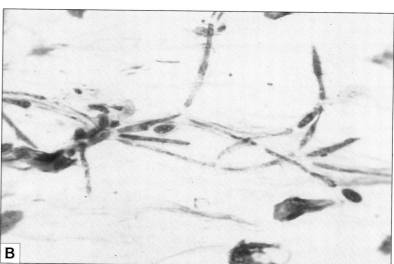

FIGURE 13-13 A, *Candida* sp. Mucocutaneous pseudomembranous candidiasis characterized by yellowish-white patches on the tongue and buccal mucosa. Patches may be scraped free and are composed of epithelial and inflammatory cells admixed with necrotic debris and with blastospores and pseudohyphae of *Candida*. (*Courtesy of Alexandra Gurtman, MD*.) B, Microscopic presentation of a scraping of oral patches shows blastospores and branching pseudohyphae characteristic of *Candida* species. (Giemsa stain, × 1000.)

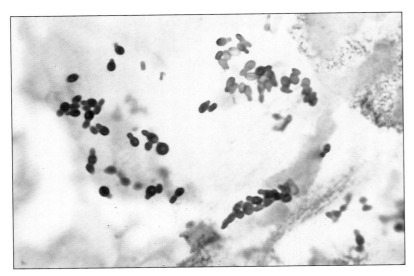

FIGURE 13-14 *Malassezia furfur.* Scraping of a facial scaling from a patient with seborrheic dermatitis shows the pale lavender, oval, budding yeast form of *Malassezia (Pityrosporon) furfur* adherent to keratinocytes. *M. furfur* is a lipophilic skin flora yeast that is unable to synthesize medium- or long-chain fatty acids and therefore requires exogenous fatty acids (C-12–C-24 carbon chain length) for growth on culture media, usually provided by an olive oil overlay or supplementation of media. *M. furfur* may be distinguished from other yeastlike organisms in stained preparations by its being devoid of any internal inclusions and showing blunted collarettes at site of yeast bud scar. (Giemsa stain, × 1000.)

PROTOZOA

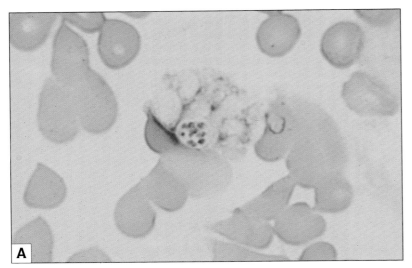

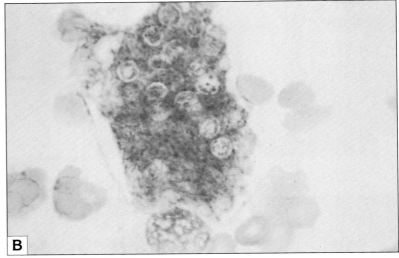

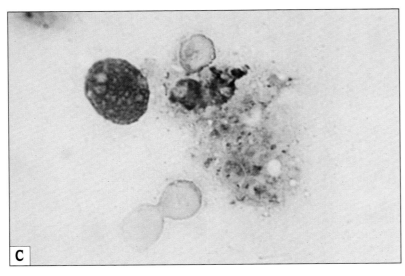

FIGURE 13-15 A, *Pneumocystis carinii.* A touch imprint of an open lung biopsy specimen shows an oval cyst of *Pneumocystis carinii* containing eight sporozoites. The cyst wall is unstained, and cytoplasm of intracystic bodies stain blue with excentric nuclei staining reddish purple. (Giemsa stain, × 1000.) **B**, A bronchoalveolar lavage specimen shows a cluster of cysts of *P. carinii* in varying stages of maturity, admixed with innumerable free trophozoites. The lavender-staining, honey-combed matrix, enveloping the organisms may be readily discerned by low power (× 100) microscopy. (Giemsa stain, × 1000.) **C**, A smear of bronchoalveolar lavage fluid shows a cyst of *P. carinii* and numerous free trophozoites. The cyst is distinguished by the clear halo surrounding it, whereas trophozoites are crescent-shaped and contain a reddish-purple nucleus. The presence of numerous trophozoites and a sparsity of cysts often characterize the microscopic presentation of acute *P. carinii* pneumonia. (Giemsa stain, × 1000.) *(continued)*

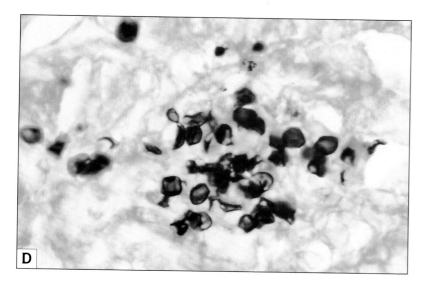

D

FIGURE 13-15 *(continued)* **D,** Gomori methenamine silver staining of a touch print from an open lung biopsy specimen shows clusters of black- to brown-staining cysts of *P. carinii.* Cysts are located within a "foamy exudate" in the alveoli and may display a variety of shapes, including collapsed sickled-shaped cysts. Thickening or indentation of the cyst wall may also occur. Intracystic bodies, unlike the cyst wall, are not stained. Budding, as in yeastlike organisms (*eg, Histoplasma, Torulopsis*), is never observed with *P. carinii.* (Gomori methenamine silver stain, × 1000.)

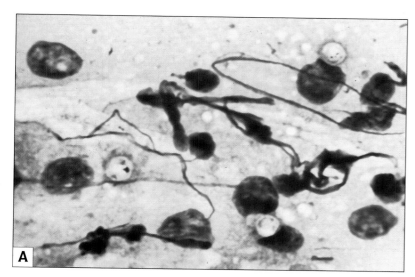

A

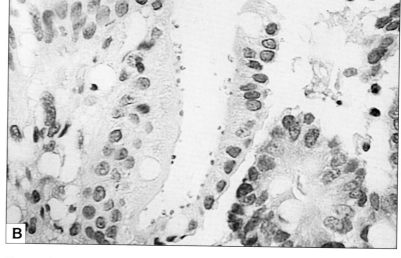

B

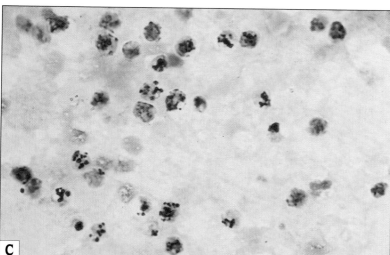

C

FIGURE 13-16 A, *Cryptosporidium* sp. Touch imprint from a colonic biopsy specimen of a patient with protracted watery diarrhea shows round oocysts of *Cryptosporidium* containing one to four intracystic sporozoites. Note the overall morphologic similarity of cryptosporidial oocysts and sporozoites to those of *Pneumocystis carinii.* (Giemsa stain, × 1000.) Differention of suspected *Cryptosporidium* oocysts from cysts of *P. carinii,* especially in respiratory specimens, is enabled by the absence of a halo around oocysts, only one to four sporozoites, and modified Kinyoun acid-fast staining. **B,** A colonic biopsy specimen shows oval, basophilic-staining, cryptosporidial bodies lining the epithelial border and protruding into the lumen. (Hematoxylin-eosin stain, × 1000.) The entire life cycle, sexual and asexual, takes place in the same host on the infected epithelial surface. Infection begins by the host's ingestion of mature oocysts containing up to four sporozoites. These sporozoites are released on passage into the intestinal tract and then associate with mucosal epithelial cells to complete their life cycle. **C,** Direct preparation of a fecal sample shows numerous oval oocysts of *Cryptosporidium.* The specimen was stained with a modified Kinyoun acid-fast procedure (10% H_2SO_4 decolorizer), rendering the oocysts bright red. Note the variability among oocysts in uptake and retention of red carbol-fuchsin stain. (Modified Kinyoun stain, × 1000.)

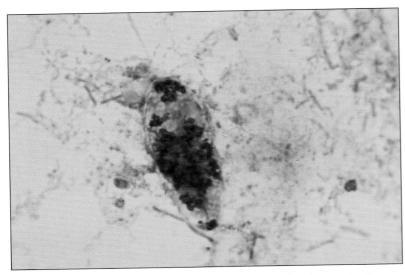

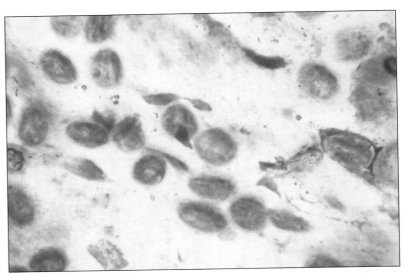

FIGURE 13-17 *Isospora belli*. Direct smear of a fecal sample shows a large elipsoidal oocyst of *Isospora belli*, a coccidian protozoa similar to *Cryptosporidium*. The oocyst stains red with the modified Kinyoun acid-fast stain and may contain two sporocysts. (Modified Kinyoun stain, × 1000.)

FIGURE 13-18 *Giardia lamblia*. Duodenal aspirate shows numerous oval to pear-shaped trophozoites of *Giardia lamblia*. Each trophozoite has four pairs of flagella (not seen) and two nuclei with a densely stained endosome in the anterior aspect of the cell. Trophozoites attach to epithelial cells in crypts of duodenum and upper jejunum through a concave sucking disk on their ventral surface. While attached to the epithelial surface, the parasite absorbs nutrients from the host. The mature cyst form is oval and has four nuclei; it is the infective unit. (Giemsa stain, × 1000.)

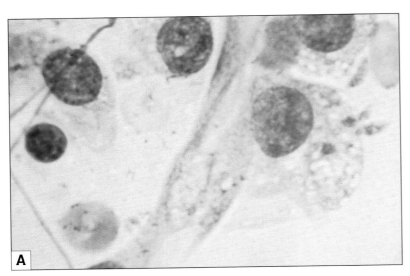

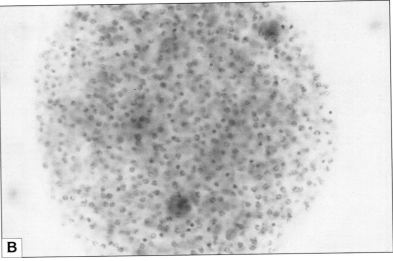

FIGURE 13-19 A, *Toxoplasma gondii*. A bronchoalveolar lavage smear shows crescent-shaped tachyzoites of *Toxoplasma gondii* within, penetrating, and adjacent to pulmonary epithelial cells. The tachyzoite is distinguished by its arc-shape, with one end tapered more than the other. The tachyzoite cytoplasm stains light blue with a reddish or purplish nucleus. (Giemsa stain, × 1000.) The tachyzoite of *Toxoplasma* is the invasive form and can enter phagocytic and nonphagocytic cells with subsequent destruction of these cells as a consequence of internal multiplication. The invasion process takes 15–45 seconds. **B**, A brain biopsy specimen shows the tissue cyst form of *T. gondii*, which can persist for years in tissue of an infected host. The cyst form is initiated by the parasite, a process that may be hastened by the host's immune response to the parasite. Tachyzoites (now called *bradyzoites*) are circular and contain a reddish-purplish nucleus; they reproduce by an internal budding process (endodyogeny), analogous to that in infected cells, and fill the cyst. (Giemsa stain, × 1000.) Persistence of the cyst form in human tissue accounts for reactivation of toxoplasmosis in the setting of immunosuppression.

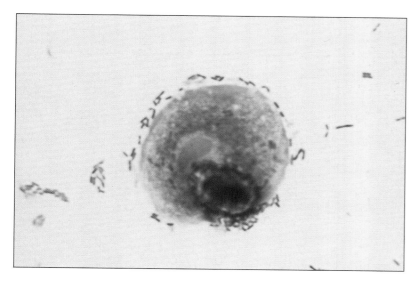

FIGURE 13-20 *Acanthamoeba* sp. A smear of ulcerative skin lesion shows the trophozoite of the free-living ameba, *Acanthamoeba*. Note the presence of bacillary forms (*Xanthomonas maltophilia*) adherent to the ameba surface, which serve as a food source for the phagocytic ameba. *Acanthamoeba* trophozoites have a dense round nucleus with a central nucleolus surrounded by a clear zone. Cytoplasmic vacuoles and inclusions may also be present. (Giemsa stain, × 1000.) In the setting of immunosuppression, an acanthamoeba etiology of a skin lesion should be suspected if there is chronicity with negative cultures and smears for diverse microorganisms. Dissemination to the central nervous system (brain) may occur from a primary skin lesion.

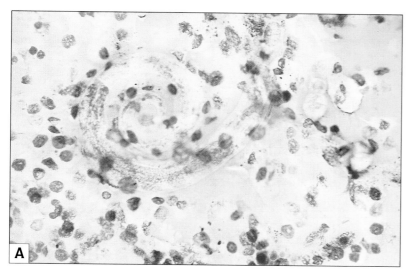

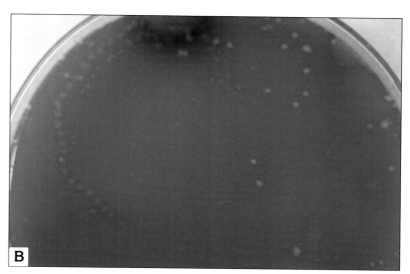

FIGURE 13-21 **A**, *Strongyloides stercoralis*. A bronchoalveolar lavage specimen shows coiled filariform larvae of *Strongyloides stercoralis*, an intestinal nematode. (Giemsa stain, × 1000.) Systemic dissemination of *S. stercoralis* from the gastrointestinal tract to other organs is rare but, if undiagnosed, produces a frequently fatal infection mainly seen in immunocompromised hosts. Because of an autoinfection cycle, *Strongyloides* may persist for many years either asymptomatically or with mild gastrointestinal symptoms. Often patients with *Strongyloides* hyperinfection have either single or recurrent episodes of gram-negative enteric species bacteremia, including polymicrobic bacteremia. **B**, Direct inoculation of a bronchoalveolar lavage specimen onto blood agar shows migration of larvae of *S. stercoralis*, manifested as "tracking" of bacteria across the agar surface from a central inoculum of the clinical specimen. Translocated bacterial colonies, because of larval migration, resemble a string of pearls. Similar translocation of colonies may be seen in stool cultures of patients with strongyloides infection.

VIRUSES

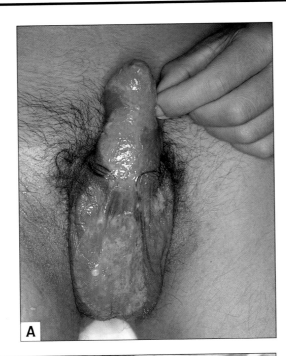

A

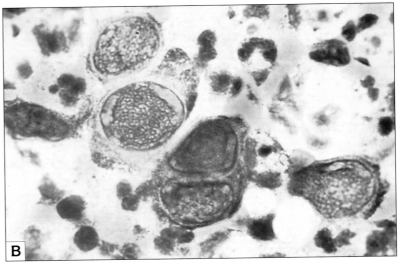

B

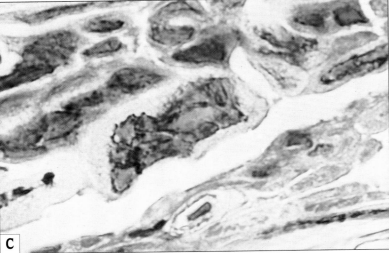

C

FIGURE **13-22** **A,** Herpes simplex virus. Severe genital herpes infection manifested by excoriating ulceration of the penile shaft and scrotum in a patient who was an intravenous drug user. The patient was treated with acyclovir with clearing of the lesion; the patient returned 6 months later with *Pneumocystis carinii* pneumonia. In this instance, severe genital herpes was the initial presentation of human immunodeficiency virus infection. **B,** A smear of scraping from a vesicular or ulcerative lesion shows a multinucleated giant cell and individual cells with intranuclear inclusion characteristic of herpes virus infection. Intranuclear inclusion may be discerned by its "ground glass" appearance, surrounded by the nuclear membrane, which may be irregular. (Giemsa stain, × 1000.) **C,** Histologic examination of a skin biopsy specimen shows a multinucleated giant cell characteristic of herpes virus infection. Multinucleated cells are formed as a consequence of the expression of herpes virus antigens on the surface of infected cells and their fusion with adjacent cells to form large syncytia of epithelial cells. (Hematoxylin-eosin stain, × 1000.)

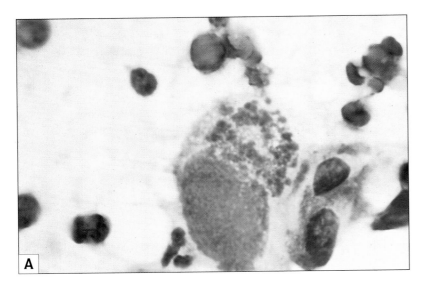

A

FIGURE **13-23** **A,** Cytomegalovirus. A smear of bronchoalveolar lavage fluid shows an enlarged pneumocyte containing numerous discrete, reddish-purple inclusions of cytomegalovirus. The large number of these discrete inclusions—some of which may also be seen in nucleus—distinguishes them from random phagocytosis by pulmonary macrophages of cellular debris or iron, which stains blue-green. Cytoplasmic inclusions are not found in herpes virus infections. (Giemsa stain, × 1000.) *(continued)*

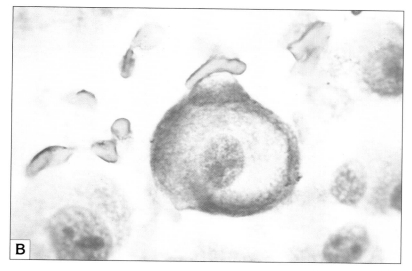

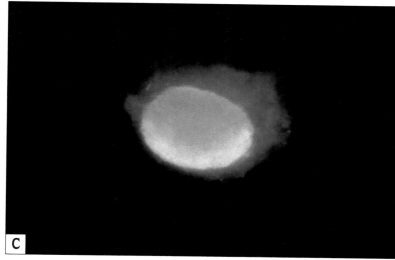

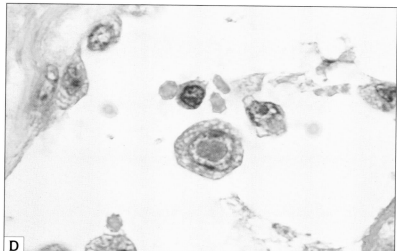

FIGURE 13-23 *(continued)* **B,** A smear of bronchoalveolar lavage fluid shows an enlarged pneumocyte with a discrete, lavender-staining intranuclear inclusion surrounded by nuclear membrane, rendering an "owl's eye" appearance to the infected cell. The inclusion is surrounded by a clear halo and thickened nuclear membrane. (Giemsa stain, × 1000.) **C,** Immunofluorescence of a pneumocyte in bronchoalveolar lavage fluid stained with fluorescein-conjugated anticytomegalovirus monoclonal antibody. Note the cytoplasmic apple-green fluorescence, which may be focal or confluent, and the orange counterstain. (× 1000.) **D,** Histologic section of lung shows characteristic intranuclear inclusion of cytomegalovirus. Note the halo surrounding the inclusion and the clearly visible, thickened nuclear membrane followed by a rim of cell cytoplasm. The infected cell is much larger than noninfected adjoining cells. Unstained oval cytoplasmic inclusions are also apparent. (Hematoxylin-eosin stain, × 1000.)

SELECTED BIBLIOGRAPHY

Bottone EJ: Spectrum and multiplicity of infectious complications in patients with AIDS: A microbiological perspective. *Compr Ther* 1990, 16:24–33.

Shulman HM, Hacilman RC, Sale LE, Meyers JD: Rapid cytologic diagnosis of cytomegalovirus interstitial pneumonia on touch imprints from open lung biopsy. *Am J Clin Pathol* 1982, 77:90–94.

Wormser GP (ed): *AIDS and Other Manifestations of HIV Infection*, 2nd ed. New York: Raven Press; 1992.

Straus WL, Ostroff SM, Jernigan DB, *et al.*: Clinical and epidemiologic characteristics of *Mycobacterium haemophilum*, an emerging pathogen in immunocompromised patients. *Ann Intern Med* 1994, 120:118–125.

Martinez AJ: *Free Living Amebas: Natural History, Prevention, Diagnosis, Pathology, and Treatment of Disease.* Boca Raton, Florida: CRC Press; 1985.

CHAPTER 14

Clinical Manifestations of Opportunistic Infections

Harold A. Kessler

VIRAL INFECTIONS

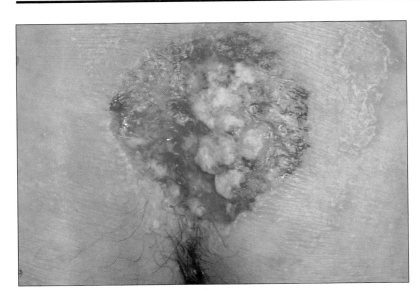

FIGURE 14-1 Chronic mucocutaneous herpes simplex infection. Recurrent mucocutaneous herpes simplex virus (HSV) infections are common in the general population. In the immune competent host, these recurrences are self-limited, but in patients with severe immune suppression, such as those with advanced HIV disease, recurrences may be progressive. These herpetic lesions are nonhealing and expand relentlessly over time if not treated with effective antiviral therapy. The drug of choice for these infections is acyclovir. In some patients with advanced immune suppression who have received repeated courses of acyclovir, an acyclovir-resistant mutant population of virus may emerge. The exact incidence of this complication in patients with AIDS is unknown, but it appears to be relatively uncommon, given the common occurrence of HSV infections in patients with AIDS and their frequent treatment with acyclovir. The patient in this slide had chronic mucocutaneous herpes simplex type 2 infection of the sacrum, which was unresponsive to oral and intravenous acyclovir. The lesion healed completely with intravenous foscarnet therapy, which is active against acyclovir-resistant strains of HSV.

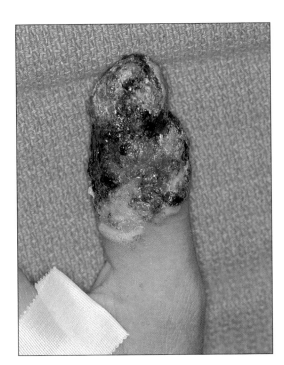

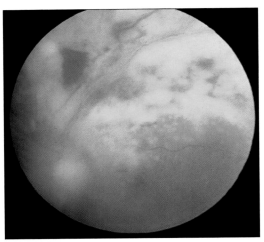

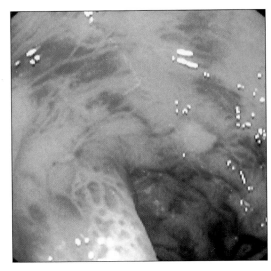

FIGURE 14-2 Herpetic whitlow of the thumb. Herpetic lesions occasionally can occur on nonorogenital sites. Herpetic whitlow probably is spread through digital contact with either HSV-infected body secretions or active HSV lesions. Lesions on the digits can be recurrent as in the orogenital locations. This patient developed herpetic whitlow due to acyclovir-resistant herpes simplex following an injury to his thumb. This was the first reported case of acyclovir-resistant HSV disease in a patient with AIDS. (Fife KH, Norris SA, Kessler HA: Severe, progressive herpetic whitlow caused by an acyclovir-resistant virus in a patient with AIDS. *J Infect Dis* 1988, 157:209–210.

FIGURE 14-3 Cytomegalovirus retinitis. Cytomegalovirus (CMV) disease occurs in approximately 20% of CMV-infected AIDS patients per year, with the most common target organ for reactivation of CMV disease being the retina. Cytomegalovirus retinitis has a very characteristic appearance, as demonstrated in this figure. Inflammatory sheathing of retinal blood vessels and associated hemorrhage are pathognomonic of the disease.

FIGURE 14-4 Cytomegalovirus colitis. CMV involvement of the gastrointestinal tract is the second most common target organ for CMV disease in patients with AIDS. The colonoscopic appearance of CMV colitis is shown in this figure. The appearance may be nonspecific, with multiple superficial hemorrhages and ulcerations of the mucosa. Biopsy is necessary to confirm the diagnosis. (*Courtesy of* John Schaffner, MD.)

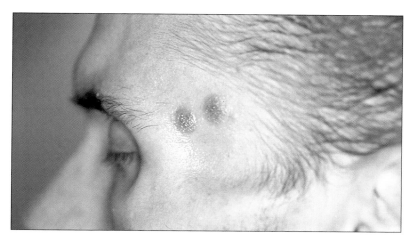

FIGURE 14-5 Cytomegalovirus skin lesions. CMV disease in patients with AIDS most commonly affects the retina, gastrointestinal tract, and nervous system. It less commonly manifests as a variety of skin lesions. This patient had two papular, inflammatory skin lesions documented on biopsy to be caused by disseminated CMV infection. The patient also had CMV retinitis and colitis. (*Courtesy of* Joel Spear, MD.)

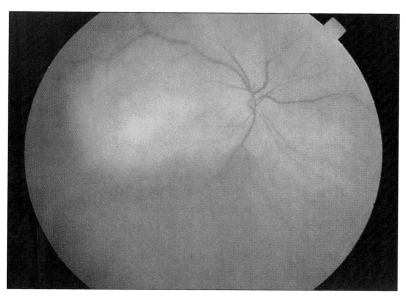

FIGURE 14-6 Acute retinal necrosis syndrome due to varicella-zoster virus. Varicella-zoster (herpes zoster) virus infections are more common in patients with HIV infection under 50 years of age than in similar age-matched persons from the general population. Acute herpes zoster in a patient under age 50 is recommended by some experts to be an indication for testing for HIV infection, in the absence of other causes of immune suppression. Herpes zoster usually presents as a typical dermatomal rash but can occasionally affect the eye. The acute retinal necrosis syndrome due to varicella-zoster virus has been reported in patients with AIDS and is a devastating infection frequently resulting in loss of vision. This patient presented with a complete retinal detachment with minimal vasculitis of the right fundus due to acute retinal necrosis; the central aspect of the macula is whitened. (*From* Hellinger WC, Bolling JP, Smith TF, Campbell RJ: Varicella-zoster virus retinitis in a patient with AIDS-related complex: Case report and brief review of the acute retinal necrosis syndrome. *Clin Infect Dis* 1993, 16:208–212; with permission of the University of Chicago.)

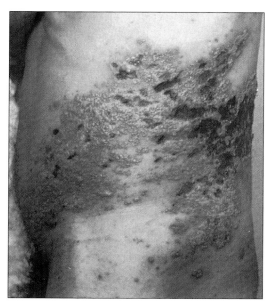

FIGURE 14-7 Disseminated herpes zoster. Multidermatomal herpes zoster in a patient with HIV infection is considered to be an AIDS-defining event. This patient has herpes zoster infection involving the left L1–L3 dermatomes with additional lesions scattered over the remainder of the body indicative of disseminated disease. (*From* Cohen PR, Beltrani VP, Grossman ME: Disseminated herpes zoster in patients with human immunodeficiency virus infection. *Am J Med* 1988, 84:1076–1080; with permission.)

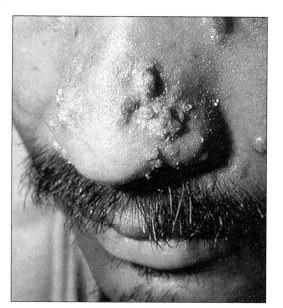

FIGURE 14-8 Acyclovir-resistant herpes zoster. Herpes zoster can become resistant to acyclovir due to mutation to a thymidine kinase–negative state, similar to that described for herpes simplex. This patient had recurrent herpes zoster lesions unresponsive to high-dose acyclovir. Herpes zoster virus was isolated from one of the hyperkeratotic papules and was shown to be acyclovir-resistant due to decreased thymidine kinase function. (*From* Jacobson MA, Berger TG, Fikrig S, *et al.*: Acyclovir-resistant varicella zoster virus infection after chronic oral acyclovir therapy in patients with the acquired immunodeficiency syndrome (AIDS). *Ann Intern Med* 1990, 112:187–191; with permission.)

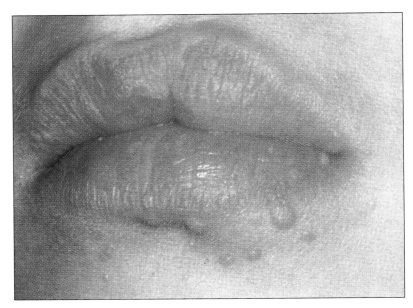

FIGURE 14-9 Common warts. Common warts due to papillomavirus infection occur with increased frequency in patients with HIV infection. The face is a common location in these patients. The oral cavity can also be involved.

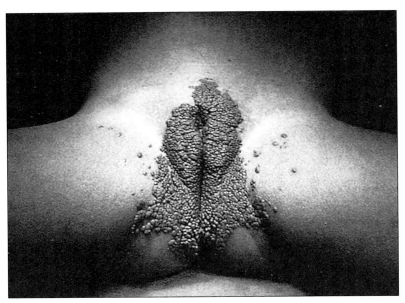

FIGURE 14-10 Anogenital warts. Exuberant anogenital papillomavirus infection in 33-month-old black girl with AIDS-related complex was refractory to topical podophyllum, fluorouracil, and recombinant interferon-α. (*From* Laraque D: Severe anogenital warts in a child with HIV infection [letter]. *N Engl J Med* 1989, 320:1220–1221; with permission.)

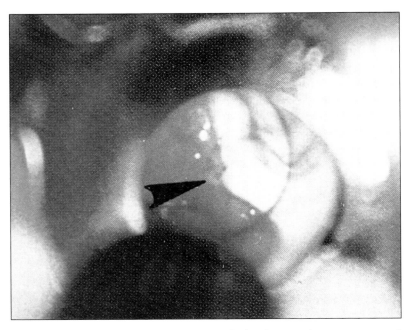

FIGURE 14-11 Anal intraepithelial neoplasia. Anoscopic appearance of anal intraepithelial neoplasia at the anorectal junction (*arrow*) in a man with symptomatic HIV disease. This lesion is well-circumscribed, raised, and leukoplakic. Infection with human papillomavirus types 16/18 and 31/33/35 is frequently associated with this neoplasia. (*From* Palefsky JM, Gonzales J, Greenblatt RM, *et al.*: Anal intraepithelial neoplasia and anal papillomavirus infection among homosexual males with group IV HIV disease. *JAMA* 1990, 263:2911–2916; with permission of the American Medical Association.)

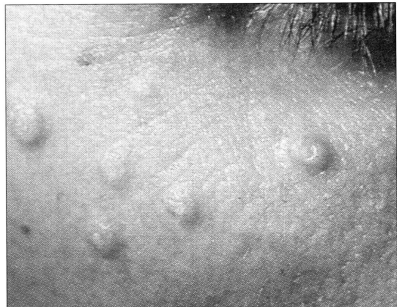

FIGURE 14-12 Molluscum contagiosum. Molluscum contagiosum is common in patients with advanced HIV disease, occurring in 8% to 15% of patients with AIDS. The face, as shown in this slide, and anogenital areas are most commonly involved. The lesions characteristically are waxy, flesh-colored, umbilicated papules. (*From* Cockerell CJ: Human immunodeficiency virus infection and the skin: A crucial interface. *Arch Intern Med* 1991, 151:1295–1303; with permission of the American Medical Association.)

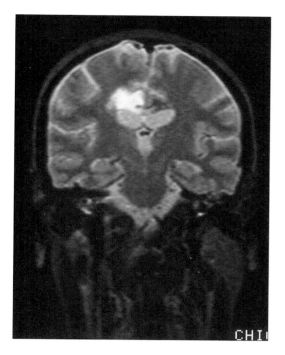

FIGURE 14-13 Progressive multifocal leukoencephalopathy (PML). PML is a rapidly progressive demyelinating disease causing mental abnormalities, aphasias, hemiparesis, and other focal signs. Magnetic resonance imaging (MRI) shows high signal intensity in the right high convexity area just adjacent to the midline. The lesion was enhancing following infusion of gadolinium. Brain biopsy revealed JC virus infection by *in situ* hybridization.

BACTERIAL INFECTIONS

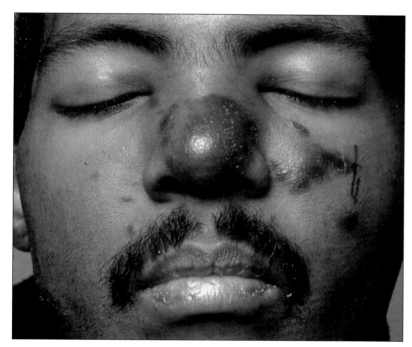

FIGURE 14-14 Epithelioid angiomatosis (cat-scratch disease) caused by *Rochalimaea henselae* or *quintana* involving the tip of the nose. The lesions may resemble those of Kaposi's sarcoma, which is also present in this patient, involving the left cheek. A biopsy specimen of the nasal lesion was positive for bacteria with the Warthin-Starry stain.

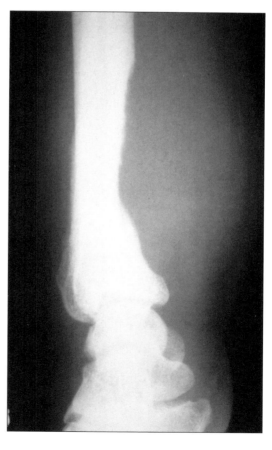

FIGURE 14-15
Disseminated cat-scratch disease. In this patient, disseminated disease involves the distal right radius, which presented as a painful right wrist mass. This radiograph shows a bony defect, which on computed tomography (CT) showed a destructive mass. (*From* Koehler JE, LeBoit PE, Egbert BM, Berger TG: Cutaneous vascular lesions and disseminated cat-scratch disease in patients with the acquired immunodeficiency syndrome (AIDS) and AIDS-related complex. *Ann Intern Med* 1988, 109: 449–455; with permission.)

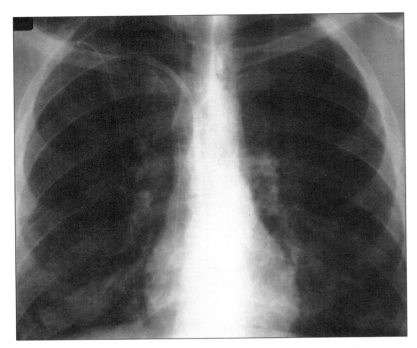

FIGURE 14-16 Hematogenous interstitial bacterial pneumonia. Patients with AIDS who require permanent-type indwelling intravenous catheter access are at increased risk of catheter-related sepsis complications. This patient developed a *Staphylococcus epidermidis* bacteremia in association with a Hickman catheter, which resulted in a bilateral lower-lobe hematogenous interstitial pneumonia.

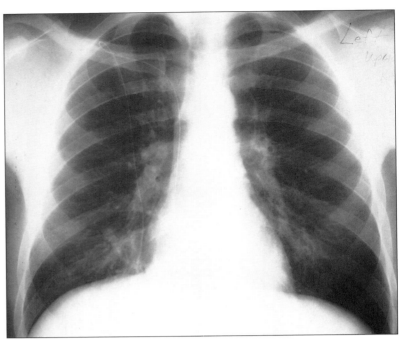

FIGURE 14-17 *Nocardia asteroides* pneumonia. Pneumonia due to *N. asteroides* has been infrequently reported in patients with AIDS. The clinical presentation in these patients has been variable. Therapy for these pneumonias may require a prolonged course of antibiotics. This patient, with a recurrent right lower lobe pneumonia due to *N. asteroides*, responded to repeated 14-day courses of third-generation cephalosporins only to relapse in the same area. Six weeks of minocycline therapy was curative.

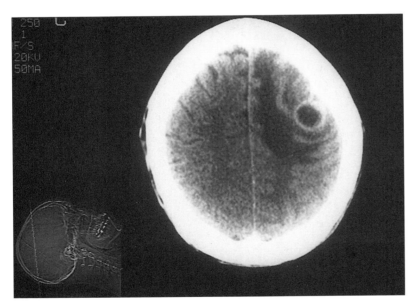

FIGURE 14-18 Brain abscess. A CT scan with infusion of the brain shows two ring-enhancing lesions in a patient presenting with seizures and right-arm paralysis. The patient also developed interstitial infiltrates, which responded to empiric trimethoprim/sulfamethoxazole therapy. *Nocardia asteroides* and *Cryptococcus neoformans* were subsequently isolated from a brain biopsy specimen. (Courtesy of D. Hines, MD.)

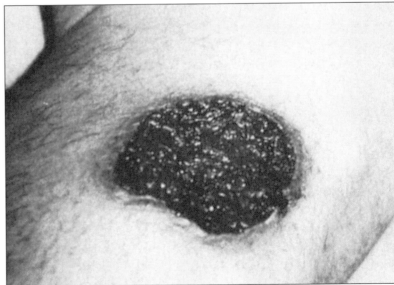

FIGURE 14-19 Chancroid. Atypical presentations of common bacterial infections are not unusual in patients with advanced HIV disease. Chancroid (*Haemophilus ducreyi*) usually occurs on the genitalia and perianal areas, with extragenital disease being rare. The cutaneous right leg ulcer in this patient with advanced HIV disease was due to chancroid. The lesion had a granulating base and undermined margins and was extremely tender. (*From* Quale J, Teplitz E, Augenbraun M: Atypical presentation of chancroid in a patient infected with the human immunodeficiency virus. *Am J Med* 1990, 88:5-43N–5-44N; with permission.)

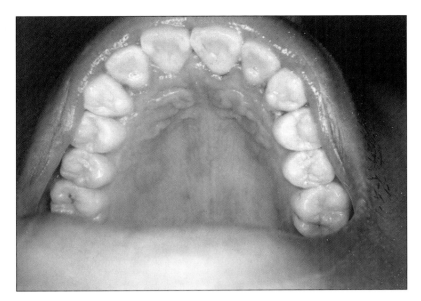

FIGURE 14-20 Recurrent secondary syphilis. An increase in the number of new cases of syphilis has been noted coincident with the AIDS epidemic. Syphilis is considered to be an important cofactor in the transmission of HIV infection, presumably due to the occurrence of chancres in primary syphilis. Other sexually transmitted diseases that cause ulcerative lesions of the genital tract, such as herpes simplex and chancroid, also have been implicated as transmission cofactors. In some cases, the symptoms of secondary syphilis and the acute retroviral syndrome of primary HIV infection can mimic one another. Treatment of the various stages of syphilis in the HIV-infected patient is similar to that in HIV-uninfected patients. HIV-infected patients may have a higher relapse rate after treatment of syphilis than noninfected patients, although this is hard to differentiate from reinfection. In this patient, mucous patches of secondary syphilis are seen on the hard palate; the patient had HIV infection and had been treated for secondary syphilis in the previous 12 months. He had continued to have high-risk sexual exposures, which made the differentiation of relapse from reinfection difficult.

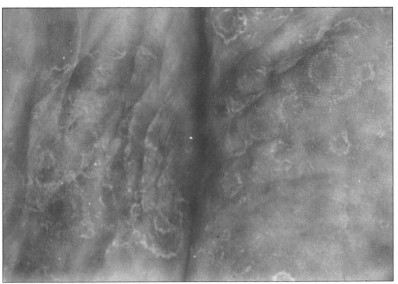

FIGURE 14-21 Secondary syphilis. The symptoms of secondary syphilis and the acute retroviral syndrome may be difficult to differentiate from each other. Both syndromes can present with fever, lymphadenopathy, mucous membrane involvement, and skin rashes. This patient recently had been diagnosed with HIV infection when he presented with fever, lymphadenopathy, hepatomegaly, liver function abnormalities, and hyperkeratotic plaques on the soles of his feet, as demonstrated on this slide. Serologic testing for syphilis showed an RPR of 1:128, consistent with secondary syphilis. Treatment with penicillin resulted in rapid clearing of the skin lesions and all associated symptoms and signs.

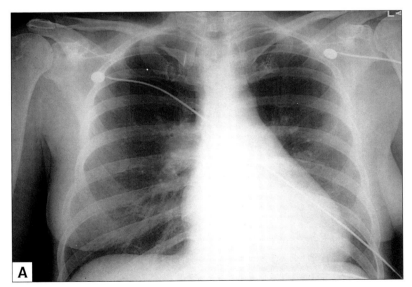

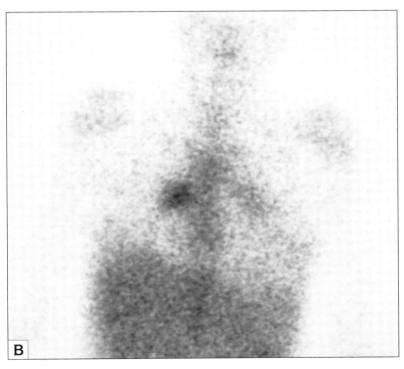

FIGURE 14-22 Disseminated *Mycobacterium kansasii* infection. **A.** In this patient, disseminated *M. kansasii* infection presented as a pericardial effusion with fever and syncope. **B.** Gallium-67 scan of the patient demonstrates coalescing, moderately intense lesions at the pulmonary hila bilaterally. *(continued)*

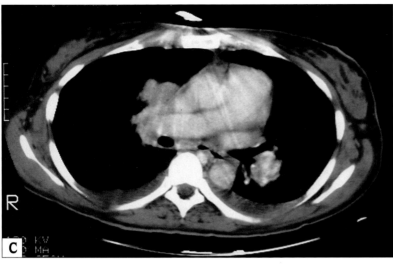

FIGURE 14-22 *(continued)* **C.** A chest CT scan shows a 3-cm x 3-cm soft tissue mass in the left hilar region and a 2.5-cm x 3-cm mass within the right mediastinum in the perihilar region. Needle aspiration showed numerous acid-fast organisms.

FIGURE 14-23 Cutaneous *Mycobacterium kansasii* infection affecting the lower extremity in association with disseminated disease. The ulcerating nodules are nonspecific and require biopsy and culture for diagnosis. (*From* Cockerell CJ: Human immunodeficiency virus infection and the skin: A crucial interface. *Arch Intern Med* 1991, 151:1295–1303; with permission of the American Medical Association.)

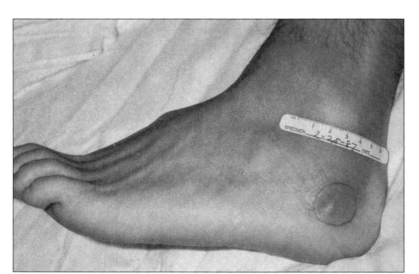

FIGURE 14-24 Disseminated *Mycobacterium haemophilum* infection. A 3-cm × 3-cm subcutaneous abscess developed below the left lateral malleolus, an aspirate of which showed numerous neutrophils and acid-fast bacilli. (*From* Rogers PL, Walker RE, Lane HC, *et al.*: Disseminated *Mycobacterium haemophilum* infection in two patients with the acquired immunodeficiency syndrome. *Am J Med* 1988, 84:640–642; with permission.)

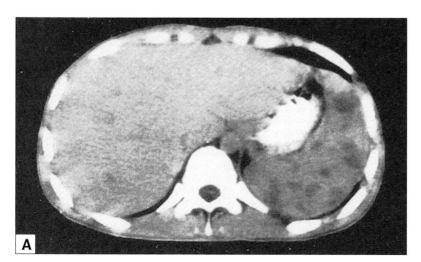

FIGURE 14-25 Extrapulmonary *Mycobacterium tuberculosis* infection affecting the spleen. **A.** Multiple hypodense nodules in an enlarged spleen and mesenteric lymphadenopathy are seen on an abdominal CT scan. (*From* Pedro-Botet J, Maristany MT, Miralles R, *et al.*: Splenic tuberculosis in patients with AIDS. *Rev Infect Dis* 1991, 13:1069-1071; with permission of the University of Chicago.)

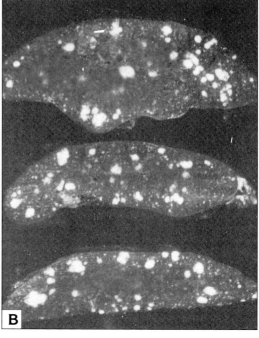

B. Gross pathologic appearance of *M. tuberculosis* abscesses. Longitudinal sections of the spleen demonstrate multiple, whitish nodules of soft caseous material strongly positive for acid-fast bacilli. (*From* Wolff MJ, Bitran J, Northland RG, Levy IL: Splenic abscesses due to *Mycobacterium tuberculosis* in patients with AIDS. *Rev Infect Dis* 1991, 13:373–375; with permission of the University of Chicago.)

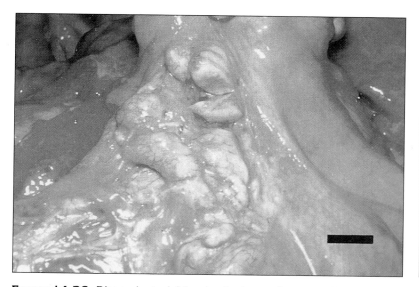

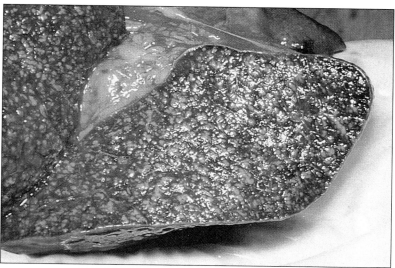

FIGURE 14-26 Disseminated *Mycobacterium avium* complex infection affecting the mesenteric lymph nodes. Gross pathologic appearance of the lymph nodes shows the characteristic yellow pigmentation (*bar* = 2 cm). (*From* Horsburgh CR Jr: *Mycobacterium avium* complex infection in the acquired immunodeficiency syndrome. *N Engl J Med* 1991, 324:1332–1337; with permission.)

FIGURE 14-27 Disseminated *Mycobacterium avium* complex infection with extensive granulomatous infiltration of the liver, as seen on gross pathologic section. (*From* Horsburgh CR Jr: *Mycobacterium avium* complex infection in the acquired immuno-deficiency syndrome. *N Engl J Med* 1991, 324:1332–1337; with permission.)

FUNGAL INFECTIONS

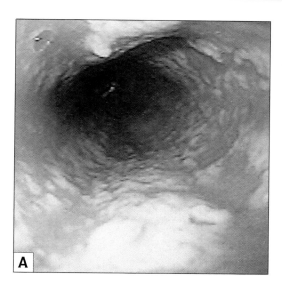

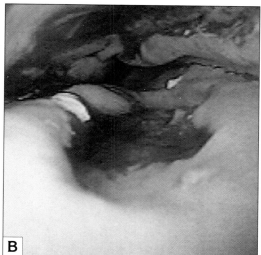

FIGURE 14-28 Invasive candida esophagitis. *Candida* is the most common opportunistic fungal pathogen affecting people with advancing HIV infection. Essentially 100% of patients with AIDS will have had some clinical manifestation of mucosal candida infection during the course of their illness. The upper gastrointestinal tract and anogenital areas are the most commonly involved. Candida esophagitis has been the most common initial AIDS-defining illness in at least two cohorts of HIV-infected women, which suggests that hormone differences may play a role in the risk of invasive disease. Involvement of the esophagus is the most common form of invasive candidal infection in patients with AIDS. **A.** The typical endoscopic appearance of candida esophagitis is shown, presenting as superficial white plaques on the mucosa. (*Courtesy of* John Schaffner, MD.) **B.** Candida involvement of the esophageal mucosa in patients with advanced HIV infection can result in either superficially invasive disease or deep discrete ulcers. In this patient, who presented with fever and odynophagia, a large deep esophageal ulcer due to *Candida* was seen endoscopically. (*Courtesy of* John Schaffner, MD.)

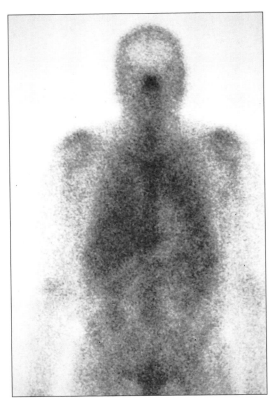

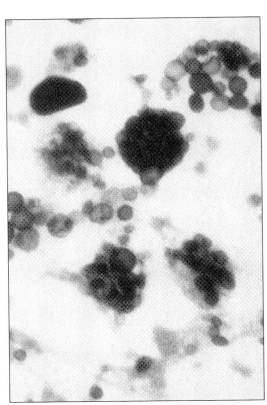

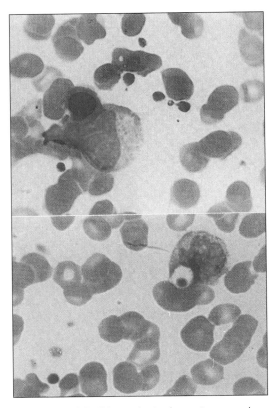

FIGURE 14-29 Disseminated *Histoplasma capsulatum* infection. A gallium-67 scan of a patient with disseminated *H. capsulatum* infection presenting as a fever of unknown origin demonstrates intense uptake throughout both lungs. The chest radiograph was without infiltrates. Blood cultures and bronchoalveolar lavage fluid were positive for *H. capsulatum*.

FIGURE 14-30 *Histoplasma capsulatum* in a bronchoalveolar lavage specimen. Abundant intracellular forms of *H. capsulatum* in alveolar macrophages are demonstrated by Gomori's methenamine stain. ($\times$ 75.) (*From* Pottage JC Jr, Sha BE: Development of histoplasmosis in a human immunodeficiency virus–infected patient receiving fluconazole [letter]. *J Infect Dis* 1991, 164:622–623; with permission of the University of Chicago.)

FIGURE 14-31 Disseminated cryptococcosis. The diagnosis is made by demonstration of budding and encapsulated yeast forms 4–8 μm in diameter on a peripheral blood smear. The *lower panel* shows a well-demarcated capsule engulfed by a monocyte. (Wright-Giemsa stain, $\times$ 1000). (*From* Yao JDC, Arkin CF, Doweiko JP, Hammer SM: Disseminated cryptococcosis diagnosed on peripheral blood smear in a patient with acquired immunodeficiency syndrome. *Am J Med* 1990, 89:100–102; with permission.)

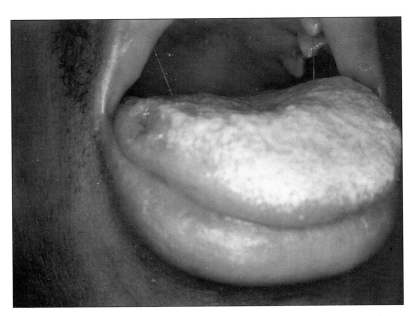

FIGURE 14-32 Oral lesions of disseminated *Histoplasma capsulatum* infection. Disseminated *H. capsulatum* infection can present as discrete painful ulcers of the upper gastrointestinal tract mucosa, particularly on the tongue and buccal mucosa. This patient presented with fever and a painful ulcer on the lateral margin of the tongue. Biopsy of the lesion showed yeast forms compatible with histoplasmosis, and cultures grew *H. capsulatum*.

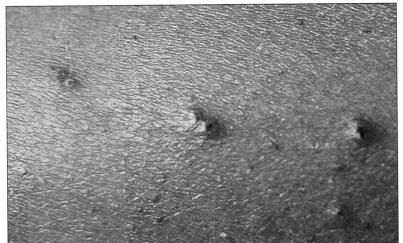

FIGURE 14-33 Cutaneous cryptococcosis presenting as waxy, translucent, umbilicated papules. The cutaneous lesions of cryptococcosis are usually nondescript and require biopsy and culture to establish the diagnosis.

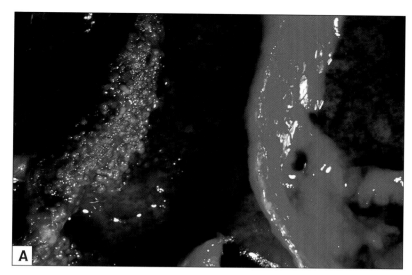

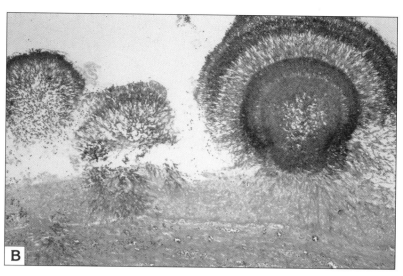

FIGURE 14-34 Necrotizing superficial tracheobronchitis due to *Aspergillus fumigatus*. Invasive *A. fumigatus* disease is being reported with increased frequency in patients with far-advanced end-stage AIDS. As in other patients at risk of this opportunistic fungal pathogen, the tracheobronchial tree is a common target organ. Invasive disease can result in invasion and thrombosis of blood vessels by *Aspergillus* hyphae with resultant infarction of surrounding tissue. In addition, a necrotizing superficial tracheo-bronchitis can occur. **A**, A gross pathologic specimen of the distal trachea showing necrotizing superficial tracheobronchitis due to *A. fumigatus*. The mucosa is diffusely studded with masses of organisms, which resulted in complete obstruction of the trachea and subsequent asphyxiation. (*Courtesy of* John Dainauskas, MD.) **B**, Histologic section with hematoxylin-eosin stain shows numerous conidial heads emanating from the necrotic superficial mucosa of the trachea. (*Courtesy of* John Dainauskas, MD.)

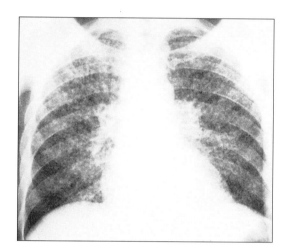

FIGURE 14-35 Coccidioidomycosis. *Coccidioides immitis* infection presented with cough, fever, night sweats, weight loss, and a diffuse reticulonodular infiltrate on the chest radiograph. The presence of diffuse bilateral reticulonodular or nodular infiltrates is one of the most consistent findings in patients with AIDS and coccidioidomycosis. (*From* Bronnimann DA, Adam RD, Galgiani JN, *et al.*: Coccidioidomycosis in the acquired immunodeficiency syndrome. *Ann Intern Med* 1987, 106:372–379; with permission.)

PROTOZOAN INFECTIONS

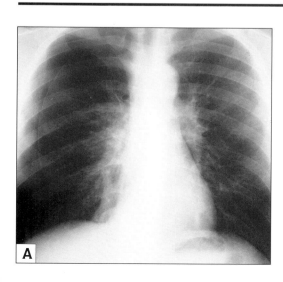

FIGURE 14-36 Disseminated *Pneumocystis carinii* infection. *P. carinii* has been the most common opportunistic pulmonary pathogen associated with AIDS. Infection outside the lungs has been reported most commonly in association with aerosolized pentamidine prophylaxis, presumably due to the uneven distribution of the aerosolized pentamidine in the lungs, which allows pneumocystis to persist in the upper lung fields and become invasive. **A**, Disseminated *P. carinii* infection can affect almost any organ. The patient in this slide presented with a fever of unknown origin, and on chest radiography, bilateral hilar adenopathy was noted. This was the only pulmonary manifestation of subsequently proven disseminated pneumocystis infection. The patient had been treated with aerosolized pentamidine therapy for secondary prophylaxis of *P. carinii* pneumonia. *(continued)*

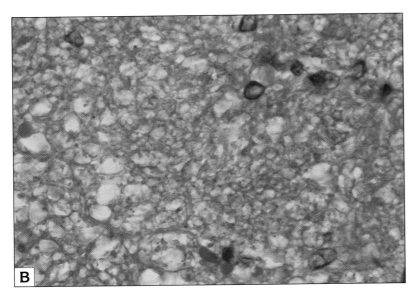

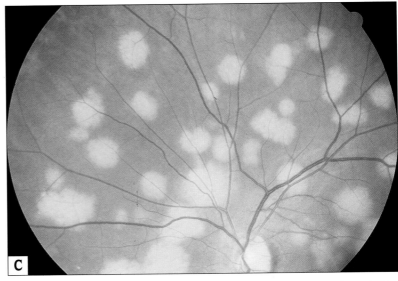

FIGURE 14-36 *(continued)* **B,** A mediastinal lymph node biopsy specimen from this patient demonstrated cysts of *P. carinii,* which established the diagnosis of disseminated pneumocystis infection. **C,** A retinal photograph of the patient shows choroiditis typical of disseminated *P. carinii* infection. The lesions appear as discrete yellow- ish-white exudates, which are differentiated from the chorioretinitis of cytomegalovirus by the lack of involvement of retinal blood vessels. These lesions are deep to the retina, and therefore the retinal vessels appear to run through the lesions.

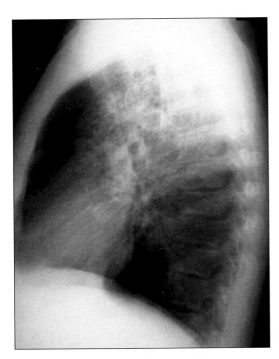

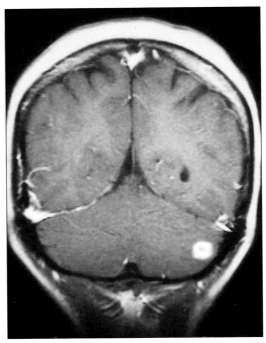

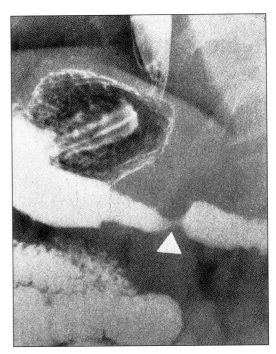

FIGURE 14-37 Bilateral upper-lobe *Pneumocystis carinii* infection. Aerosolized pentamidine prophylaxis for *P. carinii* pneumonia results in uneven distribution of the drug in the dependent portions of the lungs due to the effects of gravity. Thus, the upper lung fields are at increased risk of primary or recurrent *P. carinii* pneumonia. This patient, who presented with bilateral upper-lobe pneumonia due to *P. carinii,* had been on secondary prophylaxis with aerosolized pentamidine.

FIGURE 14-38 *Toxoplasma* encephalitis. Acute toxoplasmic encephalitis presented as fever and headache in a 36-year-old Hispanic woman who had antibodies to *Toxoplasma gondii.* Magnetic resonance imaging (MRI) demonstrated a single left cerebellar lesion, which completely resolved after several months of clindamycin and pyrimethamine therapy. Approximately 10% of patients with toxoplasmic encephalitis have solitary brain lesions visualized by MRI, as compared with the more usual appearance of multiple ring-enhancing lesions.

FIGURE 14-39 Cryptosporidiosis. The patient presented with diarrhea, dehydration, weight loss, nausea, and postprandial vomiting. An upper gastrointestinal tract radiograph following ingestion of contrast medium revealed a 4-cm-long, irregular, narrowed segment in the antrum proximal to the pylorus. A biopsy specimen of the lesion showed mild, chronic, active gastritis with several *Cryptosporidium* organisms seen. (*From* Cersosimo E, Wilkowske CJ, Rosenblatt JE, Ludwig J: Isolated antral narrowing associated with gastrointestinal cryptosporidiosis in acquired immunodeficiency syndrome. *Mayo Clin Proc* 1992, 67:553–556; with permission.)

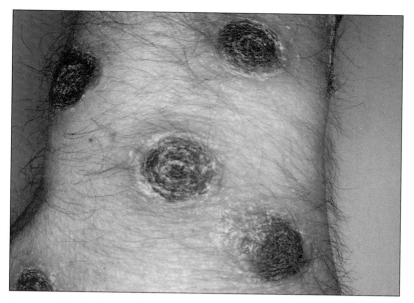

FIGURE 14-40 Disseminated *Acanthamoeba* infection. The infection presented as multiple painful papulonodular lesions, which progressed to necrotic indurated ulcers with surrounding erythema. The patient also had involvement of the sinuses and long bones of the distal extremities.

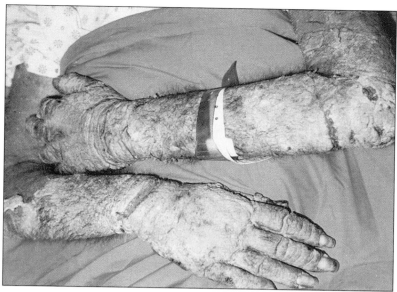

FIGURE 14-41 Norwegian scabies seen as the presenting manifestation of AIDS. The lesions covered the entire body and were characterized by severe thickening, cracking, and peeling of the skin. (*From* Hulbert TV, Larsen RA: Hyperkeratotic (Norwegian) scabies with gram-negative bacteremia as the initial presentation of AIDS. *Clin Infect Dis* 1992, 14:1164–1165; with permission of the University of Chicago.)

SELECTED BIBLIOGRAPHY

Chiasson RE, Volberding PA: Clinical manifestations of HIV infection. *In* Mandell GL, Douglas RG Jr, Bennett JE (eds): *Principles and Practice of Infectious Disease*; 3rd ed. New York: Churchill Livingstone; 1990:1059–1091.

Kessler HA, Bick JA, Pottage JP, Benson CA: AIDS: P II. *DM* 1992, 10:695–794.

Masur H: Problems in the management of opportunistic infections in patients infected with human immunodeficiency virus. *J Infect Dis* 1990, 161:858–864.

Gradon JD, Timpone JG, Schnittman SM: Emergence of unusual opportunistic pathogens in AIDS: A review. *Clin Infect Dis* 1992, 15:134–157.

Drew WL, Buhles W, Erlich KS: Management of herpes virus infections (CMV, HSV, VZV). *In* Sande MA, Volberding PA (eds): *The Medical Management of AIDS*; 3rd ed. Philadelphia: W.B. Saunders; 1992:359–382.

CHAPTER 15

Treatment and Prophylaxis of Opportunistic Infections

Judith Feinberg

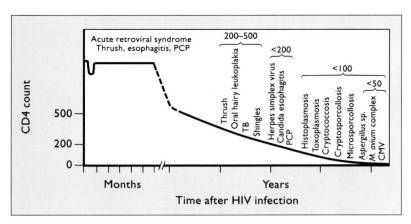

FIGURE 15-1 Opportunistic infections in HIV disease. The appearance of opportunistic infections in the course of HIV disease is primarily a function of declining CD4+ cell counts. The spectrum of opportunistic infections, however, is also dependent on the prevalence of a given infection in a given area, with an increased prevalence of some diseases being seen in hyperendemic areas, such as histoplasmosis in the Ohio and Mississippi River valleys, coccidioidomycosis in the southwest, and tuberculosis in New York City. Because of improved survival and increased use of primary prophylaxis, many opportunistic infections seem to be appearing at lower CD4+ counts now than they did in the mid-1980s. Because the immunosuppression of AIDS is chronic and progressive, lifelong suppressive therapy is generally required once a patient has had a serious opportunistic infection.

PNEUMOCYSTIS CARINII PNEUMONIA

Treatment of Acute Infection

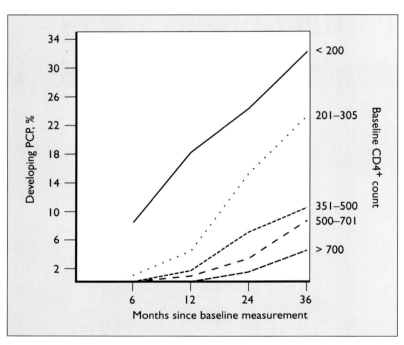

FIGURE 15-2 Risk of *Pneumocystis carinii* pneumonia (PCP) as a function of initial CD4+ count. Retrospective and prospective studies have verified that the risk of developing PCP is a function of the patient's CD4+ lymphocyte count. Over 90% of episodes occur when the total CD4+ counts are < 200 cells/mL, with most patients having counts in the range of 50 to 75 cells/mm3 when they are first diagnosed with PCP. Without prophylaxis, the risk of developing PCP is 8.4% at 6 months, 18.4% at 12 months, and 33.3% at 36 months for patients with an initial CD4+ lymphocyte count < 200 cells/mm3. (Phair J, Muñoz A, Detels R, *et al.*: The risk of *Pneumocystis carinii* pneumonia among men infected with human immunodeficiency virus type 1. *N Engl J Med* 1990, 322:161–165. Hoover DR, Saah AJ, Baceller H, *et al.*: Clinical manifestations of AIDS in the era of pneumocystis prophylaxis: Multicenter AIDS Cohort Study. *N Engl J Med* 1993, 329:1922–1926.)

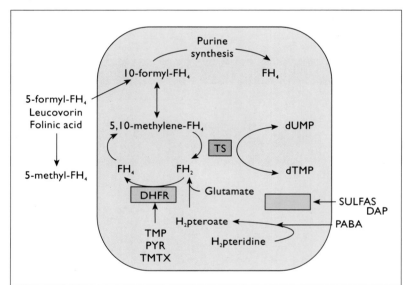

FIGURE 15-3 Intracellular folate metabolism. Inhibition of folate metabolism is a key strategy for the treatment of PCP and toxoplasmosis. Folates are an important cofactor in the biosynthesis of purines and deoxythymidine monophosphate (dTMP), which are essential components in nucleic acid synthesis, including both RNA and DNA synthesis. Rapidly dividing cells of infectious organisms are especially vulnerable to folate inhibition, which antifolate drugs accomplish by interfering at two steps in the metabolic cycle. Trimethoprim (TMP), pyrimethamine (PYR), and trimetrexate (TMTX) all inhibit the enzyme dihydrofolate reductase (DHFR), which is essential in recycling the various intracellular forms of folate. Leucovorin (folinic acid), given as an adjunct to therapy, can circumvent this blockade by providing an extracellular source of folate useful to human cells but not to pneumocystis or toxoplasma organisms, thus minimizing the adverse effects to the host. In the second pathway, sulfa drugs, such as sulfamethoxazole and sulfadiazine, and sulfones, such as dapsone (DAP), inhibit the enzyme dihydropteroate synthesis (DHPS), which incorporates *para*-aminobenzoid acid (PABA) into folic acid. (TS—thymidine synthetase.)

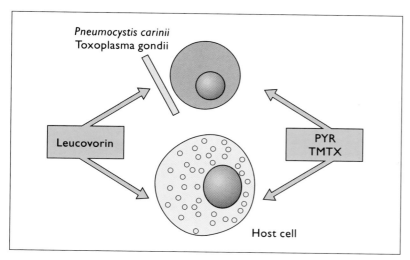

FIGURE 15-4 Leucovorin protection. The more potent DHFR inhibitors, such as pyrimethamine (PYR) and trimetrexate (TMTX), by interfering in folate metabolism, inhibit the rapid growth and division of infecting microorganisms but also host cells with high rates of division, such as bone marrow stem cells. The resulting bone marrow toxicity can be usually alleviated by concomitant administration of leucovorin. The DHFR inhibitors enter both the microorganism (*P. carinii* or *Toxoplasma gondii*) and host cells, but mammalian cells have an active transport system for uptake of extracellular folate (leucovorin, folinic acid), which is lacking in many microorganisms. Therefore, host cells can use leucovorin to bypass the antifolate effect of the DHFR inhibitors , but *P. carinii* and *T. gondii*, which synthesize *de novo*, cannot. Trimethoprim is a considerably less potent DHRF inhibitor than pyrimethamine and trimetrexate and does not require concurrent leucovorin administration.

A. Standard treatment for acute PCP

Trimethoprim/sulfamethoxazole: 15–20 mg/kg/d of TMP component IV or orally in 3–4 divided doses
Pentamidine: 4 mg/kg/d as a single IV dose
Duration: 21 days
Treatment-limiting toxicity is common to both

B. Drug-associated adverse effects of TMP/SMX vs pentamidine

	TMP-SMX, %	Pentamidine, %
Fever (> 37° C)	78	82
Hypotension	0	27
Nausea, vomiting	25	24
Rash	44	15
Anemia	39	24
Leukopenia	72	47
Thrombocytopenia	3	18
Azotemia	14	64
Alanine aminotransferase	22	15
Alkaline phosphatase	11	18
Hypoglycemia	0	21
Hypocalcemia	0	3

FIGURE 15-5 A, Standard treatment for acute PCP. Trimethoprim/sulfamethoxazole (TMP/SMX, co-trimoxazole; oral or parenteral) and pentamidine (parenteral) are the mainstays of treatment for acute PCP. TMP/SMX acts by providing sequential blockage of folate metabolism, with TMP inhibiting the DHFR enzyme and SMX blocking the DHPS enzyme. In recent studies, TMP/SMX is effective (as measured by survival) in up to 99% of patients with mild to moderate disease and in up to 84% with a moderately severe episode; unfortunately, a significant proportion of patients (30% to 50%) experience dose-limiting toxicity. Pentamidine is generally reserved for patients who cannot tolerate or do not respond to TMP/SMX. Some investigators advocate a lower dose of pentamidine, 3 mg/kg/d, as effective and less toxic. (Conte JE Jr, Hollander H, Golden JA: Inhaled or reduced-dose intravenous pentamidine for *Pneumocystis carinii* pneumonia: A pilot study. *Ann Intern Med* 1987, 107:495–498.) Pentamidine must be given as a slow infusion over 1 hour to avoid hypotension; intramuscular administration can cause painful sterile abscesses. Treatment-limiting toxicity is common with both agents. Unlike other immunocompromised patients, AIDS patients require a longer duration of therapy to be effectively treated, 21

days rather than 14. (Kovacs JA, Hiementz JW, Macher AM, *et al.*:*Pneumocystis carinii* pneumonia: A comparison between patients with the acquired immunodeficiency syndrome and patients with other immunodeficiencies. *Ann Intern Med* 1984, 100:633–641.) **B**, Drug-related toxicities of TMP/SMX and pentamidine. Toxicity is rarely life-threatening; one approach may be dosage reduction and aggressive supportive care, as described by Sattler *et al.* They found that rash and fever subsided with continued therapy, lasting on average 2 to 7 days, and could be made tolerable with acetaminophen or diphenhydramine. Leukopenia and thrombocytopenia were the most serious adverse affects associated with TMP/SMX and appeared to be dosage-dependent. The potentially serious reactions of nephrotoxicity, hypotension, and hypoglycemia occured more often with pentamidine and may relate to blood and tissue concentrations of this agent. The length of treatment did not appear to increase the frequency of adverse effects. (Sattler FR, Cowan R, Nielsen DM, Ruskin J: Trimethoprim-sulfamethoxazole compared with pentamidine for treatment of *Pneumocystis carinii* pneumonia in the acquired immunodeficiency syndrome: A prospective, noncrossover study. *Ann Intern Med* 1988, 109:280–287.)

Should pentamidine remain second drug of choice?

Prospective, randomized, noncrossover study
    Pentamidine (61% survival)
    T/S (86% survival)
Sequential blockade of folate metabolism may be best current
    model for treatment of PCP
      DMFR
        Trimethoprim
        Trimethoprim
        Trimetrexate (?)
      DHPS
        Sulfamethoxazole
        Dapsone
        Dapsone (?)

FIGURE 15-6 Should pentamidine be the second drug of choice? TMP/SMX remains the treatment of choice for acute PCP, with pentamidine generally reserved for those patients who cannot tolerate or who do not respond to TMP/SMX. However, there are limited data available that permit direct comparison of these agents, with most data being from retrospective or crossover studies. In the one prospective, randomized study that did not permit crossover between the two arms, survival for TMP/SMX recipients was 86% as compared with 61% for the pentamidine group ($P < 0.05$). (Sattler FR, Cowan R, Nielsen DM, Ruskin J: Trimethoprim–sulfamethoxazole compared with pentamidine for treatment of *Pneumocystis carinii* pneumonia in the acquired immunodeficiency syndrome: A prospective, noncrossover study. *Ann Intern Med* 1988, 109:280–287.) Although newer therapies (single agents or combinations) cause less treatment-limiting toxicity than TMP/SMX, none has demonstrated equivalent effectiveness in a study with adequate statistical power. At this time, the model of sequential blockade of key enzymes in the folate pathway (*eg*, as provided by TMP/SMX) offers the best approach to the treatment of acute PCP. No data are available comparing newer agents with parenteral pentamidine; therefore, its use derives largely from historical practice.

A. Adjunctive corticosteroids in antipneumocystis therapy

Indicated in patients with $PaO_2 < 70$ mm Hg or A–a gradient
    > 35 mm Hg on room air
Corticosteroids begun within 72 hrs of initiating PCP treatment
    improve clinical outcome and reduce mortality by 50%
No benefit shown for milder episodes or salvage therapy
Recommended approach: oral prednisone given
40 mg twice daily × 5 days, then
40 mg once daily × 5 days, then
20 mg once daily × 11 days

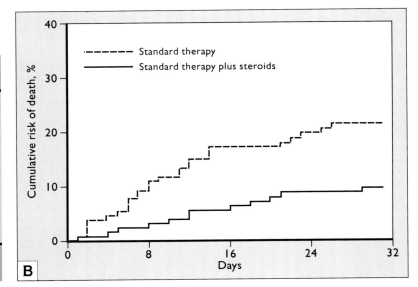

FIGURE 15-7 Adjunctive corticosteroids in antipneumocystis therapy. Survival in PCP depends primarily on the patient's level of oxygenation, with increased mortality seen in patients with significant impairment of oxygenation. To control the lung inflammation accompanying PCP, the use of corticosteroids has been proposed. Four controlled studies have demonstrated that adjunctive corticosteroids begun within 72 hours of specific antipneumocystis therapy have a significant effect on clinical outcome, including survival. **A,** The results of these studies form the basis of a National Institutes of Health–University of California consensus panel recommendation to use adjunctive corticosteroids in all AIDS patients with PCP and significant impairment of oxygenation. An arterial $PO_2 < 70$ mm Hg or an arteriolar–arterial (A–a) difference of > 35 mm Hg on room air identifies the group at highest risk for mortality from PCP and for whom adjunctive corticosteroids are indicated. Because steroids can have a detrimental effect in patients with tuberculosis, fungal pneumonia, or pulmonary Kaposi's sarcoma, caution should be exercised in these patients and vigorous attempts to confirm a diagnosis of PCP should be made rather than initiating adjunctive corticosteroids empirically. **B,** A Kaplan-Meier plot from the largest and most compelling of the four studies demonstrates a 50% improvement in survival for patients given early adjunctive prednisone as compared with standard therapy alone for moderate to severe episodes of PCP. A regimen of oral prednisone, as employed by Bozzette *et al.*, is recommended because of its ease of use and low cost; no further tapering of dosage is needed after the 20-mg dose segment is completed. (National Institutes of Health–University of California Expert Panel for Corticosteroids as Adjunctive Therapy for Pneumocystis Pneumonia: Consensus statement on the use of corticosteroids as adjunctive therapy for pneumocystis pneumonia in the acquired immunodeficiency syndrome. *N Engl J Med* 1990, 323:1500–1504. *Figure from* Bozzette SA, Sattler FR, Chiu J, *et al.*: A controlled trial of early adjunctive treatment with corticosteroids for *Pneumocystis carinii* pneumonia in the acquired immunodeficiency syndrome. *N Engl J Med* 1990, 323:1451–1457; with permission.)

Trimethoprim/dapsone vs TMP/SMX for PCP

	TMP/dapsone	TMP/SMX
Dosage	Dapsone, 100 mg/d, plus TMP, 20 mg/kg/d	TMP/SMX, 20 mg/kg/d of TMP component orally in divided doses every 6 hrs
Patients	30	30
Clinical response	28(93%)	27(90%)
Treatment-limiting toxicity	9(30%)	17(57%) (*P* < 0.025)

FIGURE 15-8 Trimethoprim/dapsone vs TMP/SMX. In a small prospective study, 60 patients were randomized to receive TMP/dapsone or TMP/SMX for mild to moderate PCP (PaO$_2$ > 60 mm Hg on room air). Although laboratory abnormalities were more common in the TMP/SMX group, clinical side effects such as intolerable rash and vomiting were similar in both groups. This trial was too small to establish whether TMP/dapsone was equivalent to TMP/SMX in terms of clinical outcome, although it suggested that TMP/dapsone was certainly worthy of further study. On the basis of this limited study, TMP/dapsone has been used widely for treatment of acute PCP. (Medina I, Mills L, Leoung G, *et al.*: Oral therapy for Pneumocystis carinii pneumonia in the acquired immunodeficiency syndrome: A controlled trial of trimethoprim-sulfamethoxazole versus trimethoprim-dapsone. *N Eng J Med* 1990, 323:776–782.)

A. Trimetrexate vs TMP/SMX for PCP: Design

Double-blind (to day 10), randomized, multicenter trial
Hospitalized patients with moderately severe PCP
 (A–a gradient > 30 mm Hg on room air)
Dosages:
 Trimetrexate, 45 mg/m^2/d IV, plus leucovorin, 20 mg/m^2
 every 6 hrs
 vs
 TMP/SMX, 20 mg/kg/wk of TMP component divided
 every 6 hrs
No adjunctive corticosteroids permitted
Goal: Survival at day 21 (end of therapy)
Assumption: Trimetrexate is at least 15% better than TMP/SMX

B. Trimetrexate vs TMP/SMX for PCP: Results

	Trimetrexate *n* = 106	TMP/SMX *n* = 109	*P* value
Lack of therapeutic efficacy			
Day 10	28(27%)	17(16%)	0.064
Day 21	38(38%)	21(20%)	0.008
Treatment-limiting toxicity			
By day 21	9(9%)	30(28%)	< 0.001
Mortality			
Day 21	20%	12%	0.088
Day 49	31%	16%	0.028

FIGURE 15-9 Trimetrexate vs TMP/SMX. Trimetrexate is a highly potent folate antagonist, with activity against pneumocystis DHFR that is 1000-fold better than that of pyrimethamine and 1500-fold better than that of trimethoprim. (Allegra CJ, Kovacs JA, Drake JC, *et al.*: Activity of antifolates against *Pneumocystis carinii* dihydrofolate reductase and identification of a potent new agent. *J Exp Med* 1987, 165:926–931.) **A,** After a pilot study that included AIDS patients treated with trimetrexate as initial or salvage treatment for PCP showed promising results (Allegra CJ, Chabner BA, Tuazon CH, *et al.*: Trimetrexate for the treatment of *Pneumocystis carinii* pneumonia in patients with acquired immunodeficiency syndrome. *N Engl J Med* 1987, 317:978–985), a comparative study in patients sick enough to require hospitalization was undertaken, as trimetrexate

must be given intravenously. Because of trimetrexate's potency as a DHFR inhibitor, leucovorin must be coadministered. Trimetrexate has a relatively long half-life (approx 11 hrs), which permits once-daily dosing. **Outcome: B,** Despite its potency as a DHFR inhibitor, trimetrexate was not shown to be superior to TMP/SMX in terms of clinical response. It was, however, considerably less toxic. Although there was no significant difference in mortality at day 21 (the primary study endpoint), there was a significant difference in favor of TMP/SMX by day 49. (Sattler FR, Frame P, Davis R, *et al.*: Comparison of trimetrexate with leucovorin versus trimethoprim-sulfamethoxazole for moderate-to-severe episodes of *Pneumocystis carinii* pneumonia in patients with AIDS. *J Infect Dis* 1994, in press.)

A. Atovaquone vs TMP/SMX for PCP: Design

Double-blind, randomized, multicenter trial
Mild (A–a gradient < 35 mm Hg) to moderate (A–a gradient 35–45 mm Hg) PCP (adjunctive corticosteroid therapy given also for moderate PCP)
Dosage: atovaquone, 750 mg orally 3 × daily with food
vs
TMP/SMX, 2 double-strength tablets orally 3 × daily with food
Goal: Proportion with mild disease who are "successfully treated"
Assumption: Atovaquone not more than 15% worse than TMP/SMX

FIGURE 15-10 Atovaquone vs TMP/SMX. Atovaquone represents a novel class of antipneumocystis agents, the hydroxynaphthoquinones. It acts by interrupting mitochondrial electron transport, an entirely new mechanism of action. In an animal model of PCP, atovaquone is the only agent to have apparent "cidal" activity (Hughes WT, Gray VL, Gutteridge WE, *et al.*: Efficacy of hydroxynaphthoquinone, 566C80, in experimental *Pneumocystis carinii*. *Antimicrob Agents Chemother* 1990, 34:225–228.) Bioavailability is limited and shows considerable variability. **A,** However, after a pilot study showed clinical activity against PCP in AIDS patients (Falloon J, Kovacs J, Hughes W, Gray VL, Gutteridge WE, *et al.*: Efficacy of hydroxynaphthoquinone, 566c80, in experimental *Pneumocystis carinii* pneumocystis. A preliminary evaluation of 566C80 for the treatment of pneumocystis pneumonia in patients with the acquired immunodeficiency syndrome. *N Engl J Med* 1991, 325:1534–1538), a definitive comparative study was undertaken. *(continued)*

B. Atovaquone vs TMP/SMX: for PCP: Results

	Atovaquone $n = 160$	TMP/SMX $n = 162$	P value
Lack of therapeutic efficacy	28(20%)	10(7%)	0.002
Treatment-limiting toxicity	11(7%)	33(20%)	0.001
"Successful therapy" (clinical response + lack of toxicity)	99(62%)	103(64%)	0.82
Mortality	11(7%)	1(0.6%)	0.003

Clindamycin/primaquine for PCP

Pilot study in previously untreated patients with mild PCP
Dosages:
    Clindamycin, 900 mg IV every 8 hrs or 450 mg orally every 8 hrs
    plus
    Primaquine, 30 mg/d
Response rate: 92% (55/60 patients showed clinical improvement by day 7)
Toxicity: rash, neutropenia
    15% (9/16 patients) discontinued due to toxicity

FIGURE 15-10 *(continued)* **Outcome**: **B**, Despite the promise of the work in the animal model, atovaquone was shown to be less effective than TMP/SMX in terms of clinical response of the PCP by day 49. It was, however, considerably less toxic. When these two aspects of treatment are combined as a single endpoint, termed *successful therapy*, the inferior response rate for atovaquone balanced against its better tolerability yields an outcome that is not more than 15% worse than that of TMP/SMX. Low plasma atovaquone levels were associated with a poorer clinical outcome; diarrhea at baseline was predictive of low drug levels and was associated with reduced effectiveness and increased mortality. (Hughes W, Leoung G, Kramer F, et al.: Comparison of atovaquone (566C80) with trimethoprim–sulfamethoxazole to treat *Pneumocystis carinii* pneumonia in patients with AIDS. *N Engl J Med* 1993, 328:1521–1527.)

FIGURE 15-11 Clindamycin/primaquine for PCP. Clindamycin/primaquine is a promising combination for the treatment of acute PCP that has found wide acceptance by clinicians, although only uncontrolled, limited data have appeared in the literature thus far. (Black JR, Feinberg J, Murphy RL, et al.: Clindamycin and primaquine therapy for mild-to-moderate episodes of *Pneumocystis carinii* pneumonia in patients with AIDS: AIDS Clinical Trials Group 044. *Clin Infect Dis* 1994, 18:905–913.) The combination has been shown to be effective in an animal model of PCP, but the mechanism of action remains unclear (neither agent is active against PCP alone). The most common toxicity is a morbilliform rash that typically appears in the second week of dosing and, in many cases, can be "treated through." Definitive studies are needed to establish the role of this combination as compared with TMP/SMX and TMP/dapsone. Toma *et al.* have had similar success using slightly different doses as initial therapy and have explored its use as salvage therapy after TMP/SMX. (Toma E, Fournier, Poisson M, et al.: Clindamycin with primaquine for *Pneumocystis carinii* pneumonia. *Lancet* 1989, 1:1046–1048.)

Indications for PCP prophylaxis

Prior episode of PCP
CD4$^+$ count < 200/mm^3
Earlier initiation warranted for patients with:
    Oral candidiasis
    Unexplained fever > 100° F for ≥ 2 wks
    Rapid fall in CD4$^+$ count

FIGURE 15-12 Indications for PCP prophylaxis. The Multicenter AIDS Cohort Study has provided the best information on the population at risk for developing PCP. (Phair J, Muñoz A, Detels R, et al.: The risk of *Pneumocystis carinii* pneumonia among men infected with human immunodeficiency virus type 1. *N Engl J Med* 1990, 322:161–165.) Individuals with HIV infection are at greatest risk for an initial episode of PCP when their absolute CD4$^+$ count drops below 200 cells/mm^3 (although the risk is not zero at counts above 200). Additional factors that are independently associated with PCP development and warrant earlier prophylaxis include unexplained fever and thrush (the predictive value of vaginal candidiasis in women is unknown). Patients with a recent rapid decline in CD4$^+$ count also should be monitored closely for initiation of prophylaxis. All patients with a prior documented episode are at increased risk of recurrence and should receive prophylaxis. PCP prophylaxis should be continued for life. These guidelines are the updated recommendations of the US Public Health Service Task Force on Antipneumocystis Prophylaxis. (Centers for Disease Control: Guidelines for prophylaxis against *Pneumocystis carinii* pneumonia for persons infected with human immunodeficiency virus. *MMWR* 1992, 41:1–11. Masur H, Feinberg J, et al.: Guidelines for prophylaxis of *Pneumocystis carinii* pneumonia for persons infected with the human immunodeficiency virus. *J Acquir Defic Syndr* 1993, 6:46–55.)

US Public Health Service Task Force on PCP prophylaxis: Revised recommendations 1992

Trimethoprim/sulfamethoxazole is preferable to AP if tolerated

Dose: One double-strength tablet/day

FIGURE 15-13 Recommended dosage of TMP/SMX for PCP prophylaxis. Data that have emerged since the 1989 recommendations of the US Public Health Service Task Force indicate that TMP/SMX is the preferred form of prophylaxis in patients who can tolerate it. (Centers for Disease Control: Guidelines for prophylaxis against *Pneumocystis carinii* pneumonia for persons infected with human immunodeficiency virus. *MMWR* 1992, 41[RR-4]:1–11. Masur H, Feinberg J, *et al.*: Guidelines for prophylaxis of *Pneumocystis carinii* pneumonia for persons infected with the human immunodeficiency virus. *J Acquir Immune Defic Syndr* 1993, 6:46–55.) This conclusion is based primarily on the results of a prophylaxis study comparing TMP/SMX and aerosolized pentamidine in patients who had recovered from a documented episode of PCP ("secondary prophylaxis") within 10 weeks prior to study entry. In this study, patients receiving TMP/SMX (160 mg/800 mg once daily) had significantly fewer recurrences by 18 months than did patients treated with aerosolized pentamidine (300 mg every 4 weeks by jet nebulizer)—11.4% vs 27.6% ($P < 0.001$). By 24 months, the rates were 14.7% and 36.1%, respectively. (*From* Hardy WD, Feinberg J, Finkelstein DM, *et al.*: A controlled trial of trimethoprim–sulfamethoxazole or aerosolized pentamidine for secondary prophylaxis of *Pneumocystis carinii* pneumonia in patients with the acquired immunodeficiency syndrome: AIDS Clinical Trials Group protocol 021. *N Engl J Med* 1992, 327:1842–1848; with permission.) TMP/SMX has also proven to be more effective than aerosolized pentamidine in a European study of primary prophylaxis. (Schneider MME, Hoepelman AIM, Eeftinck-Schattenkerk JKM, *et al.*: A controlled trial of aerosolized pentamidine or trimethoprim–sulfamethoxazole as primary prophylaxis against *Pneumocystis carinii* pneumonia in patients with human immunodeficiency virus infection. *N Engl J Med* 1992, 329:1836–1841.) The recommended prophylactic dosage of TMP/SMX is one double-strength tablet daily, continued for life, and should be administered to patients for both primary and secondary prophylaxis.

A. Aerosolized pentamidine vs TMP/SMX for secondary PCP prophylaxis (ACTG 021): Design

Randomized, open-label, multicenter trial
310 patients:
 Recovered from initial episode of PCP within 10 wks before
  study entry
 No dose-limiting toxicity to study drugs
Dosage:
 TMP/SMX, one double-strength tablet/day
 vs
 Aerosolized pentamidine, 300 mg/mo via jet nebulizer
Standard dose zidovudine provided by study

B. Aerosolized pentamidine (AP) vs TMP/SMX for secondary PCP prophylaxis (ACTG 021): Results

	AP	TMP/SMX
Mean (median) follow-up	17.1 (17.4) mo	17.1 (17.4) mo
Recurrences		
Intent to treat	36	14 ($P = 0.0005$)
As treated	43	7
12-mo estimated recurrence rate	18.5%	3.5%
Serious bacterial infections	38	19
Survival	22.8 mo	25.8 mo

FIGURE 15-14 Aerosolized pentamidine vs TMP/SMX for secondary PCP prophylaxis. **A,** The AIDS Clinical Trials Group (ACTG) study 021 assessed the strategy of providing secondary prophylaxis in the form of daily oral TMP/SMX or monthly aerosolized pentamidine to patients receiving zidovudine. **Outcome**: **B,** Although there was no significant difference in survival, there was an enhanced protective effect of TMP/SMX over aerosolized pentamidine that led to the early termination of the study. TMP/SMX prophylaxis also conferred a protective effect against serious bacterial infections (50% reduction), which is an expected benefit of systemic prophylaxis with an agent that also has broad-spectrum antibacterial activity. There were too few cases of toxoplasmosis to discern a significant advantage for TMP/SMX, but a trend was noted indicating that it may have a protective effect for toxoplasmic encephalitis as well. (*From* Hardy WD, Feinberg J, Finkelstein DM, *et al.*: A controlled trial of trimethoprim–sulfamethoxazole or aerosolized pentamidine for secondary prophylaxis of *Pneumocystis carinii* pneumonia in patients with the acquired immunodeficiency syndrome: AIDS Clinical Trials Group protocol 021. *N Engl J Med* 1992, 327:1842–1848; with permission.)

A. Aerosolized pentamidine vs TMP/SMX for primary PCP prophylaxis (Dutch ATG): Design

Randomized, open-label, multicenter trial
Patients:
  HIV⁺ with CD4⁺ count < 200/mm³
  No prior therapy with pentamidine or TMP/SMX within 2 mo
  Adequate performance status and hematologic, hepatic, and renal function
Three treatment arms:
  TMP/SMX, one single-strength (480 mg) tablet/day, or
  TMP/SMX, one double-strength (960 mg) tablet/day, or
  Aerosolized pentamidine, 300 mg/mo via jet nebulizer with albuterol pretreatment

B. Aerosolized pentamidine vs TMP/SMX for primary PCP prophylaxis (Dutch ATG): Results

	TMP/SMX (480 mg)	TMP/SMX (960 mg)	AP
Mean follow-up	288 d	277 d	264 d
PCP episodes	0	0	6 (*P*=0.002)
12-mo estimated incidence rate	0%	0%	11%
Toxoplasmosis episodes*	0	0	3

*All cases fatal.

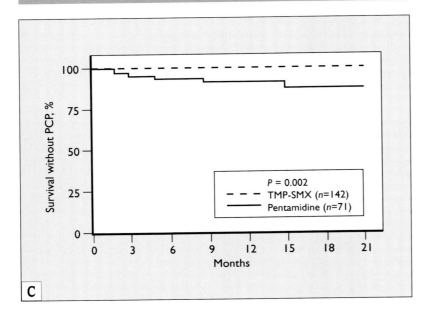

FIGURE 15-15 Aerosolized pentamidine vs TMP/SMX for primary PCP prophylaxis. Compelling evidence for the superiority of TMP/SMX prophylaxis over aerosolized pentamidine also exists for patients at high risk who have not yet had an episode of PCP ("primary prophylaxis"). **A.** The Dutch AIDS Treatment Group (ATG) assessed two different doses of TMP/SMX—one double-strength (960-mg) tablet and one single-strength (480-mg) tablet daily—versus monthly aerosolized pentamidine. **Outcome: B,** There were 71 patients enrolled in each of the study's three arms. The groups were well matched at entry except that there was more zidovudine (*P*=0.04) and antifungal (*P*=0.08) use in the pentamidine arm. **C,** This study was also terminated early because of the significant protection against PCP conferred by TMP/SMX prophylaxis, based on a comparison of the two TMP/SMX groups taken together vs the pentamidine group; the cumulative incidence of PCP was 0 in the combined TMP/SMX groups vs 11% in the aerosolized pentamidine group (*P*=0.002, *panel 15C*). Once again, there were too few cases of toxoplasmic encephalitis to assess the prophylactic efficacy of TMP/SMX. (*From* Schneider MME, Hoepelman AIM, Eeftinck-Schattenkerk JKM, *et al.*: A controlled trial of aerosolized pentamidine or trimethoprim–sulfamethoxazole as primary prophylaxis against *Pneumocystis carinii* pneumonia in patients with human immunodeficiency virus infection. *N Engl J Med* 1992, 327:1836–1841; with permission.)

A. TMP/SMX vs dapsone vs aerosolized pentamidine for primary PCP prophylaxis (ACTG 081): Design

Randomized, open-label, multicenter trial

All patients received zidovudine as part of trial design

Dosages:
  TMP/SMX, one double-strength tablet twice daily
  vs
  Dapsone, 50 mg twice daily
  vs
  Aerosolized pentamidine, 300 mg/mo

B. TMP/SMX vs dapsone (D) vs aerosolized pentamidine (AP) for primary PCP prophylaxis (ACTG 081): PCP endpoints (intent to treat)

	AP	D	TMP/SMX
PCP episodes	54	48	42 (*P*=0.22)
Estimated 24-mo incidence	14%	8.6%	9.8%

	AP/D	AP/TMP/SMX	D/TMP/SMX
PCP hazard	0.139	0.126	0.88
Baseline CD4⁺-adjusted hazard	0.112	0.091	0.932

FIGURE 15-16 TMP/SMX vs dapsone vs aerosolized pentamidine for primary PCP prophylaxis. A major prospective trial (ACTG 081) comparing proven effective agents for PCP prophylaxis, TMP/SMX and aerosolized pentamidine, to dapsone was completed in 1993. Like sulfa drugs, dapsone is a folate antagonist that inhibits the enzyme dihydropteroate synthetase (DHPS). **A,** When this study was undertaken, there were animal model and anecdotal data to suggest it would be effective as a single agent for PCP prophylaxis. **Outcome:**

B, Of 842 participants enrolled between May 1989 and June 1990 and followed for a median of 39.1 months, only 137 patients (16.3%) developed PCP (105 proven, 32 presumptive), affirming the overall effectiveness of primary PCP prophylaxis. In the intent-to-treat analysis, which analyzes patients according to the way they were randomized (includes withdrawals due to toxicity, failure to respond, and other reasons), there were no significant differences among the three groups, even when adjusted for baseline CD4⁺ count.(*continued*)

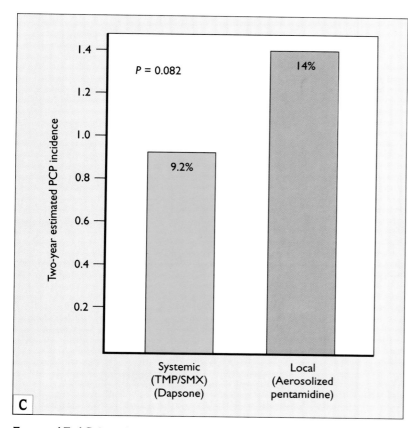

D. TMP/SMX vs dapsone vs aerosolized pentamidine (AP) for primary PCP prophylaxis (ACTG 081): PCP endpoints (as treated)

	AP	Dapsone	TMP/SMX
No. of patients with PCP while still receiving assigned prophylaxis	53/54 (98%)	36/48 (75%)	3/42 (7%)
Total PCP events while receiving prophylaxis	74	61	9

FIGURE 15-16 (continued) **C,** An intent-to-treat analysis comparing the two approaches—systemic (dapsone or TMP/SMX) vs local (aerosolized pentamidine)—showed a marginally significant trend toward a protective effect for systemic prophylaxis (*P*=0.082). **D,** Because the study allowed for crossover to another arm due to treatment-limiting toxicity or the development of PCP, a secondary analysis based on what patients were actually receiving at the time they developed PCP was performed ("as treated" analysis). Among patients who could tolerate the agent to which they were originally assigned, TMP/SMX conferred the best protection against PCP, with dapsone providing intermediate protection and aerosolized pentamidine providing the least. The same pattern is seen when the total number of episodes of PCP are counted, including those episodes that occurred after patients had crossed over to another arm. (Bozzette SA, *et al.*: [abstract]. Presented at the First National Conference on Human Retroviruses and Associated Conditions, Washington, DC, 1993.)

1992 recommendations for aerosolized pentamidine prophylaxis

Acceptable for patients who cannot take TMP/SMX
Dosages:
Jet nebulizer: 300 mg/mo
Ultrasonic nebulizer: 60 mg every 2 wks (give 5 loading doses over first 2 wks)

FIGURE 15-17 1992 Revised recommendations for aerosolized pentamidine prophylaxis. For an aerosol approach to be effective, enough drug must be nebulized into particles of appropriate size for deposition throughout the lung. Particle size depends on the characteristics of the nebulizer employed. From the results of studies using different doses of pentamidine delivered by different nebulizers, the USPHS Task Force has broadened its recommendations concerning the use of aerosolized pentamidine as second-line prophylaxis for patients who cannot take TMP/SMX (Centers for Disease Control: Guidelines for prophylaxis against *Pneumocystis carinii* pneumonia for persons infected with human immunodeficiency virus. *MMWR* 1992, 41[RR-4]:1–11. Masur H, Feinberg J, *et al.*: Guidelines for prophylaxis of *Pneumoncystis carinii* pneumonia for persons infected with the human immunodeficiency virus. *J Acquir Immune Defic Syndr* 1993, 6:46–55.)

Alternatives for PCP prophylaxis

Intermittent TMP/SMX, every other day or M-W-F
Dapsone, 25–50 mg/d, or any dose intermittently
Dapsone, 50 mg/d, plus pyrimethamine, 50 mg/wk

FIGURE 15-18 Alternatives for PCP prophylaxis. Various alternative regimens have shown effectiveness for PCP prophylaxis and are used by some clinicians in efforts to limit toxicity or cost associated with the standard TMP/SMX regimen. The data supporting intermittent use of TMP/SMX, daily doses of dapsone < 100 mg, or intermittent use of dapsone (at any dose) are less compelling, coming from studies that were retrospective, uncontrolled, or small. No data regarding appropriate doses and schedules are yet available for clindamycin/primaquine, trimetrexate, or atovaquone, although their use has been described in anecdotal reports in patients unable to take other proven forms of prophylaxis.

Unproven alternatives for PCP prophylaxis

Parenteral pentamidine
Trimethoprim/dapsone
Clindamycin/primaquine
Atovaquone
Trimetrexate

FIGURE 15-19 Unproven alternatives for PCP prophylaxis. Agents active against acute PCP are potential candidates for prophylaxis as well. However, only anecdotal data exist at this time, and no clear comparative data regarding appropriate dose and schedule are yet available.

TOXOPLASMIC ENCEPHALITIS

Standard therapy for toxoplasmic encephalitis

Dosage:
Pyrimethamine, 25–100 mg/d, after an initial loading dose
plus
Sulfadiazine, 4–8 g/d
plus
Leucovorin, 10 mg/d
Initial response rate 80% to 90%
Treatment-limiting toxicity frequent

FIGURE 15-20 Standard therapy for toxoplasmic encephalitis. Standard therapy with pyrimethamine/sulfadiazine is initially successful in 80% to 90% of patients. However, as with TMP/SMX for acute PCP, treatment-limiting toxicity occurs frequently, in up to 40% of patients, and consists mainly of hematologic toxicity and rash. This has led to a search for alternative forms of therapy. (Leport C, Raffi F, Matheson S, *et al*.: Treatment of central nervous system toxoplasmosis with pyrimethamine/sulfadiazine combination in 35 patients with the acquired immunodeficiency syndrome: Efficacy of long-term therapy. *Am J Med* 1988, 84:94–100.)

A. Pyrimethamine/sulfadiazine vs pyrimethamine/clindamycin for toxoplasmic encephalitis: Design

Randomized, open-label, European multicenter trial
Patients with first episode of toxoplasmic encephalitis
Acute therapy:
Pyrimethamine, 50 mg/d
plus
Oral clindamycin, 2.4 g/d, or oral sulfadiazine, 4 g/d
Maintenance:
Pyrimethamine, 25 mg/d
plus
Clindamycin, 1.2 g/d, or sulfadiazine, 2 g/d

B. Pyrimethamine/sulfadiazine (P/S) vs pyrimethamine/clindamycin (P/C) for toxoplasmic encephalitis: Results

	P/S	P/C	*P* value
Overall response	77%	68%	NS
Complete response	55%	47%	NS
Switch to other arm	31%	24%	
	(45 patients)	(37 patients)	
Toxicity	44/45	17/37	< 0.00001
Failure	1/45	20/37	< 0.00001
Adverse effects			
Rash	20%	13%	
Fever	20%	13%	
Diarrhea	0.7%	19%	< 0.0001

FIGURE 15-21 Pyrimethamine/sulfadiazine vs pyrimethamine/clindamycin for toxoplasmic encephalitis. Again, as with acute PCP, the combination of pyrimethamine and clindamycin, effective in animal models, has been investigated as an alternative to pyrimethamine/sulfadiazine. A small comparative study demonstrated equivalent clinical and radiographic results (although mortality occurred in 19% of patients randomized to pyrimethamine/clindamycin as opposed to 6% among those randomized to pyrimethamine/sulfadiazine. (Dannemann B, McCutchan JA, Israelski D, *et al*.: Treatment of toxoplasmic encephalitis in patients with AIDS: A randomized trial comparing pyrimethamine plus clindamycin to pyrimethamine plus sulfadiazine. *Ann Intern Med* 1992, 116:33–43.) **A**, A large, prospective, comparative study was conducted in Europe among

299 patients. **Outcome**: **B**, As in the earlier study, the larger trial did not demonstrate a significant difference between the two regimens when analyzed on an intent-to-treat basis. However, crossover to the other arm was significantly more common among pyrimethamine/sulfadiazine recipients for treatment-limiting toxicity and, conversely, significantly more common among pyrimethamine/clindamycin recipients for failure to respond clinically. (Katlama C, De Wit S, Guichard A, *et al*.: A randomized European trial comparing pyrimethamine-clindamycin to pyrimethamine-sulfadiazine in AIDS toxoplasmix encephalitis. [abstract 1215]. Presented at the 32nd Interscience Conference on Antimicrobial Agents and Chemotherapy, Anaheim, CA, 1992.)

Alternative therapies for toxoplasmosis

Several new agents have *in vitro* activity:
  Atovaquone
  Trimetrexate
  Clarithromycin
  Azithromycin
	Single-agent use has been primarily for "salvage"
	Studies, particularly in combination with pyrimethamine or sulfadiazine, are ongoing

FIGURE 15-22 Alternative therapies. Use of newer agents in uncontrolled studies, primarily aimed at patients intolerant of or refractory to established therapies, has demonstrated some clinical activity. Current studies are exploring the use of some of these agents in combination with either pyrimethamine or sulfadiazine in an attempt to achieve a better outcome.

Primary prophylaxis for toxoplasmosis

Single-agent prophylaxis: Pyrimethamine
Combination studies: Dapsone plus pyrimethamine
TMP/SMX is likely effective, though the the evidence is indirect

FIGURE 15-23 Primary prophylaxis for toxoplasmosis. Single-agent pyrimethamine and various combinations have been evaluated for their effectiveness as primary prophylaxis against toxoplasmic encephalitis. Contradictory results have emerged from two recently completed placebo-controlled studies of single-agent pyrimethamine prophylaxis for toxoplasmosis. Although there were differences in the designs of these two studies, one showed a small protective effect for pyrimethamine in the individuals at highest risk, whereas the other showed an unexplained poorer survival for pyrimethamine recipients. Combination therapy has shown more positive results. In a study by Girard *et al.*, dapsone plus pyrimethamine (and leucovorin) was protective against both toxoplasmosis and PCP, especially toxoplasmosis. (Girard P-M, Landman R, Gaudebout C, *et al.*: Dapsone-pyrimethamine compared with aerosolized pentamidine as primary prophylaxis against *Pneumocystis carinii* pneumonia and toxoplasmosis in HIV infection. *N Engl J Med* 1993, 328:1514–1520.) Retrospective data by Carr and prospective data from PCP prophylaxis trials by several groups, which yielded small numbers of toxoplasmosis cases, suggest that TMP/SMX is likely to be effective in preventing toxoplasmosis as well as PCP. (Carr A, Tindall B, Brew BJ, *et al.*: Low-dose trimethoprim-sulfamethoxazole prophylaxis for toxoplasmic encephalitis in patients with AIDS. *Ann Intern Med* 1992, 117:106–111. Hardy WD, Feinberg J, Finkelstein DM, *et al.*: A controlled trial of trimethoprim–sulfamethoxazole or aerosolized pentamidine for secondary prophylaxis of *Pneumocystis carinii* pneumonia in patients with the acquired immunodeficiency syndrome: AIDS Clinical Trials Group protocol 021. *N Engl J Med* 1992, 327:1842–1848. Schneider MME, Hoepelman AIM, Eeftinck-Schattenkerk JKM, *et al.*: A controlled trial of aerosolized pentamidine or trimethoprim–sulfamethoxazole as primary prophylaxis against *Pneumocystis carinii* pneumonia in patients with human immunodeficiency virus infection. *N Engl J Med* 1992, 327:1836–1841. Mallolas J, Lamora L, Gatell IM, *et al.*: Primary prophylaxis for *Pneumocystis carinii* pneumonia: A randomized trial comparing cotrimazole, aerosolized pentamidine, and dapsone plus pyrimethamine. *AIDS* 1993, 7:69–64.)

A. Dapsone/pyrimethamine vs aerosolized pentamidine for primary prophylaxis: Design

Randomized, open-label, multicenter trial
Patients:
  Symptomatic
  CD4+ count < 200/mm^3
  No prior episodes of toxoplasmosis or PCP
349 patients evaluable/362 enrolled
Dosages:
  Dapsone, 50 mg/d, plus pyrimethamine, 50 mg/wk (and leucovorin, 25 mg/wk)
vs
Aerosolized pentamidine, 300 mg/mo

B. Dapsone/pyrimethamine (D/P) vs aerosolized pentamidine (AP) for primary prophylaxis: Results

	D/P	AP	*P* Value
Mean follow-up at early discontinuation	476 + 37 d	476 + 37 d	—
Toxoplasmosis events			
Intent to treat	15	29	0.015
As treated	6	36	
PCP events	7	9	NS
Treatment-limiting toxicity	40	3	0.001

FIGURE 15-24 Dapsone/pyrimethamine vs aerosolized pentamidine as primary prophylaxis of toxoplasmosis and PCP. Because toxoplasmosis is one of the most common opportunistic infections in western Europe, and because some agents are likely to confer cross-protection for both toxoplasmosis and PCP, a number of studies have been designed to explore simultaneous protection against both diseases. **A,** The most successful of these to date compared daily dapsone plus weekly pyrimethamine with aerosolized pentamidine as primary prophylaxis in patients at high risk for both PCP and toxoplasmic encephalitis. **Outcome: B** and **C,** The study was terminated early because of the statistically significant protective effect of dapsone/pyrimethamine for toxoplasmosis. (continued)

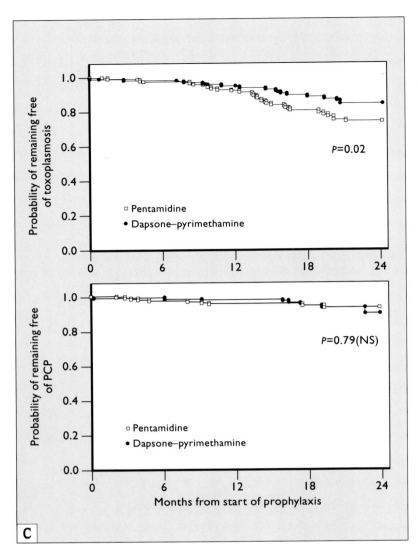

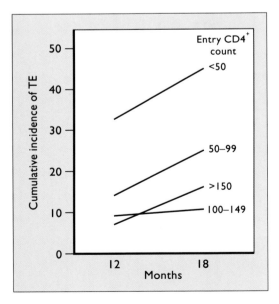

FIGURE 15-24 (continued) All episodes of toxoplasmic encephalitis occurred in patients with anti-*Toxoplasma gondii* IgG antibody. At the time the study was closed, there was no difference in prophylactic benefit against PCP between the two arms (*panel 24C, bottom*). As expected, systemic prophylaxis proved to more toxic than local aerosol administration. (*From* Girard P-M, Landman R, Gaudebout C, *et al.*: Dapsone-pyrimethamine compared with aerosolized pentamidine as primary prophylaxis against *Pneumocystis carinii* pneumonia and toxoplasmosis in HIV infection. *N Engl J Med* 1993, 328:1514–1520; with permission.)

FIGURE 15-25 Incidence of toxoplasmic encephalitis. Valuable information about the natural history of toxoplasmosis emerged from the placebo group in the ACTG/ANRS study. An increased risk of toxoplasmic encephalitis was clearly associated with lower CD4+ lymphocyte counts, as had previously been demonstrated for PCP. The development of toxoplasmosis was relatively uncommon at CD4+ counts > 100, with a 10% incidence or less at 12 months, but the rate rose sharply with lower CD4+ counts. A cumulative incidence of 33% at 12 months and 45% at 18 months was noted for participants whose entry CD4+ was < 50. The risk was 2.3 times greater for patients with CD4+ counts < 50 and with an AIDS diagnosis. (Leport C, Morlat P, Chene G, *et al.*: Pyrimethamine for primary prophylaxis of toxoplasmosis in HIV patients. A double-blind randomized trial. [abstract 36.] Presented at the First National Conference on Human Retroviruses and Related Infections, Washington, DC, Dec 12–16, 1993.)

A. Pyrimethamine vs placebo for toxoplasmosis prophylaxis: Design

	CPCRA study	ACTG/ANRS study
Pyrimethamine dosage	25 mg 3×/wk	50 mg 3×/wk
Leucovorin	None	15 mg 3×/wk
PCP prophylaxis	Any	Aerosolized pentamidine
Patient ratio (pyrimethamine:placebo)	2:1	1:1

B. Pyrimethamine vs placebo for toxoplasmosis prophylaxis: Results

	CPCRA $n = 396$	ACTG/ANRS $n = 540$
Survival	Worse for pyrimethamine	No difference
Toxoplasmosis All patients	Event rate too low to discern difference	No difference
Subgroup	Patients getting TMP/SMX for PCP prophylaxis had lowest rate	Pyrimethamine more effective in patients with entry CD4+ < 100/mL

FIGURE 15-26 Pyrimethamine prophylaxis. Two large, double-blind, placebo-controlled trials of single-agent pyrimethamine prophylaxis have been conducted. Both studies enrolled patients with low CD4+ lymphocyte counts (< 200/mm³) and IgG antibody to *T. gondii*. **A,** They differed, however, in some significant ways: the dose of pyrimethamine employed, concurrent use of leucovorin, and type of PCP prophylaxis. The Community Program for Clinical Research in AIDS (CPCRA) study was begun as a three-arm study comparing clindamycin (300 mg twice daily) and pyrimethamine with placebo. However, the clindamycin arm was terminated early because of excessive toxicity (diarrhea, rash). (Jacobson MA, Besch CL, Child C, *et al*.: Toxicity of clindamycin as prophylaxis for AIDS-associated toxoplasmic encephalitis. *Lancet* 1992, 339:333–334.) The trial then continued as a pyrimethamine-vs-placebo study with a 2:1 patient ratio. In the ACTG/ANRS study, all patients, whether randomized to pyrimethamine or placebo, received leucovorin three times a week. **Outcome: B,** In the CPCRA study, the number of toxoplasmosis endpoints was so low that the study was terminated early. However, an unexplained higher mortality rate (*P*=0.005) among the 264 pyrimethamine recipients was seen. The low rate of toxoplasmosis was probably due to widespread use of systemic PCP prophylaxis; only 1 of 218 (0.5%) participants taking TMP/SMX for PCP prophylaxis at study entry developed toxoplasmic encephalitis, compared with 7 of 117 (6.0%) receiving aerosolized pentamidine. (Jacobson MA, Besch CL, Child C, *et al*.: Primary prophylaxis with pyrimethamine for toxoplasmic encephalitis in patients with advanced human immunodeficiency virus disease: Results of a randomized trial. *J Infect Dis* 1994, 169:384–394.) The excess mortality for pyrimethamine recipients was not confirmed by the larger ACTG/ANRS study. In the intent-to-treat analysis, there was no significant difference in the 12-month toxoplasmic encephalitis rates—12% for pyrimethamine vs 13% for placebo (*P*=0.75). However, an analysis of those at highest risk (entry CD4+ count < 100) indicated a trend toward a protective effect for pyrimethamine (11% vs 21% for placebo, *P*=0.08). For patients who could tolerate pyrimethamine, the "as-treated" analysis showed a clear benefit (12-month toxoplasmic encephalitis rate, 4%, 12% for placebo, *P*=0.006). Patients who had to discontinue pyrimethamine because of rash appeared to have an enhanced risk of subsequent toxoplasmosis. (Leport C, Morlat P, Chene G, *et al*.: Pyrimethamine for primary prophylaxis of toxoplasmosis in HIV patients: A double-blind randomized trial. [abstract 36.] Presented at First National Conference on Human Retroviruses and Related Infections, Washington, DC, 1993.)

Indications and regimens for toxoplasmosis prophylaxis

Indicated for patients with IgG antibody to *T. gondii* and CD4+ < 200 cells/mm³

TMP/SMX given for PCP prophylaxis is probably protective

For patients given dapsone (≥ 50 mg/d) for PCP, add pyrimethamine, 50 mg/wk (plus leucovorin, 25 mg/wk)

For patients intolerant of TMP/SMX and dapsone, use pyrimethamine, 50 mg 3×/wk (plus leucovorin, 15 mg 3×/wk), when CD4+ is < 50–100/mL

FIGURE 15-27 Indications and regimens for toxoplasma prophylaxis. There are as yet no consensus guidelines for prevention of toxoplasmosis. A reasonable course of action based on the available data is to target patients who are seropositive for *T. gondii* and whose CD4+ lymphocyte counts are < 200 cells/mm³ (especially those with very low counts). Patients who are receiving TMP/SMX for PCP prophylaxis are probably also protected against toxoplasmosis, and so additional prophylaxis may be unnecessary. Likewise, those receiving dapsone for PCP probably will be protected against toxoplasmosis if a weekly dose (50 mg) of pyrimethamine is added, although it may not be necessary to add pyrimethamine until CD4+ counts are < 50–100/mm³. For patients who tolerate neither TMP/SMX nor dapsone for PCP, it may be reasonable to administer pyrimethamine, 50 mg three times per week (if they are able to tolerate this regimen).

MUCOCUTANEOUS CANDIDIASIS

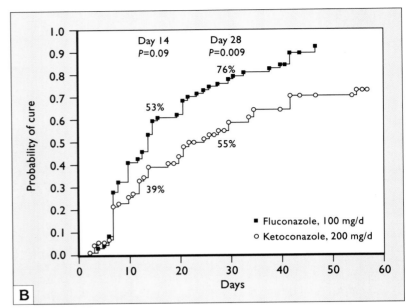

A. Standard therapy for candidiasis

Mucocutaneous (pharyngitis, vaginitis)
Topical: Nystatin, clotrimazole
Oral: Ketoconazole, fluconazole, itraconazole
Esophagitis
Oral: Fluconazole, 100 mg/d, is superior to ketoconazole, 200 mg/d

FIGURE 15-28 Standard therapy for candidiasis. Candida is the most common opportunistic pathogen in HIV disease. **A**, Many drugs are effective for management of mucocutaneous candidiasis. Oral azoles are comparable or superior to topical agents. Because of the growing problem of fluconazole resistance, topical agents should probably be used preferentially for thrush and vaginitis. **B**, Oral agents are clearly preferred for esophagitis, and fluconazole has been shown to be superior to ketoconazole for

this indication. The role of itraconazole in esophagitis is less clear. Achlorhydria noted in many patients with advanced HIV disease may impair absorption of ketoconazole, which requires an acid environment for bioavailability; administration with acidic foods such as orange juice may be helpful. (*From* Laine L, Dretler RH, Conteas CN, *et al.*: Fluconazole compared with ketoconazole for the treatment of candida esophagitis in AIDS: A randomized trial. *Ann Intern Med* 1992, 117:665–660; with permission.)

Fluconazole-resistant candidiasis

Mechanisms of refractory infection:
　Reduced susceptibility to fluconazole
　Selection of yeast outside the spectrum of fluconazole:
　　Torulopsis glabrata
　　Candida tropicalis
　　Candida krusei
　　Candida parapsilosis
Alternative treatments:
　? Itraconazole
　Amphotericin B

FIGURE 15-29 Fluconazole resistance. A growing problem arising from widespread use of long-term suppressive therapy for candidiasis with fluconazole is the development of fluconazole-resistant disease. On *in vitro* susceptibility testing, some fluconazole-resistant isolates retain sensitivity to ketoconazole and/or itraconazole. Alternatively, there may be selection for yeasts that are not in the spectrum of fluconazole. Itraconazole may be useful in these fluconazole-resistant infections both because some *Candida albicans* strains resistant to fluconazole remain susceptible to itraconazole and because it has some intrinsic activity *in vitro* against selected non-*albicans* species. Amphotericin B can be used in fluconazole-resistant infection, although the response may be slow. (Boken DJ, Swindens S, Rinaldi MC: Fluconazole-resistant *Candida albicans* in HIV infection, [abstract PO-B09-1358.] Presented at the IX International Conference on AIDS, Berlin, 1993. Baily GG, Perry FM, Denning DW, Mandal BR: Fluconazole-resistant candidiasis in an HIV cohort [abstract PO-B09-1375.] Presented at the IX International Conference on AIDS, Berlin, 1993.)

CRYPTOCOCCAL MENINGITIS

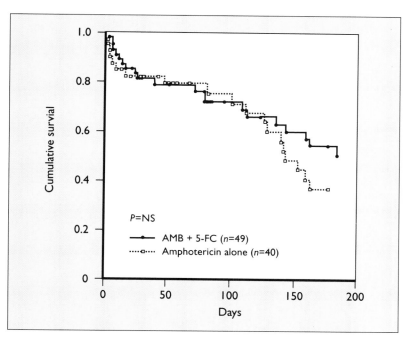

FIGURE 15-30 Amphotericin plus flucytosine for cryptococcal meningitis. In the pre-AIDS era, amphotericin B was the standard of care for cryptococcal meningitis. Later, amphotericin B in combination with flucytosine (5-FU) was shown to be more effective than amphotericin B alone, achieving a more rapid sterilization of cerebrospinal fluid (CSF), more cures, fewer relapses, less nephrotoxicity, and equivalent mortality. (Bennett JE, Dismukes WE, Duma RJ, *et al.*: A comparison of amphotericin B alone and combined with flucytosine in the treatment of cryptococcal meningitis. *N Engl J Med* 1979, 301:126–131.) However, controversy exists about the utility and tolerability of flucytosine in AIDS patients, with evidence offered both in support of (Larsen RA, Leal MAE, Chan LS: Fluconazole compared with amphotericin B plus flucytosine for cryptococcal meningitis in AIDS: A randomized trial. *Ann Intern Med* 1990, 113:183–187) and against its use (Chuck SL, Sande MA: Infections with *Cryptococcus neoformans* in the acquired immunodeficiency syndrome. *N Engl J Med* 1989, 321:794–799). Ongoing investigation will elucidate the role of flucytosine in the treatment of acute cryptococcal meningitis in AIDS.

A. Fluconazole vs amphotericin B for acute cryptococcal meningitis in AIDS: Design

Randomized, open-label, multicenter trial
Acute cryptococcal meningitis diagnosed by CSF culture
Patients randomized 2:1 fluconazole:amphotericin B
Dosages:
  Fluconazole, 400-mg bolus IV or orally, then 200 mg/d, vs
  Amphotericin B, at least 0.3 mg/kg/d IV
Duration of treatment 10 wks
Definition of outcomes
  Clinical response: Two negative CSF cultures by week 10, plus clinical improvement
  "Quiescent disease": Culture positive at week 10 (or < 2 negative cultures), plus clinical improvement

B. Fluconazole vs amphotericin B for acute cryptococcal meningitis: Results

	Fluconazole	Amphotericin B
Total patients	131	63
Responders	44 (33.6%)	25 (39.7%)
Nonresponders	87 (66.4%)	38 (60.5%)
Failure	47	15
Quiescent	35	18
Toxicity	3	5
Noncompliant	2	0

FIGURE 15-31 Fluconazole vs amphotericin B for acute cryptococcal meningitis. The advent of fluconazole opened the possibility of oral treatment of cryptococcal meningitis with minimal toxicity. **A,** A multicenter, open-label study compared fluconazole, 200 mg/d, with amphotericin B alone (minimum daily dose, 0.3 mg/kg/d; median dose, 0.5 mg/kg/d). Eligible patients had to have a positive CSF culture at study entry. Responders were defined as patients who had both clinical improvement and two negative CSF cultures by the end of therapy (week 10). Patients with "quiescent disease" had clinical improvement but failed to have sterilization of their CSF by the end of therapy. **Outcome: B,** The response did not differ significantly between the two arms, nor did overall mortality during the 10-week treatment period. **C,** However, there was a trend toward increased early mortality (in the first 2 weeks) in the fluconazole group and for earlier culture conversion in the amphotericin B arm. Fluconazole was the better tolerated therapy. The overall response rate for the study was disappointingly low, despite the fact that the criteria for response were strict. This study has been criticized because the dose of amphotericin was too low and the failure rate in this arm unacceptably high (60.3%). (*From* Saag MS, Powderly WG, Cloud GA, *et al.*: Comparison of amphotericin B with fluconazole in the treatment of acute AIDS-associated cryptococcal meningitis. *N Engl J Med* 1992, 326:83–89; with permission.)

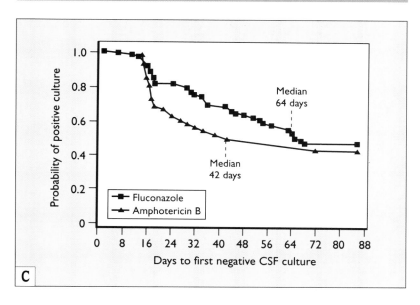

C

Factors associated with mortality in acute cryptococcal meningitis

Altered mental status at diagnosis
CSF cryptococcal antigen titer > 1:1024
CSF leukocyte count < 20/mm³
Age < 35 yrs

FIGURE 15-32 Predictors of mortality in acute cryptococcal meningitis. In the Saag trial comparing fluconazole and amphotericin B, a multivariate analysis indicated that several factors were associated with decreased survival: decreased level of consciousness at diagnosis, large organism burden (elevated CSF antigen titer), poor inflammatory response in the central nervous system (CNS) (low CSF leukocyte count), and younger age. At a minimum, these characteristics help to define patients who should be treated more aggressively (with a higher dose of amphotericin B, with or without flucytosine), at least for the first 2 weeks. (Saag MS, Powderly WE, Cloud GA, *et al.*: Comparison of amphotericin B with fluconazole in the treatment of acute AIDS-associated cryptococcal meningitis. *N Engl J Med* 1992, 326:83–89.)

Triazoles as initial therapy for acute cryptococcal meningitis

	Response rate		
	Saag *n* = 194	Larsen *n* = 21	DeGans *n* = 28
Amphotericin B	40%	100%	100%
Fluconazole	34%	43%	—
Itraconazole	—	—	50%

FIGURE 15-33 Are triazoles acceptable initial therapy for acute cryptococcal meningitis? The effectiveness of the triazoles fluconazole and itraconazole for use as initial therapy in acute cryptococcal meningitis is controversial. Some clinicians accept fluconazole as adequate initial therapy (at acute treatment doses of 400 mg/d) for patients with favorable prognostic findings (normal mental status, low CSF cryptococcal antigen titer, and CSF leukocytosis). The study by Saag *et al.* that showed comparable benefit of fluconazole and amphotericin B is flawed because of its use of a relatively low dose of amphotericin B. (Saag MS, Powderly WE, Cloud GA, *et al.*: Comparison of amphotericin B with fluconazole in the treatment of acute AIDS-associated cryptococcal meningitis. *N Engl J Med* 1992, 326:83–89.) Two smaller studies comparing amphotericin B to either fluconazole or itraconazole again raise the question of whether any AIDS patient with cryptococcal meningitis should be treated with a fungistatic triazole from the outset, as the amphotericin B recipients had a much better outcome. (Larsen RA, Leal MAE, Chan LS: Fluconazole compared with amphotericin B plus flucytosine for cryptococcal meningitis in AIDS: A randomized trial. *Ann Intern Med* 1990, 113:183–187. de Gans J, Portegies P, Tiessens, *et al.*: Itraconazole compared with amphotericin B plus flucytosine in AIDS patients with cryptococcal meningitis. *AIDS* 1992, 6:185–190.)

A. Suppressive therapy for cryptococcal meningitis: Design

Randomized, open-label, multicenter trial
AIDS patients who have successfully completed acute treatment
  with amphotericin B plus flucytosine
    Minimum total dose of 15 mg/kg
    At least two negative CSF cultures
189 evaluable/219 enrolled
Dosages:
    Fluconazole, 200 mg/d orally, vs
    Amphotericin B, at least 1 mg/kg/wk
Failure:
    Culture-or biopsy-proven relapse at any site other than uri-
      nary tract or
    Dose-limiting toxicity

FIGURE 15-34 Suppressive therapy for cryptococcal meningitis. Relapse of cryptococcal meningitis in the absence of chronic suppressive ("maintenance") therapy was 50% to 60% in three retrospective studies. In a placebo-controlled trial with a median follow-up of 125 days, the relapse rate was 37% among placebo recipients (Bozzette SA, Larsen RA, Chiu J, *et al.*: A placebo-controlled trial of maintenance therapy with fluconazole after treatment of cryptococcal meningitis in the acquired immunodeficiency syndrome. *N Engl J Med* 1991, 324:580–584), and a persistent urinary focus of cryptococcosis was reported in 20% of patients who completed a course of amphotericin B therapy (Larsen RA, Bozzette SA, McCutchan JA, *et al.*: Persistent cryptococcus neoformans infection of the prostate after successful treatment of meningitis. *Ann Intern Med* 1989, 111:125–128). **A**, A study comparing fluconazole, 200 mg/d, with amphotericin B, 1 mg/kg/wk, was designed with the hypothesis that amphotericin B suppression would result in at least a 15% lower relapse rate than fluconazole. *(continued)*

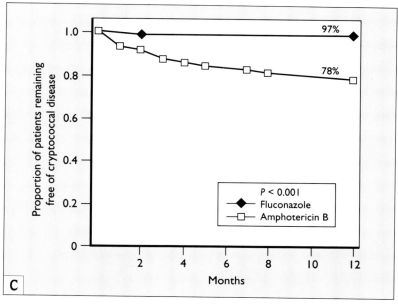

B. Suppressive therapy for cryptococcal meningitis: Results

	Amphotericin B	Fluconazole
Total patients	78	111
Suppressive therapy failure	26 (33%)	8 (8%)
Relapse	14	2 (*P*=0.0009)
Toxicity	12	6

FIGURE 15-34 *(continued)* **Outcome**: **B** and **C**. The study was terminated early (median follow-up of 217 days) because fluconazole maintenance therapy was significantly more effective in preventing meningitis relapse than amphotericin B. Although surveillance lumbar punctures were performed at 3-month intervals, no "silent" relapses were detected by periodic CSF examination (all relapses were symptomatic). As a result, fluconazole is the preferred maintenance therapy. Clinical assessment of such patients is sufficient; recrudescent symptoms require a lumbar puncture for evaluation by the usual studies, including culture for cryptococcus. (*From* Powderly WG, Saag MS, Cloud GA, et al.: A controlled trial of fluconazole or amphotericin B to prevent relapse of cryptococcal meningitis in patients with the acquired immunodeficiency syndrome. *N Engl J Med* 1992, 326:793–798; with permission.)

HISTOPLASMOSIS

Treatment of histoplasmosis

Amphotericin B is standard therapy (especially for patients with sepsis syndrome, CNS disease)

Itraconazole is effective in uncontrolled studies for:

Acute therapy in less severe disease (300 mg 2×/d ×3 days, then 200 mg 2×/d ×12 wks)

Chronic maintenance therapy (200 mg twice daily) after initial amphotericin B treatment

FIGURE 15-35 Treatment of histoplasmosis. Amphotericin B was standard therapy for histoplasmosis before the development of the oral triazoles, and it remains the preferred therapy for AIDS patients who present with severe disease (a sepsislike syndrome or CNS involvement). (Wheat LJ, Connolly-Stringfield PA, Baker RL, et al.: Disseminated histoplasmosis in the acquired immunodeficiency syndrome: Clinical findings, diagnosis and treatment, and review of the literature. *Medicine* 1990, 69:361–374.) Two uncontrolled studies have indicated that itraconazole is effective for both initial treatment of milder disease and for chronic suppressive therapy after an initial course of amphotericin B. (Wheat LJ, Hafner RE, Ritchie M, Schneider D: Itraconazole is effective treatment for histoplasmosis in AIDS: Prospective multicenter non-comparative trial. [abstract 1206.] Presented at the 32nd Interscience Conference on Antimicrobial Agents and Chemotherapy, Anaheim, CA, 1992. Wheat J, Hafner R, Wulfsohn M, et al.: Prevention of relapse of histoplasmosis with itraconazole in patients with acquired immunodeficiency syndrome. *Ann Intern Med* 1993, 118:610–616.)

VIRAL INFECTIONS

A. Foscarnet vs vidarabine for acyclovir-resistant herpes simplex: Design

Small, randomized, open-label multicenter trial
HSV unresponsive to at least 10 days of IV acyclovir
Confirmed *in vitro* resistance to acyclovir and susceptibility to study drugs
Dosages:
　　Foscarnet, 40 mg/kg IV every 8 hrs
　　vs
　　Vidarabine, 15 mg/kg IV once daily
Goal: Time to complete healing (epithelialization)

B. Foscarnet vs vidarabine for acyclovir-resistant herpes simplex: Results

	FOS $n = 8$	VID $n = 6$	*P* value
Median lesion size, cm^2	29	101	0.07
Median CD4, *cells/mm³*	17.5	13.5	NS
Time to healing, d^*	13.5	38.5	0.01

*Controlled for lesion size.

FIGURE 15-36 A and **B**, Shingles (reactivated varicella zoster infection) is a common manifestation of early HIV disease, when CD4 counts are typically between 300–500. Acyclovir, in a dosage sufficient to treat zoster, is standard therapy. Foscarnet, which is the current treatment of choice for acyclovir-resistant herpes simplex infection, has also been used successfully for acyclovir-resistant zoster. (Safrin S, Crumpacker C, Chatis P, *et al.*: A controlled trial comparing foscarnet with vidarabine for acyclovir-resistant mucocutaneous herpes simplex in the acquired immunodeficiency syndrome: The AIDS Clinical Trials Group. *N Engl J Med* 1991, 325:551–555. Safrin S, Berger TG, Gilson I, *et al.*: Foscarnet therapy in five patients with AIDS and acyclovir-resistant varicella-zoster virus infection. *Ann Intern Med* 1991, 115:19–21.)

A. Treatment of CMV retinitis: Design

Study design: Immediate vs deferred treatment for peripheral (non–sight-threatening) disease

Therapy initiated in deferred group at first sign of progression (border advancement by ≥ 750 μm or new lesion)

Dosages:
　　Ganciclovir, 5 mg/kg IV 2×/d × 14 d, then 5 mg/kg IV daily
　　vs
　　Foscarnet, 60 mg/kg IV 2×/d × 21 d, then 90 mg/kg IV daily

B. Treatment of CMV retinitis: Results

	Immediate treatment	Deferred treatment	*P* value
Ganciclovir			
Patients, *n*	13	22	—
Median time to progression, *d*	49.5	13.5	0.001
Foscarnet	13	11	—
Patients, *n*	13.3	3.2	< 0.001
Mean time to progression, *wks*			

FIGURE 15-37 Treatment of cytomegalovirus (CMV) retinitis. Two separate studies with the same design provide controlled data on the usefulness of single-agent therapy for CMV retinitis. Patients with peripheral retinitis were randomized to receive immediate or deferred treatment; in the deferred group, therapy was begun at the first sign of progression. Endpoints were documented by retinal photographs, which were interpreted by an experienced ophthalmologist who was unaware of treatment assignment. **A.** Peripheral retinitis refers to lesions that are not considered immediately sight-threatening and are located at least 1500 μm from the optic disk margin and 3000 μm from the fovea. **Outcome: B.** Uncontrolled data had indicated that treatment with either the nucleoside analogue ganciclovir or the pyrophosphate analogue foscarnet was effective in slowing the inexorable progression of CMV retinitis by inhibiting viral DNA polymerase, which prevented viral DNA elongation. Two separate, randomized, open-label studies of immediate vs deferred therapy demonstrated clear clinical (and virustatic) benefit. (Spector SA, Weingeist T, Pollard RB, *et al.*: A randomized, controlled study of intravenous ganciclovir therapy for cytomegalovirus peripheral retinitis in patients with AIDS: AIDS Clinical Trials Group and Cytomegalovirus Cooperative Study Group. *J Infect Dis* 1993, 168:557–563. Palestine AG, Polis MA, DeSmet MD, *et al.*: A randomized controlled trial of foscarnet in the treatment of CMV retinitis in patients with AIDS. *Ann Intern Med* 1991, 115:665–673.)

A. Foscarnet vs ganciclovir for CMV retinitis: Design

Randomized, open-label multicenter trial
Previously untreated CMV retinitis
Ganciclovir 5 mg/kg 2×/d 14 d, then 5 mg/kg daily
vs
Foscarnet 60 mg/kg 3×/d 14 d, then 90 mg/kg daily
Patients reinduced for progression
Cross-over for dose-limiting toxicity permitted
Antiretroviral therapy permitted as tolerated
Goals: Time to retinitis progression, visual loss, mortality

B. Foscarnet vs ganciclovir for CMV retinitis: Results

	FOS $n = 107$	GCV $n = 127$	P value
Time to retinitis progression (median, days)	59	56	NS
Any antiretroviral TX	84%	66%	0.02
Cross-over (any reason) for toxicity	39	14	0.001
	22	1	0.006
Mortality	36(34%)	65(51%)	
Median survival, *mo*	12.6	8.5	

FIGURE 15-38 **A,** Ganciclovir and foscarnet were compared as initial therapy of CMV retinitis in a collaborative study of the Studies of Ocular Complications of AIDS (SOCA) and the AIDS Clinical Trial Group (ACTG). **Outcome: B,** Ganciclovir and foscarnet monotherapy were equivalent for control of CMV retinitis (Meinert C, *et al, N Engl J Med* 1992; 326:213–220). Ganciclovir was better tolerated, with only one patient switching to foscarnet because of dose-limiting toxicity, but 22 patients switching from foscarnet to ganciclovir because of toxicity. There was, however, an unexplained survival advantage of approximately 4 months for the group assigned to foscarnet, which also has anti-HIV activity at the dosages used for retinitis. In an analysis of baseline covariates, only the subgroup with impaired renal function at entry had a higher risk of mortality with foscarnet therapy.

MYCOBACTERIUM AVIUM COMPLEX

A. Rifabutin vs placebo for *M. avium* complex (MAC) prophylaxis: Design

Two identical randomized, double-blind, placebo-controlled, multicenter studies

Entry criteria:
  Diagnosis of AIDS and CD4$^+$ count ≤ 200 cells/mm^3
  Negative blood and stool cultures for *M. avium* complex
  Patients receiving antiretroviral therapy and PCP prophylaxis

Dosages:
  Rifabutin, 300 mg once daily, vs placebo

Goal: Time to development of MAC bacteremia

B. Rifabutin vs placebo for *M. complex* (MAC) prophylaxis: Results

1146 total patients enrolled in two studies
Study duration (mean): 218 days
Mean CD4$^+$ count at onset of MAC bacteremia = 14 cells/mm^3

	Rifabutin	Placebo	P value
Patients, *n*	566	580	—
MAC bacteremia			
Intent-to-treat	48	102	< 0.001
As-treated	35	89	< 0.001
Treatment-limiting toxicity	16%	8%	—

FIGURE 15-39 Rifabutin vs placebo for *Mycobacterium avium* complex prophylaxis. **A,** Thus far, only one drug has been studied prospectively for *M. avium* complex prophylaxis. Two identical studies were performed to investigate single-agent prophylaxis with rifabutin, a new rifamycin, which is active against *M. avium* complex *in vitro* and shown to have modest activity in some animal models. Participants had to have an AIDS diagnosis as well as a CD4$^+$ count < 200/mm^3 and continued to receive standard-of-care management for their HIV disease. **Outcome: B,** Rifabutin prophylaxis reduced the frequency of *M. avium* complex bacteremia by approximately 50% in both intent-to-treat and as-treated analyses. Although the rate of study drug discontinuation due to toxicity was twice as high among rifabutin recipients, in general toxicities were mild, consisting primarily of neutropenia, rash, arthralgias, and myalgias. No significant difference in survival was seen, but the study was not designed to assess this endpoint. (Nightingale SD, Cameron DW, Gordin FM, *et al.*: Two controlled trials of rifabutin prophylaxis against *Mycobacterium avium* complex in AIDS. *N Engl J Med* 1993, 329:828–833.)

1993 USPHS recommendations for *M. avium* complex prophylaxis and therapy

CD4$^+$ count < 100 cells/mm^3
No active disease due to:
  M. avium complex
  Tuberculosis
  Other mycobacteria
Assess potential risks/benefits on an individual basis
Rifabutin, 300 mg/d

FIGURE 15-40 1993 Recommendations for prophylaxis and treatment of *M. avium* complex. Based on the results of the two rifabutin studies and additional analyses performed by the US Food and Drug Administration, a US Public Health Service Task Force recommended the use of rifabutin prophylaxis in patients with a CD4$^+$ count < 100 cells/mm^3 and no active mycobacterial disease. The threshold of 100 cells was chosen because the benefit of prophylaxis was almost entirely limited to participants with CD4$^+$ count < 75/mm^3 and no benefit accrued to those with entry CD4$^+$ counts > 100/mm^3. Seventy-two percent of all *M. avium* complex bacteremias occurred in individuals with CD4$^+$ < 25 at the time of diagnosis. (Centers for Disease Control: Recommendations on prophylaxis and therapy for disseminated *Mycobacterium avium* complex for adults and adolescents infected with the human immunodeficiency virus. *MMWR* 1993, 42[RR-9]:14–19. Masur H, *et al.*: Recommendations on prophylaxis and therapy for disseminated *Mycobacterium avium* complex disease in patients infected with the human immunodeficiency virus. *N Engl J Med* 1993, 329:898–904.) Rifabutin prophylaxis for *M. avium* complex infection is more problematic than TMP/SMX prophylaxis for PCP. The potential for rifabutin resistance in areas with high rates of tuberculosis and for drug–drug interactions with other commonly used agents (such as fluconazole, clarithromycin, and methadone) means that the decision to initiate prophylaxis must be individualized. Moreover, uncertainty about the duration of the preventive effect, the possible development of drug-resistant *M. avium* complex, and the substantial number of patients who experience breakthrough bacteremia must be considered and studied further.

SELECTED BIBLIOGRAPHY

Bartlett JG, Feinberg J: Update on management of opportunistic infections in patients with HIV infection. *Infect Dis Clin Pract* 1993, 2:233–246.

Crowe SM, *et al.*: Predictive value of CD4 lymphocyte numbers for the development of opportunistic infections and malignancies in HIV-infected persons. *J Acquir Immune Defic Syndr* 1991, 4:770.

Feinberg J: Biology, treatment and prophylaxis of *Pneumocystis carinii* pnuemonia. *Am J Med* 1994 (suppl), in press.

Girard P-M, Feinberg J: Progress and problems in AIDS-associated opportunistic infections. (*In* AIDS 1993—A Year in Review). *AIDS* 1994, in press.

CHAPTER 16

AIDS-Associated Malignancies

Josephine Paredes
Susan E. Krown

Malignancies associated with HIV infection
Kaposi's sarcoma*
Non-Hodgkin's lymphoma*
Systemic high or intermediate grade lymphomas
Primary central nervous system lymphomas
Hodgkin's disease
Anogenital squamous cancer
Invasive cervical cancer*
Anal cancer

*AIDS-defining diagnosis.

FIGURE 16-1 Several neoplasms occur with increased frequency or behave in an uncharacteristically aggressive manner in patients who are infected with HIV. The original surveillance definition of AIDS included Kaposi's sarcoma and primary lymphomas of the central nervous system. In 1985, systemic high- or intermediate-grade lymphomas were added to the case-definition, and in 1993, invasive cervical cancer was added as well. Although increased incidences of anal cancer and Hodgkin's disease have not been demonstrated unequivocally, both behave more aggressively in HIV-infected patients. In addition, HIV-infected people show an increased incidence of noninvasive anogenital dysplasia associated with human papillomavirus infection.

KAPOSI'S SARCOMA

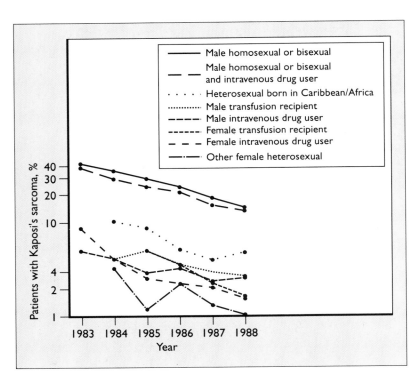

FIGURE 16-2 Over the past several years, the incidence of Kaposi's sarcoma (KS) as an AIDS-defining diagnosis has been declining. At the beginning of the AIDS epidemic, KS was second only to *Pneumocystis carinii* pneumonia as the initial presentation of AIDS. By 1990, it ranked fourth among AIDS-defining diagnoses. (Centers for Disease Control: HIV/AIDS Surveillance Report. 1991, (Jan):1.) Among the factors contributing to its apparent decline in incidence are changes in the risk categories of newly diagnosed patients to include a higher proportion of heterosexual men and women and changes in the surveillance definition of AIDS. For example, the HIV wasting syndrome, which was added to the AIDS surveillance definition in 1987, was the second most common AIDS-defining illness in 1992. For patients who develop KS after another AIDS-defining illness, KS is not reported. (Centers for Disease Control and Prevention: HIV/AIDS Surveillance Report. 1993, (Feb):1–23.) Epidemiologic studies indicate that, whereas the risk of developing KS remains constant in homosexual men beginning about 2 years after HIV infection, the risk of developing an opportunistic infection or non-Hodgkin's lymphoma continues to increase with increasing duration of infection and progressive immunosuppression. With improvements in the care of patients with advanced HIV infection, more patients survive to develop these late complications. There is evidence, however, that the impact of KS on late morbidity and mortality is increasing, at least in some subsets of patients, as the treatment and prophylaxis of opportunistic infections improve. (Rabkin CS, Goedert JJ: Risk of non-Hodgkin's lymphoma and Kaposi's sarcoma in homosexual men. *Lancet* 1990, 336:248–249. Peters BS, Beck EJ, Coleman DG, *et al.*: Changing disease patterns in patients with AIDS in a referral centre in the United Kingdom: The changing face of AIDS. *BMJ* 1991, 302:203–207.)

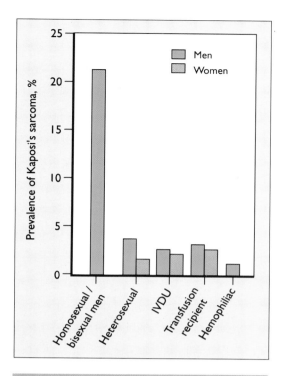

FIGURE 16-3 Kaposi's sarcoma is, by far, the most common HIV-associated neoplasm. Among HIV-infected people, the risk of developing KS is estimated to be about 20,000 times greater than in age- and sex-matched controls from the general US population. Sexual transmission of KS has been suggested by its approximately 10-fold higher frequency of this neoplasm in homosexual or bisexual men than in heterosexual men with HIV infection and by its approximately fourfold higher frequency in women who acquired their infection from bisexual men than in HIV-infected women with exclusively heterosexual partners (intravenous drug users [IVDU]). (Beral V, Peterman TA, Berkelman RI, *et al.*: Kaposi's sarcoma among persons with AIDS: A sexually transmitted infection. *Lancet* 1990, 335:123–128. *Figure from* Roth WK, Brandstetter H, Stürzl M: HIV-associated KS: Cellular and molecular features. *J Cancer Res Oncol* 1991, 117:186–191; with permission.)

Factors involved in development of Kaposi's sarcoma

Growth factors and cytokines
  Oncostatin M
  Interleukin-6
  Interleukin-1
  Basic fibroblast growth factor
  Vascular endothelial growth factor
  Tumor necrosis factor
  Platelet-derived growth factor
  Granulocyte—macrophage colony
    stimulating factor
Viral products
  HIV *tat* gene product (Tat)

FIGURE 16-4 Studies of the pathogenesis of KS were made possible by the discovery that conditioned media from CD4+ T lymphocytes infected with human retroviruses, including HTLV-I, HTLV-II, and HIV, could support the *in vitro* growth of spindle cells from Kaposi's sarcoma lesions. The active factor in these media was later identified as oncostatin M. Various cytokines and growth factors secreted by immune-activated T lymphocytes, or by the KS cells themselves, also stimulate the *in vitro* proliferation of KS-derived spindle cells via autocrine or paracrine pathways. Some of these factors, which are prototypic angiogenic factors, are thought to contribute to the neovascularization that is a histologic characteristic of KS lesions. (Nakamura S, Salahuddin SZ, Biberfeld B, *et al.*: Kaposi's sarcoma cells: Long-term culture with growth factor from retrovirus infected CD4+ T cells. *Science* 1988, 242:426–430. Miles SA, Martinez-Maza O, Rezai A, *et al.*: Oncostatin M as a potent mitogen for AIDS-Kaposi's sarcoma derived cells. *Science* 1992, 255:1432–1434). Although there is no evidence that HIV is present within KS lesions, transgenic mice bearing the HIV *tat* gene develop multicentric skin tumors resembling human KS. These lesions occur only in male mice; interestingly, both testosterone and glucocorticoids have been shown to stimulate the *in vitro* growth of human KS-derived spindle cells. *In vitro*, the *tat* gene product (Tat) stimulates KS spindle cell proliferation, an effect enhanced in the presence of cytokines secreted by activated T lymphocytes. (Vogel J, Hinrichs SH, Reynolds RK, *et al.*: The HIV *tat* gene induces dermal lesions resembling Kaposi's sarcoma in transgenic mice. *Nature* 1988, 335:606–611. Gill PS, Naidu Y, Nakamura S, *et al.*: IL-6 regulation by steroid hormones and autocrine activity in Kaposi's sarcoma. *AIDS Res Hum Retroviruses* 1991, 7:220. Ensoli B, Barillari G, Salahuddin SZ, *et al.*: Tat protein of HIV-1 stimulates growth of cells derived from Kaposi's sarcoma lesions of AIDS patients. *Nature* 1990, 345:84–86. Barillari G, Buonaguro L, Fiorelli V, *et al.*: Effects of cytokines from activated immune cells on vascular cell growth and HIV-1 gene expression. *J Immunol* 1992, 149:3727–3734.)

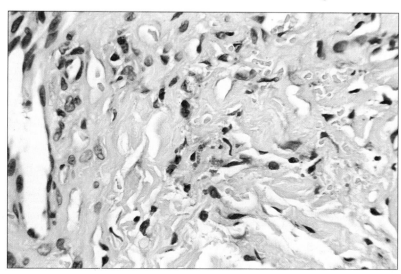

FIGURE 16-5 Pathologically, KS lesions are characterized by proliferation of spindle cells with slitlike vascular spaces, extra-vasated erythrocytes, and a variable inflammatory cell infiltrate. (Hematoxylin-eosin.)

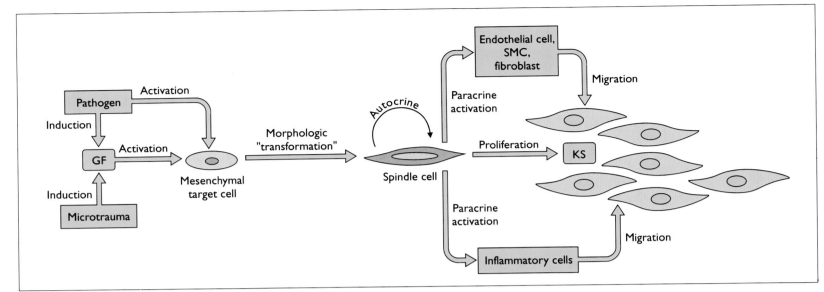

FIGURE 16-6 Pathogenesis of Kaposi's sarcoma. *Bold arrows* indicate main sequence of events. Growth factors (platelet-derived growth factor [PDGF], transforming growth factor [TGF]-β, TGF-α, interleukin [IL]-1, [IL]-6, oncostatin M) induced by a pathogen (unknown infectious agent, virus) activate mesenchymal target cells (pluripotent undifferentiated mesenchymal cells, endothelial cells, SMC, fibroblasts), leading to morphologic transformation into spindle cells. Activated spindle cells induce their own growth via autocrine acting factors (unknown and known fibroblast growth factor [FGF]-like factor). Secretion of paracrine acting factors (*eg*, TGF-β, PDGF, macrophage chemotactic protein-1, FGF-like factors, tumor necrosis factor-α) by spindle cells induces migration and activation of inflammatory cells, endothelial cells, SMC, and fibroblasts; KS is therefore a reactive tumor composed of histogenetically different cell types. Initially, growth factors could also be induced by microtrauma, leading to platelet degranulation with subsequent release of PDGF, TGF-β, and other cytokines involved in inflammation and granulation tissue induction. It is also conceivable that a pathogen directly activate mesenchymal target cells (by infection), which induces morphologic "transformation" and generation of KS. In late stages of KS, permanent activation of spindle cells could lead to malignant genetic transformation. (*From* Roth WK, Brandstetter H, Stürzl M: Cellular and molecular features of HIV-associated Kaposi's sarcoma. *AIDS* 1992, 6:895–913; with permission.)

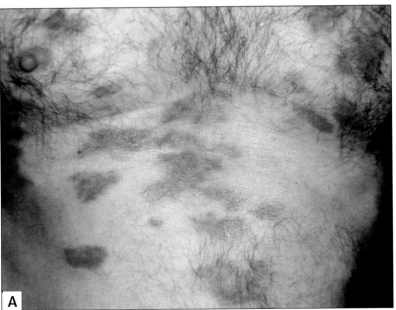
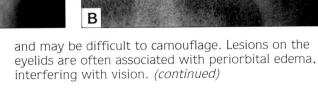

FIGURE 16-7 Clinically, KS has a variety of presentations. **A**, Skin lesions may be few and small or may be widespread and large. **B**, Cosmetically disfiguring lesions are common on the face, particularly the nose, and may be difficult to camouflage. Lesions on the eyelids are often associated with periorbital edema, interfering with vision. *(continued)*

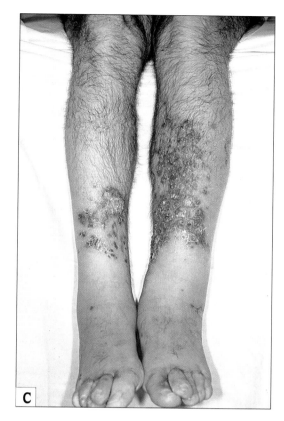

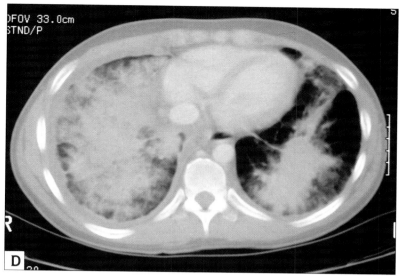

FIGURE 16-7 *continued* **C,** Lymphedema of the lower extremities is common and may occur in the absence of extensive cutaneous involvement or enlarged proximal lymph nodes. **D,** Visceral involvement, particularly when it involves the gastrointestinal tract, may be asymptomatic. When KS involves other viscera, particularly the lungs, it may be symptomatic and life-threatening. This figure shows the chest CT scan of a patient with extensive pulmonary KS.

TREATMENT OF KAPOSI'S SARCOMA

Determinants of treatment of AIDS-related Kaposi's sarcoma

Clinical severity of KS
  Cosmetically unacceptable lesions
  Localized bulky or painful KS lesions
  Extensive cutaneous KS
  Tumor-associated edema
  Symptomatic visceral KS
Severity of underlying HIV infection
  Concomitant opportunistic infections
  Wasting
  Neutropenia
  Severity of immunosuppression
  Organ dysfunction

FIGURE 16-8 Both the clinical severity of KS and the severity of the underlying HIV infection must be considered in deciding when to treat KS and which type of treatment to use.

Therapies for AIDS-related Kaposi's sarcoma

Observation
Local therapies
Systemic therapies
New therapeutic approaches

FIGURE 16-9 For patients with minimal, asymptomatic, and/or nondisfiguring Kaposi's sarcoma or for those with multiple other HIV-related medical conditions and a very short estimated survival, a decision may be made to defer treatment until the KS causes symptoms and to treat only the underlying HIV infection and its nonneoplastic complications. For other patients, however, treatment may be indicated, and the available treatments may be broadly categorized as local (directed at specific lesions or body areas) or systemic. In addition, a number of new approaches are under investigation, many of which are based on recent developments in the understanding of KS pathogenesis.

Local Therapies

Local treatment options for Kaposi's sarcoma
Surgical excision
Laser therapy/cryotherapy
Intralesional chemotherapy
Intralesional IFN-α
Intralesional TNF-α
Radiotherapy

FIGURE 16-10 Among available local therapies, surgical excision of lesions is the least often used, being most frequently employed for diagnostic purposes. Although laser therapy may be effective, there is concern about aerosolization of infected tissue. Liquid nitrogen cryotherapy is widely employed, especially for small, lightly pigmented lesions. Because this treatment destroys melanocytes, it results in hypopigmentation, making it most suitable cosmetically for fair-skinned people. Several forms of intralesional therapy have shown activity against KS, including vinblastine, interferon-α (IFN-α), and tumor necrosis factor (TNF-α). Often, intralesional therapies require multiple injections to be effective, and the injection procedure may be painful. For TNF, systemic toxicities, indicative of TNF absorption, have been reported. Although local cosmetic results may be satisfactory with intralesional therapy, only those lesions that are directly injected respond to treatment, making this therapy suitable only for patients with a limited number of lesions. Radiation therapy has been used widely to treat KS, particularly for localized, bulky lesions and for isolated, cosmetically disfiguring lesions, such as those on the nose and ears. Radiotherapy has been used with some success to treat KS-associated edema of the legs and in the periorbital area. Although oral mucosal lesions may respond very well to radiation therapy, severe mucositis is a frequent complication. Although radiation therapy is considered the treatment of choice in classic KS, with long response durations being the rule, in AIDS-associated KS lesions recur within a few months.

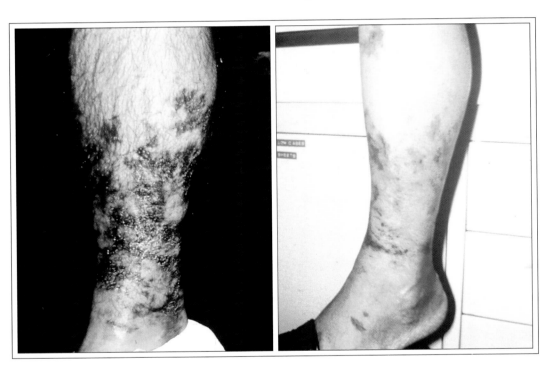

FIGURE 16-11 An excellent response to radiation therapy (*right panel*) is shown in a patient with extensive, confluent KS lesions and edema prior to treatment (*left panel*).

Systemic Chemotherapy

Chemotherapeutic agents used to treat Kaposi's sarcoma		
Single agents	**Combination regimens**	**Alternating regimens**
Doxorubicin	Bleomycin + vincristine	Vincristine/vinblastine
Bleomycin	Doxorubicin + bleomycin + vincristine	Doxorubicin + bleomycin + vinblastine/vincristine + dactinomycin + dacarbazine
Vinblastine	Doxorubicin + bleomycin + vinblastine	Bleomycin/vinblastine
Vincristine	Vinblastine + methotrexate	Doxorubicin/bleomycin + vincristine
Etoposide	Doxorubicin + bleomycin + vinblastine + etoposide	

FIGURE 16-12 Chemotherapy is the most widely used approach to the systemic treatment of KS. Although tumor regression has been reported after the use of single agents, more commonly agents are used in multidrug combinations administered every 2–4 weeks. To decrease toxicity, some investigators use alternating sequences of drugs, giving one or more drugs at one time and a different drug or drug combination at weekly or longer intervals. (Krown SE, Myskowski PL, Paredes J: Kaposi's sarcoma: Management of Kaposi's sarcoma in HIV-infected patients. *Med Clin North Am* 1992, 76:235–252.)

Results of chemotherapy for Kaposi's sarcoma

Single agents: response rates of 10% to 76%
Combinations/alternating regimen: response rates of 45% to 88%
Comparative efficacy of different regimens difficult to assess
  Nonuniformity of response criteria
  Patients selection criteria vary
Median response duration approx 6–8 months

FIGURE 16-13 The reported results of chemotherapeutic regimens against KS have varied tremendously, but overall response rates generally have been higher for combination or alternating regimens than for single agents. There is no unanimity about the most effective regimen (the criteria used to define response have varied widely, as have the criteria used to select patients). On average, responding patients show response durations of 6–8 months, but these figures also vary. Many patients can be expected to have symptomatic improvement with chemotherapy (*eg*, improvement or resolution of edema, improvement in respiratory symptoms of pulmonary KS) or slowing of disease progression without showing objective partial or complete tumor regression. Methods are under development to characterize better the impact of chemotherapy on quality of life in patients with AIDS and KS.

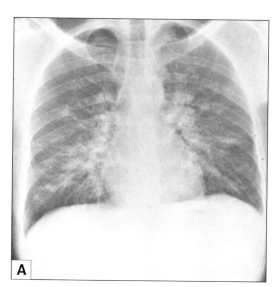

A

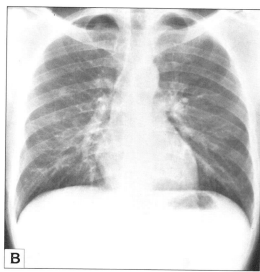

B

FIGURE 16-14 Patients with symptomatic visceral KS may benefit significantly from chemotherapy. **A**, A chest roentgenogram from a patient with extensive pulmonary Kaposi's sarcoma before chemotherapy is shown. **B**, After treatment with bleomycin and vincristine, the patient shows marked improvement of bilateral pulmonary lesions.

Toxicity of chemotherapy for Kaposi's sarcoma

Hematologic
Neutropenia most common
Impact on concomitant antiretroviral treatment and infection
  prophylaxis
Usually responsive to G/GM-CSF
Thrombocytopenia/anemia less common

Alopecia
Most common with doxorubicin, etoposide

Agent-specific
Doxorubicin: cardiac
Bleomycin: pulmonary, cutaneous, fever
Vinca alkaloids: neuropathy (especially vincristine)
Etoposide: neuropathy (less frequent than with vincas)

Gastrointestinal/mucositis
May occur with all agents
Ileus with vincristine

FIGURE 16-15 Chemotherapy for KS is associated with a variety of side effects. Hematologic toxicity is most common, especially with doxorubicin and etoposide, but hematologic suppression also occurs to some extent with bleomycin and vincristine. Until the development of hematopoietic colony-stimulating factors, chemotherapy-induced neutropenia often impaired both the ability to treat successfully with chemotherapy and the ability to treat the underlying HIV infection and opportunistic infections. The availability of granulocyte and granulocyte-macrophage colony-stimulating factors (G/GM-CSF) and less-myelosuppressive antiretroviral agents has significantly alleviated these problems. The choice of chemotherapeutic agents is often dictated or modified by the patient's wish to avoid hair loss and by specific toxicities of different chemotherapeutic agents.

Interferon-α

Potential mechanisms of inhibition of Kaposi's sarcoma by interferons

Direct antiproliferative/antineoplastic
Antiviral
Immune modulation
Cytokine/growth factor inhibition
Angiogenesis inhibition

FIGURE 16-16 Among the newer therapeutic approaches to KS are various biologic agents, including interferons, which have proven effective in some patients. The rationale for using interferons has evolved over the last decade. Interferon-α was first proposed as a treatment for KS because of its antiproliferative and immunomodulatory activities. However, with the discovery of HIV and demonstration that interferons can inhibit HIV replication *in vitro*, antiviral activity became a potential basis for their use. More recent studies demonstrate that interferons 1) can affect the production of growth factors by tumor cells; 2) increase the production of cytokine inhibitors (*eg*, the interleukin-1 receptor antagonist and soluble tumor necrosis factor receptor); and 3) inhibit both experimentally induced angiogenesis and life-threatening angiomatous lesions in patients (*ie*, pulmonary hemangiomatosis and giant hemangiomas of infancy). (Ho DD, Hartshorn KL, Rota TR, *et al.*: Recombinant human interferon alpha-A suppresses HTLV-III replication *in vitro. Lancet* 1985, 1:602–604. Tilg H, Mier JW, Vogel W, *et al.*: Induction of circulating IL-1 receptor antagonist by IFN treatment. *J Immunol* 1993, 150:4687–4692. Ezekowitz RAB, Mulliken JB, Folkman J: Interferon alfa-2a for life-threatening hemangiomas of infancy. *N Engl J Med* 1992, 326:1456–1463.)

FIGURE 16-17 Clinical studies in HIV-infected patients with KS have shown that relatively high doses of interferon-α (IFN-α) are capable of inducing tumor regression in approximately 30% of patients. Most studies have documented the efficacy of interferon doses in excess of 20×10^6 U/m² body surface area and the absence of substantial single-agent activity with doses $< 10 \times 10^6$ U/m². Relatively few studies have investigated intermediate dosage levels, and these have shown varying results, ranging from activity approaching that of high-dose interferon to minimal activity. (Krown SE, Myskowski PL, Paredes J: Kaposi's sarcoma: Management of Kaposi's sarcoma in HIV-infected patients. *Med Clin North Am* 1992, 76:235–252.)

Factors associated with response to interferons

Immune functional status
High CD4 lymphocyte counts (>200 cells/mm³)
High lymphoproliferative responses
Preserved delayed hypersensitivity skin-test reactions
Absent endogenous serum IFN-α
Low serum β₂-microglobulin/neopterin levels

HIV disease status
Absent "B" symptoms (fever, weight loss, night sweats)
Absent opportunistic infections

FIGURE 16-18 The pretreatment characteristics associated with responsiveness of KS to interferon-α include evidence for preserved cell-mediated immunity (*ie*, CD4 counts > 200 cells/mm³, relatively high lymphoproliferative responses to mitogens and antigens, and absence of cutaneous anergy), low levels of immune activation markers (*eg*, endogenous serum interferon, β₂-microglobulin and neopterin), and absence of HIV-associated wasting, fevers, and opportunistic infections. (Krown SE, Myskowski PL, Paredes J: Kaposi's sarcoma: Management of Kaposi's sarcoma in HIV-infected patients. *Med Clin North Am* 1992, 76:235–252.)

Side effects of interferon-α therapy

Flulike symptoms:
  Low-grade fevers
  Myalgia
  Malaise
  Anorexia
Labile blood pressure
Hematologic:
  Neutropenia
  Anemia
  Thrombocytopenia
Hepatic enzyme elevations
Neurologic:
  Headache
  Minor cognitive impairment
  Distal paresthesias
Reversible congestive cardiomyopathy

FIGURE 16-19 Of the many side effects ascribed to high-dose interferon-α treatment, chronic flulike symptoms are the most frequently dose-limiting. Because there is considerable overlap between symptoms of interferon toxicity and those associated with advancing HIV disease and opportunistic infections, care must be taken in distinguishing the two.

Rationale for IFN-α/nucleoside reverse transcriptase inhibitor combinations

Distinct loci of antiviral activity
Antiviral synergy *in vitro* vs HIV-1
Antiviral synergy *in vivo* vs murine retrovirus
Decreased potential for selection of resistant virus
RT inhibitors modify immune markers associated with responsiveness to IFN-α

FIGURE 16-20 Until the development of nucleoside reverse transcriptase (RT) inhibitors, interferon-α was used either alone or in combination with chemotherapy. Interferon-chemotherapy combinations, in general, have proven no more effective than interferon alone but usually have induced more toxicity. Combinations of interferons with RT inhibitors were suggested by several observations. Whereas interferons inhibit HIV primarily at a late stage of virus replication, RT inhibitors act at an early phase of virus replication. *In vitro*, antiviral synergy has been reported for interferons in combination with zidovudine, didanosine, and zalcitabine, and antiviral synergy has been demonstrated *in vivo* in a murine retrovirus model. Combinations of drugs may have the potential to inhibit the selection of drug-resistant viral strains. Finally, the factors associated with responsiveness to interferon-α monotherapy have been favorably influenced by treatment with RT inhibitors. (Pitha P: Multiple effects of interferon on HIV-1 replication. *J Interferon Res* 1991, 11:313–318. Hartshorn KL, Vogt MW, Chou TC, *et al.*: Synergistic inhibition of human immunodeficiency virus *in vitro* by azidothymidine and recombinant interferon-alpha A. *Antimicrob Agents Chemother* 1987, 31:168–172. Johnson VA, Merrill DP, Videler JA, *et al.*: Two-drug combinations of zidovudine, didanosine, and recombinant interferon-alpha A inhibit replication of zidovudine-resistant human immunodeficiency virus type 1 synergistically *in vitro*. *J Infect Dis* 1991, 164:646–655. Vogt MW, Durno AG, Chou TC, *et al.*: Synergistic interaction of 2′,3′-dideoxycytidine(ddCyd) and recombinant interferon alpha A (rIFN-alpha A) on HIV-1 replication. *J Infect Dis* 1988, 158:378–385.)

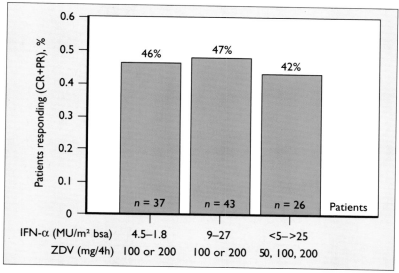

FIGURE 16-21 Phase I studies of the interferon-α (IFN-α) and zidovudine combination in patients with KS have all documented tumor response rates > 40%. Responses have been observed in some patients with CD4 counts < 200/mm³ and in patients treated with interferon doses < 10×10^6 U/m². The optimal dosage combination and the minimal effective doses have yet to be defined. (Krown SE, Gold JWM, Niedzwiecki D, *et al.*: Interferon-alpha with zidovudine: Safety, tolerance, and clinical and virologic effects in patients with Kaposi's sarcoma associated with the acquired immunodeficiency syndrome (AIDS). *Ann Intern Med* 1990, 112:812–821. Fischl MA, Uttamchandani RB, Resnick L, *et al.*: A phase I study of recombinant human interferon-alfa-2a or human lymphoblastoid interferon alfa-n1 and concomitant zidovudine in patients with AIDS-related Kaposi's sarcoma. *J Acquir Immune Defic Syndr* 1991, 4:1–10. Kovacs JA, Deyton L, Davey R, *et al.*: Combined zidovudine and interferon-alpha therapy in patients with Kaposi' sarcoma and the acquired immunodeficiency syndrome (AIDS). *Ann Intern Med* 1989, 111:280–287.)

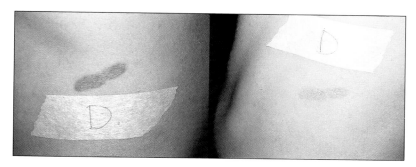

FIGURE 16-22 The response of a cutaneous KS lesion in a patient with a CD4 cell count < 200/mm³ who was treated with a combination of low-dose interferon-alpha (1×10^6 U/d) and a standard didanosine dose. The *left panel* shows the lesion before treatment, and the *right panel*, after 16 weeks of treatment.

Dose-limiting side effects of IFN-α + zidovudine combinations

Hematologic	Nonhematologic
Neutropenia	↑ Transaminases
Anemia	↑ Lactate dehydrogenase
Thrombocytopenia	↑ Alkaline phosphatase

FIGURE 16-23 The major side effect of combined interferon-α and zidovudine treatment has been neutropenia. Although several studies have indicated that hematopoietic colony-stimulating factors can prevent or reverse neutropenia, newer studies are investigating combinations of interferon with less myelosuppressive nucleoside analogs. (Scadden DT, Bering HA, Levine JD, *et al.*: Granulocyte-macrophage colony-stimulating factor mitigates the neutropenia of combined interferon alfa and zidovudine treatment of acquired immune deficiency syndrome-associated Kaposi's sarcoma. *J Clin Oncol* 1991, 9:802–808. Krown SE, Paredes J, Bundow D, *et al.*: Interferon-alpha, zidovudine, and granulocyte-macrophage colony-stimulating factor: A phase I AIDS Clinical Trials Group study in patients with Kaposi's sarcoma associated with AIDS. *J Clin Oncol* 1992, 10:1344–1351.)

Overview of Standard Treatments

Treatment guidelines for Kaposi's sarcoma

Status of KS	Status of HIV disease	KS treatment options
Few, small cutaneous KS lesions, not in exposed areas	CD4 + count <200/μL	No treatment
	Prior opportunistic infection or "B" symptoms	Local treatment
		No treatment
	CD4 + count >200/>μL	Local treatments
	No prior opportunistic infection or "B" symptoms	IFN-α ± zidovudine
		Local treatments
Cosmetically unacceptable lesions	Any	Radiation therapy
Extensive cutaneous KS ± asymptomatic visceral KS	CD4 + count <200/μL	Single or multiagent chemotherapy
	Prior opportunistic infection or "B" symptoms	? IFN-α ± zidovudine
	CD4 + count > 200/μL	IFN-α ± zidovudine
	No prior opportunistic infection or "B" symptoms	Single or multiagent chemotherapy
Localized bulky or painful KS lesions	Any	Radiation therapy
Tumor-associated edema	Any	Radiation therapy
		Single or multiagent chemotherapy
Symptomatic visceral KS	Any	Multiagent chemotherapy

FIGURE 16-24 Treatment guidelines for KS An overview of the standard treatments for KS outlines the choice of options based on the status of KS and the severity of HIV disease. In some cases, combinations of these approaches may be appropriate (*eg,* radiation to a site of bulky disease along with systemic chemotherapy), and treatment must be individualized according to the needs of the patient. (Krown SE, Myskowski PL, Paredes J: Kaposi's sarcoma: Management of Kaposi's sarcoma in HIV-infected patients. *Med Clin North Am* 1992, 76:235–252.)

Investigational Treatments

A. Investigational approaches to treatment of Kaposi's sarcoma

Liposomal anthracyclines
Decreased toxicity
Prolonged serum half-life
Increased tumor concentration

Retinoids
Topical
Systemic (± interferon)
Down-regulation of IL-6 receptors

FIGURE 16-25 Several investigational approaches have been suggested on the basis of recent insights into KS pathogenesis. **A,** Liposomally encapsulated anthracyclines (doxorubicin and daunorubicin) induce less systemic toxicity than the free drug, while remaining in the circulation longer and preferentially concentrating in tumor tissue. (Northfelt DW, Martin FJ, Kaplan LD, *et al.*: Pharmacokinetics (PK), tumor localization (TL), and safety of Doxil™ (liposomal doxorubicin) in AIDS patients with Kaposi's sarcoma (AIDS-KS). *Proc Am Soc Clin Oncol* 1993, 12:51.) Retinoids are under investigation, alone and in combination with interferon. There is a report of partial tumor regression after topical application of *trans*-retinoic acid, whereas systemic administration has led to tumor regression in some patients but increased tumor growth in others. There is evidence for synergy between interferon and retinoids *in vitro*, and high tumor response rates have been reported in advanced human epithelial cancers when interferon-α and *cis*-retinoic acid were combined. In myeloma cells, retinoic acid has been reported to down-regulate interleukin-6 (IL-6) receptors, an observation of potential relevance in KS. (Bonhomme L, Fredj G, Averous S, *et al.*: Topical treatment of epidemic Kaposi's sarcoma with all-*trans*-retinoic acid. *Ann Oncol* 1991, 2:234. Von Roenn J, von Gunten C, Mullane M, *et al.*: All-*trans*-retinoic acid (TRA) in the treatment of AIDS-related Kaposi's sarcoma: A phase II Illinois Cancer Center study. *Proc Am Soc Clin Oncol* 1993, 12:51. Sidell N, Taga T, Hirano T, *et al.*: Retinoic acid-induced growth inhibition of a human myeloma cell line via down-regulation of IL-6 receptors. *J Immunol* 1991, 146:3809–3814.) *(continued)*

B. Investigational approaches to treatment of Kaposi's sarcoma

Cytokine inhibitors
Interleukin-6 inhibition
  Interleukin-4
TNF inhibition
  Pentoxifylline
  Thalidomide
  TNF receptor
Interleukin-1 inhibition
  Interleukin-1 receptor
  Interleukin-1 receptor antagonist

Angiogenesis inhibitors
DS-4152
TNP-470 (AGM-1470)
Platelet factor 4

C. Investigational approaches to treatment of Kaposi's sarcoma

Tat antagonists
Antiestrogens
Tyrosine kinase/protein kinase C
  inhibitors
Metalloproteinase inhibitors

FIGURE 16-25 *continued* **B**, Cytokine and angiogenesis inhibitory strategies have been suggested by studies of KS pathogenesis. Various agents (some already in early clinical trials) inhibit the production or action of IL-6, IL-1, and tumor necrosis factor (TNF), cytokines which stimulate the *in vitro* proliferation of KS-derived spindle cells. Several angioinhibitory compounds, including DS-4152 (a sulfated polysaccharaide-peptidoglycan compound derived from *Arthrobacter* cell wall) and TNP-470 (a fumagillin analog, derived from *Aspergillus fumigatus fresnesius*), are under investigation. Both inhibit basic fibroblast growth factor-induced endothelial cell proliferation, angiogenesis, and proliferation of KS-derived spindle cells *in vitro*. Recombinant platelet factor 4, a platelet α-granule protein, inhibits vascular endothelial cell migration and proliferation. It may play a physiologic role in blood vessel development along with platelet-derived growth factor. (Nakamura S, Sakaruda SS, Salahuddin SZ, *et al.*: Inhibition of development of Kaposi's sarcoma-related lesions by a bacterial cell wall complex. *Science* 1992, 255:1437–1440. Kusaka M, Sudo K, Fujita T, *et al.*: Potent anti-angiogenic action of AGM-1470: Comparison to the fumagillin parent. *Biochem Biophys Res Commun* 1991, 174:1070–1076. Malone TE, Gray GS, Petro J, *et al.*: Inhibition of angiogenesis by recombinant human platelet factor-4 and related peptides. *Science* 1990, 247:77–79.) **C**, Other proposed therapies, not yet in clinical trials, include Tat antagonists (based on the ability of the *tat*-induced protein to stimulate KS-derived spindle cell proliferation *in vitro*). Antiestrogens, such as tamoxifen, can inhibit angiogenesis in the chick chorioallantoic membrane assay, an effect that is not inhibited by estrogens but which may be mediated by inhibition of protein kinase C. Both protein kinase C and tyrosine kinase may be involved in the intracellular signal transduction pathways through which angiostimulatory molecules, such as oncostatin M and vascular endothelial growth factor, exert their effects. The metalloproteinases are a group of enzymes important in the regulation of tumor growth, metastasis, and neovascularization. Naturally occurring inhibitors of these enzymes have been shown to inhibit tumor cell invasion and angiogenesis. (Gagliardi A, Collins DC: Inhibition of angiogenesis by antiestrogens. *Cancer Res* 1993, 53:533–535. de Vries C, Escobedo JA, Ueno H, *et al.*: The *fms*-like tyrosine kinase, a receptor for vascular endothelial growth factor. *Science* 1992, 255:989–991. Finkenzeller G, Marme D, Welch HA, *et al.*: Platelet-derived growth factor-induced transcription of the vascular endothelial growth factor gene is mediated by protein kinase C. *Cancer Res* 1992, 52:4821–4823. Albini A, Melchiori A, Santi L, *et al.*: Tumor cell invasion inhibited by TIMP-2. *J Natl Cancer Inst* 1991, 83:775–779.)

NON-HODGKIN'S LYMPHOMA

AIDS-associated non-Hodgkin's lymphoma

Approximately 3% of AIDS-defining illnesses
Up to 10% of patients with AIDS develop NHL during the course
  of disease
Risk of NHL increases with increasing survival from diagnosis of
  HIV infection
Histology
  Large-cell lymphomas (60% to 80%)
    Immunoblastic
    Diffuse large cell
  Small noncleaved (20% to 40%)
Primary CNS lymphomas comprise approx 15% to 17% of all
  HIV-associated lymphomas
All HIV risk groups at risk for NHL

FIGURE 16-26 The non-Hodgkin's lymphomas (NHL) account for approximately 3% of initial AIDS-defining diagnoses, but 10% or more of patients with AIDS develop NHL at some point in their disease. Unlike Kaposi's sarcoma, in which the annual risk of new onset remains constant through most of the disease course, the risk of developing NHL increases with time, particularly for patients with primary lymphomas of the central nervous system (CNS). HIV-associated lymphomas are usually of large-cell (high-grade immunoblastic or intermediate-grade diffuse large cell) or small noncleaved (high-grade Burkitt or non-Burkitt type) histology. Unlike Kaposi's sarcoma, NHL affects all HIV risk groups, although the incidence may be higher in homosexual or bisexual men and hemophiliacs than in intravenous drug users.

A. Biologic features of AIDS-associated NHL

Vast majority are B-cell neoplasms
Clonal Ig heavy- and light-chain gene rearrangements
No evidence that HIV is directly involved in malignant transformation of B cells
EBV in found in 40% to 50% of all AIDS-associated NHLs
  100% of NHLs in body cavities and primary CNS are EBV-
    positive
  100% of immunoblastic NHLs are EBV-positive
  25% to 30% of large cell or small noncleaved NHLs are EBV-
    positive
Possible role for IL-6 as growth factor for immunoblastic NHL

B. Genetic features of AIDS-associated NHL

Proto-oncogenes
  c-*myc* rearrangements occur in approx 80% of systemic
    AIDS-associated NHLs
    100% of small noncleaved NHLs
    ≤1/3 of immunoblastic plasmacytoid and large-cell NHLs
  N-*ras* or K-*ras* mutations occur in approx 15% of systemic
    AIDS-associated NHLs
  No *bcl*-1 or *bcl*-2 gene rearrangements

Tumor-suppresser genes
  p53 mutations occur in approx 1/3 of systemic AIDS-associ-
    ated NHLs
    Approx 2/3 of small noncleaved NHLs
    Rare or absent in immunoblastic plasmacytoid and large-
      cell NHLs
  No *RB* gene mutations

FIGURE 16-27 A, Biologic characteristics of NHL. The vast majority of AIDS-associated NHLs are B-cell tumors, most of which express monotypic surface Ig or B-cell-associated antigens and lack T-cell-associated antigens, similar to B-cell NHLs occurring in the absence of HIV infection. Some lymphomas, particularly those involving body cavities (eg, gastrointestinal tract), have an indeterminate immunophenotype that is typical of late stages of B-cell activation or differentiation and is similar to that of Epstein-Barr virus (EBV)-infected B cells. AIDS-associated NHLs of either immunophenotype show clonal Ig heavy- and light-chain gene rearrangements and lack clonal T-cell receptor β-chain rearrangements. (Knowles DM, Inghirami G, Ubriaco A, *et al.*: Molecular genetic analysis of three AIDS-associated neoplasms of uncertain lineage demonstrates their B-cell derivation and the possible pathogenetic role of the Epstein-Barr virus. *Blood* 1989, 73:792–799.) HIV sequences have not been identified in the genome of AIDS-associated NHLs, and there is no evidence that HIV is directly involved in the malignant transformation of B cells in these patients. In contrast, EBV sequences or EBV nuclear antigens have been identified in 40% to 50% of all AIDS-associated NHLs. There is evidence that EBV infection occurs prior to clonal expansion, leading to proliferation of genetically unstable immortalized B-cell clones that may undergo subsequent malignant transformation. The presence of EBV within AIDS-associated NHLs varies according to the anatomic site of origin and histologic type of NHL. For EBV-negative NHLs, other infectious agents may lead to the same sort of nonspecific B-cell activation that predisposes to malignant transformation. Recent data indicate that IL-6 may act as a growth factor for certain forms of high-grade NHL. (Ballerini P, Gaidano G, Gong JZ, *et al.*: Multiple genetic lesions in AIDS-related non-Hodgkin lymphoma. *Blood* 1993, 81:166–176.) **B,** Genetic characteristics of NHL. Several proto-oncogenes are associated with specific chromosomal translocations that are, in turn, associated with specific types of lymphoid neoplasia in patients without HIV infection. Among patients with HIV-associated systemic NHLs, approximately 80% show rearrangements of the c-*myc* gene. Rearrangements in c-*myc*, of the type associated in the general population with sporadic Burkitt's lymphoma, have been found in virtually 100% of small-noncleaved-cell NHLs, but in only a minority of large cell NHLs in HIV-infected patients. About 15% of systemic AIDS-associated NHLs show point mutations involving either the N-*ras* or K-*ras* gene, whereas in the general population such mutations are rarely associated with high- or intermediate-grade lymphomas. AIDS-associated NHLs consistently lack *bcl*-1 and *bcl*-2 gene rearrangements, which are associated in the general population with mantle cell and follicular center cell-derived NHLs. (Ballerini P, Gaidano G, Gong JZ, *et al.*: Multiple genetic lesions in AIDS-related non-Hodgkin lymphoma. *Blood* 1993, 81:166–176. Knowles DM, Inghirami G, Ubriaco A, *et al.*: Molecular genetic analysis of three AIDS-associated neoplasms of uncertain lineage demonstrates their B-cell derivation and the possible pathogenetic role of the Epstein-Barr virus. *Blood* 1989, 73:792–799.) Mutation or loss of the tumor suppressor genes *p53* and *RB* are believed to play an important role in the development and progression of various human tumors. Among AIDS-associated lymphomas, *p53* mutations have been demonstrated in almost two thirds of small-noncleaved-cell NHLs but are rare or absent among the large-cell NHLs. *RB* gene mutations or deletions, which occur in a small proportion of intermediate- and high-grade NHLs in the general population, have not been identified in AIDS-associated NHLs. (Ballerini P, Gaidano G, Gong JZ, *et al.*: Multiple genetic lesions in AIDS-related non-Hodgkin lymphoma. *Blood* 1993, 81:166–176.)

Clinical characteristics of systemic NHL

High frequency of extranodal involvement
  Meninges, bone marrow, GI tract, mucocutaneous sites
Advanced stage (III-IV) at presentation
Occurs at any point in HIV infection
Median survival 6–7 months for all patients, 12–15 months for
  complete responders to therapy
Longer survival associated with
  Karnofsky performance score > 70
  Localized disease (stage I or II)
  Absence of bone marrow involvement
  Absence of B symptoms
  No prior AIDS-defining diagnoses
  CD4 count > 100/mm³

FIGURE 16-28 Clinical characteristics. Clinically, the systemic NHLs associated with HIV infection are distinguished by their frequent extranodal presentation and advanced clinical stage at presentation. They may occur at any timepoint in the course of HIV infection. Although the overall median survival after diagnosis is only 6 to 7 months, patients whose tumors respond completely to chemotherapy show median survivals of 1 year or more.

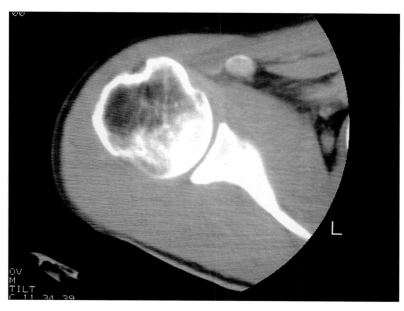

FIGURE 16-29 Extranodal presentation of an AIDS-associated NHL. A CT scan of the bone shows lymphomatous involvement of the head of the humerus.

Therapy for non-Hodgkin's lymphoma

Increased hematologic toxicity with full-dose, standard
  chemotherapy regimens
Reduced-dose regimens better tolerated
  46% complete response rate with reduced-dose m-BACOD
Dose-intensification possible with hematopoietic CSF
  Standard-dose m-BACOD tolerated with GM-CSF support
  5 of 8 complete responses at standard-dose m-BACOD, 3 with
    sustained remission at 19, 22, and 23 mos
Study in progress to compare low-dose m-Bacod vs standard-
  dose m-BACOD + GM-CSF (ACTG 142)

FIGURE 16-30 Treatment of systemic AIDS-associated NHLs has been complicated by the poor tolerance of many patients to chemotherapeutic regimens considered standard for treatment of NHLs in the general population. Modified-dose chemotherapeutic regimens have been reasonably well tolerated and have induced complete tumor regression in close to 50% of patients. The availability of myeloid colony-stimulating factors (CSF) made it possible to safely administer standard chemotherapeutic dosage regimens to the majority of patients with AIDS-associated NHLs. Prospective, randomized studies are in progress (ACTG142) to determine whether use of the more intensive regimens, made possible by the use of CSFs, will result in more frequent or prolonged remissions (Kaplan L, *et al.*: unpublished data). (m-BACOD—methotrexate, bleomycin, doxorubicin, cyclophosphamide, vincristine, dexamethasone.) (Levine AM, Wernz JC, Kaplan L, *et al.*: Low dose chemotherapy with CNS prophylaxis and zidovudine maintenance in AIDS-related lymphomas: A prospective multi-institutional trial. *JAMA* 1991, 266:84–88. Walsh C, Wernz JC, Levine AM, *et al.*: Phase I trial of m-BACOD and granulocyte macrophage colony stimulating factor in HIV-associated non-Hodgkin's lymphoma. *J Acquir Immune Defic Syndr* 1993, 6:265–271.)

Predictors of therapeutic response in non-Hodgkin's lymphoma

Response correlates with factors that reflect severity of immunodeficiency
  65% complete response rate with dose-intensive chemother-
    apy in patients with good PS, no OI
  50% 2-year survival in patients with CD4 >100/mm³, good PS,
    no B symptoms, nonimmunoblastic histology
  14% complete response and 3.5-month median survival in
    patients with poor PS and/or history of OI treated with low-
    dose chemotherapy and zidovudine

FIGURE 16-31 Response to treatment in AIDS-associated NHLs is correlated with factors reflective of the degree of HIV-induced immunodeficiency. Among patients with a high performance status (PS) and no history of opportunistic infection (OI), an intensive chemotherapy regimen was reported to induce a complete response rate of 65%, with 50% of patients showing a 2-year survival. In contrast, among patients with a poor performance status or history of opportunistic infection, a less intensive chemotherapy regimen (chosen to avoid severe toxicity) induced only a 14% complete response rate and a median survival of only 3.5 months. (Gisselbrecht C, Oksenhendler E, Tirelli U, *et al.*: Non-Hodgkin's lymphoma associated with human immunodeficiency virus: Treatment with NHL84 regimen in a selected group of patients. *Leukemia* 1992, 6(suppl 3):105–115. Tirelli U, Errante D, Oksenhendler E, *et al.*: Prospective study with combined low-dose chemotherapy and zidovudine in 37 patients with poor-prognosis AIDS-related non-Hodgkin's lymphoma. *Ann Oncol* 1992, 3:843–847.)

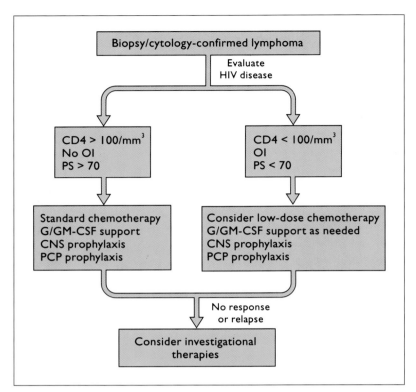

FIGURE 16-32 Management schema for systemic lymphomas in HIV-infected patients. Whereas patients with good prognostic features may benefit from standard chemotherapy with growth factor support, central nervous system (CNS) prophylaxis for meningeal lymphoma, and opportunistic infection (OI) prophylaxis, those with far-advanced HIV disease may realistically be offered the option of no treatment or cautious treatment with modified-dose chemotherapy. Newer, investigational therapies may be considered for some patients who fail to respond to standard agents or who relapse after an initial response. (PCP—*Pneumocystis carinii* pneumonia; PS—performance scale.)

Investigational approaches to treatment of non-Hodgkin's lymphoma

Radiolabeled or toxin-conjugated monoclonal antibodies
Interleukin-4
Interleukin-2 + zidovudine
MGBG
Topoisomerase inhibitors

FIGURE 16-33 Investigational treatment approaches to AIDS-associated lymphomas include a variety of radiolabeled or toxin-conjugated monoclonal antibodies that may selectively target neoplastic B cells; interleukin-4 (which may down-regulate the production of IL-6, a growth factor for some AIDS-associated NHLs); the combination of interleukin-2 with zidovudine (in a small clinical trial, it induced complete responses in 2 of 12 patients); and chemotherapeutic agents including methyl-glyoxal-*bis*-guanylhydrazone (MGBG) and topoisomerase inhibitors. (Mazza P, Bocchia M, Tumietto F, *et al.*: Recombinant interleukin-2 in acquired immunodeficiency syndrome: Preliminary report in patients with lymphoma associated with HIV infection. *Eur J Haematol* 1992, 49:1–6.)

PRIMARY CNS LYMPHOMA

Clinical features of primary CNS lymphoma

Associated with advanced-stage HIV disease
Prior AIDS-defining illness
Low CD4 count
Clinical presentations may be subtle
Multiple visions common
Frequent delays in diagnosis
Short survival (2–3 months) without treatment
Improved neurologic function, quality-of-life, and survival after whole-brain radiotherapy

FIGURE 16-34 AIDS-associated primary CNS lymphomas generally are diagnosed in patients at advanced stages of HIV infection, usually after one or more AIDS-defining illnesses have been diagnosed. Although the primary CNS lymphomas may present with typical signs of a space-occupying lesion of the brain (*eg*, seizures, hemiparesis), the clinical presentation is often subtle, with confusion, memory loss, or lethargy as the only sign of disease. Radiographically, single or multiple lesions may be present on CT or MRI scans, and the lesions often show ring-enhancement after administration of intravenous contrast. Often, because of the subtlety of clinical signs, the similarity of the radiographic picture to that of toxoplasmosis, and the reluctance of many physicians to recommend biopsy of intracranial lesions in patients with advanced HIV disease, the diagnosis is delayed. Without treatment, survival after a diagnosis of primary CNS lymphoma is short, averaging a few months. With whole-brain radiation therapy, improved neurologic function, quality of life, and survival have been reported in several studies. Because the success of treatment is likely to depend on the duration of neurologic dysfunction, early diagnosis is essential to improving treatment outcomes. (Baumgartner JE, Rachlin JR, Beckstead JH, *et al.*: Primary central nervous system lymphoma: Natural history and response to radiation therapy in 55 patients with acquired immunodeficiency syndrome. *J Neurosurg* 1990, 73:206–211. Nisce LZ, Metroka C: Radiation therapy in patients with AIDS-related central nervous system lymphoma. *JAMA* 1992, 267:1921–1922.)

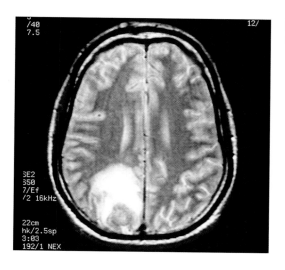

FIGURE 16-35 The CT scan appearance of a large lymphoma lesion, with ring enhancement after contrast administration, in a patient with AIDS.

Differential diagnosis of brain masses in HIV-infected people

Toxoplasmosis
Usually ring-enhancing
Usually multiple
Mass effect
Antibody (IgG) present

Primary CNS lymphoma
Ring-enhancing or homogeneous
Single or multiple (50:50)
Mass effect

Progressive multifocal leukoencephalopathy
Nonenhancing
Usually multiple
Lesions confined to subcortical white matter
No mass effect

FIGURE 16-36 Differential diagnoses. Although other conditions, such as pyogenic abscesses, tuberculosis, and cryptococcosis, may cause brain masses in HIV-infected people, the most common causes are toxoplasmosis, primary CNS lymphoma, and progressive multifocal leukoencephalopathy (PML). PML lesions are usually distinguishable by their location and lack of contrast enhancement. In distinguishing between toxoplasmosis and primary CNS lymphoma, the absence of IgG antitoxoplasma antibodies should prompt early attempts at obtaining a definitive tissue diagnosis.

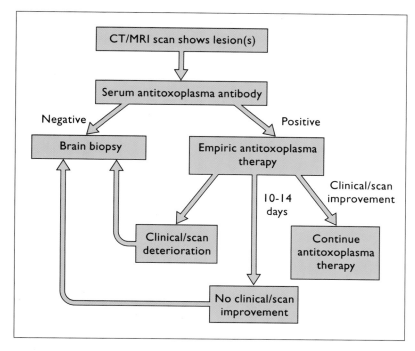

FIGURE 16-37 Evaluation of a patient with ring-enhancing brain lesions. In such patients, empiric antitoxoplasma therapy may be attempted before proceeding with brain biopsy, which can often be obtained through CT-guided stereotactic methods. Patients who deteriorate or in whom no improvement occurs after a 10–14 day course of treatment should be referred promptly for biopsy. The use of corticosteroids to treat brain edema may lead to temporary clinical and radiographic improvement of primary CNS lymphoma in a toxoplasma-seropositive individual, obscuring the true diagnosis. It should also be kept in mind that coexistent primary CNS lymphoma and toxoplasmosis has been reported.

HODGKIN'S DISEASE

Hodgkin's disease in association with HIV infection

Increased incidence in association with HIV is controversial
High incidence of advanced-stage (III or IV) disease
Frequent bone marrow involvement
Predominance of mixed cellularity phenotype
Median survival <1 year
Decreased response rates to standard chemotherapy
  50% complete response to MOPP or MOPP/ABVD
Decreased duration of complete response

FIGURE 16-38 Although controversy exists about whether Hodgkin's disease occurs with increased incidence among HIV-infected patients, among the nearly 200 cases of Hodgkin's disease reported in patients known to be or considered at high risk for HIV infection, the disease clearly behaves in an atypical and aggressive manner. These features are all unusual among non–HIV-infected patients with Hodgkin's disease.

ANOGENITAL SQUAMOUS CANCER

Human papilloma virus infection and anogenital neoplasia

Anogenital neoplasia associated with chronic immunosuppression in organ transplant recipients
  100 times increase in valvar and anal cancers
  144 times increase in cervical cancers
  High prevalence of detectable anogenital HPV infection
HPV genotypes 16, 18, and 31 associated with cervialc and anal cancers
  E6 gene of HPV-16 binds to p53 protein
  E7 gene of HPV-16 binds to RB protein

FIGURE 16-39 There is a clear association between immunodeficiency and the development of anal and cervical malignancies. Among organ transplant recipients, a marked increase is seen in the incidence of cancers of the entire anogenital tract. Anogenital tract infection with human papillomavirus (HPV) is also found with increased frequency in such patients, and particular HPV genotypes have been strongly associated with intraepithelial and invasive neoplasia. Several HPV gene products bind to the tumor-suppressor genes *p53* and *RB*, which are believed to be essential regulators of normal cell growth. (Werness BA, Levine AJ, Howley PM: Association of human papillomavirus types 16 and 18 E6 proteins with p53. *Science* 1990, 248:76–79. Dyson N, Howley PM, Munger K, *et al.*: The human papilloma virus-16 E7 oncoprotein is able to bind the retinoblastoma gene product. *Science* 1989, 243:934–937.)

A. Invasive cervical cancer and HIV infection

Classified as an AIDS-defining condition in 1993
Increased frequency of advanced disease at presentation
Increased frequency of persistent or recurrent disease after standard therapy

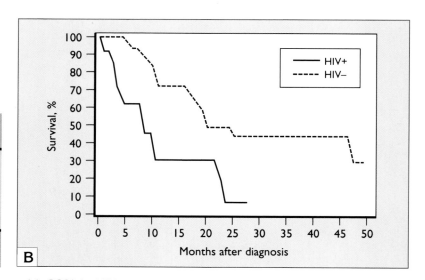

B

FIGURE 16-40 A, Invasive cervical cancer in HIV-positive women was classified as an AIDS-defining condition in 1993, based on studies showing that the clinical presentation and response to treatment differed in HIV-infected women compared with HIV-negative women. Women with HIV infection were significantly more likely to present with advanced-stage disease (bulky stage IB or greater); almost 70% had stage III or IV disease, compared with 28% in HIV-seronegative women. **B,** After standard treatment, women with HIV infection were also significantly more likely to show persistent or recurrent disease than HIV-seronegative subjects, and they also showed a shorter time to recurrence and death. (Maiman M, Fruchter RG, Guy L, *et al.*: Human immunodeficiency virus infection and invasive cervical carcinoma. *Cancer* 1993, 71:402–406.)

Invasive anal cancer and HIV infection

Incidence increasing in young unmarried men in San Francisco
 Odds ratio 2.6 for 1986 to 1987 compared with 1973 to 1978
Surgical excision associated with poor treatment outcome and
 short survival

FIGURE 16-41 Few data are available about the presentation and outcome of invasive anal cancer in HIV-infected individuals. Epidemiologic evidence has confirmed an increased odds ratio for the detection of anal cancers in young, unmarried men in San Francisco between 1986 and 1987 compared with a pre-HIV time period. Poor treatment outcomes after surgery and short survivals, similar to that seen with invasive cervical cancer, have been reported in small series. (Lorenz HP, Wilson W, Leigh B, *et al.*: Squamous cell carcinoma of the anus and HIV infection. *Dis Colon Rectum* 1991, 34:336–338. Rabkin CS, Biggar RJ, Horn J: Cancer trends associated with increasing AIDS. In the Proceedings of the VI International Conference on AIDS, San Francisco, 1990, 1:295. Svensson C, Kaigas M, Lindbrink E, *et al.*: Carcinoma of the anal canal in a patient with AIDS. *Acta Oncol* 1991, 30:8986–8991.)

Screening for anogenital neoplasia in HIV-infected individuals

Cervical neoplasia
Annual Pap smear (every 6 months for women at high risk for
 HPV infection)
Consider colposcopy, especially in women at high risk for HPV

Anal neoplasia
Anal Pap smear
Anoscopy with biopsy of abnormal areas

FIGURE 16-42 Given the poor results of treatment of invasive anogenital neoplasia in HIV-infected people and the possibility of cure if lesions are detected at a preinvasive stage, regular screening is recommended. For all HIV-infected women, an annual Papanicolaou (Pap) smear should be performed. The frequency of Pap smears should probably be increased in women at high risk for dysplasia and HPV infection (CD4 count <200/mm^3, multiple sexual partners, or partner with HIV infection). Some investigators advocate routine colposcopy, as the routine Pap smear may not detect cervical neoplasia in some patients. Although there are no general agreed-upon guidelines for screening for anal neoplasia, techniques are available to perform anal Pap smears, and some investigators advocate their use in conjunction with routine anoscopy. (Maiman M, Tarricons N, Viera J, *et al.*: Colposcopic evaluation of human immunodeficiency virus seropositive women. *Obstet Gynecol* 1991, 78:84–88.)

Cancers after organ transplantation: Lesions for HIV infection

Cancers develop in approx 6% of all transplant recipients
Increase confined to
 NHLs
 KA
 Squamous cell cancers of lip of skin
 Carcinomas of vulva and perineum
 Cancers of kidney and hepatobiliary system
Variation in mean time to development of tumors after transplantation

KS	20 mos
NHL	33 mos
Vulva/perineum tumors	107 mos

Increased incidence and earlier appearance of NHLs and KS
 with use of immunosuppressive regimens containing
 cyclosporine and/or antilymphocyte antibodies (OKT3)

FIGURE 16-43 The increased frequency and aggressive behavior of certain cancers in HIV-infected people show strong parallels to findings in organ transplant recipients. Overall, 6% of such patients go on to develop malignancies. Although there is no apparent increase in the frequency of cancers that are common in the general population, the incidence of rarer tumors, including Kaposi's sarcoma (KS) and non-Hodgkin's lymphomas (NHLs), is increased, and such tumors often show the aggressive behavior seen in patients with HIV-associated neoplasia. As has been observed in the AIDS epidemic, KS generally presents relatively soon after the institution of immunosuppressive therapy, followed by NHLs and, much later, by female genital tract cancers. Other tumors in transplant recipients have appeared after a mean of 5–6 years. Thus, as advances lead to longer survival in profoundly immunosuppressed patients with HIV infection, it is conceivable that the incidence of other cancers will increase. In addition, the use of more intensive immunosuppressive regimens—which have led to improved transplant survival and which have been proposed to counter the immune system activation in HIV infection—has the potential to increase the frequency and speed the appearance of both NHL and KS. (Penn I: Cancer complicating organ transplantation. *N Engl J Med* 1990, 323:1767–1769.)

SELECTED BIBLIOGRAPHY

Knowles DM: Biologic aspects of AIDS-associated non-Hodgkin's lymphoma. *Curr Opin Oncol* 1993, 5:845–851.

Pluda JM, Parkinson DR, Feigal E, Yarchoan R: Noncytotoxic approaches to the treatment of HIV-associated Kaposi's sarcoma. *Oncology* 1993, 7(12):25–33.

Krown SE, Myskowski PL, Paredes J: Kaposi's sarcoma. *Med Clin North Am* 1992, 76:235–252.

Northfelt DW: Cervical and anal neoplasia and HPV infection in persons with HIV infection. *Oncology* 1994, 8(1):33–37.

Levine AM: Acquired immunodeficiency syndrome-related lymphoma. *Blood* 1992, 80:8–20.

CHAPTER 17

Antiviral Treatments

Margaret A. Fischl

ANTI-HIV DRUG DEVELOPMENT

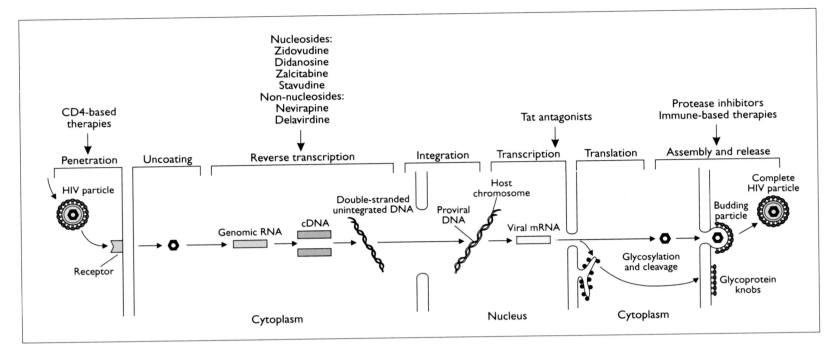

FIGURE 17-1 The life cycle of HIV and targets for antiretroviral therapy. Development of anti-HIV drugs hinges on knowledge of the replication cycle of HIV. Infection with HIV begins with the binding of the envelope protein gp120 to the cellular receptor CD4. The viral core can then enter cells, and the RNA genome is converted to a DNA copy via reverse transcription. A linear, dou- ble-stranded provirus is subsequently integrated into host chro- mosomes and transcribed into messenger RNA (mRNA). mRNA is translated to make precursor proteins, which are cleaved to form mature viral particles via a protease enzyme. (*Adapted from* Hirsch MS, D'Aquila RT: Therapy for human immunodeficiency virus. *N Engl J Med* 1993, 328:1686–1695.)

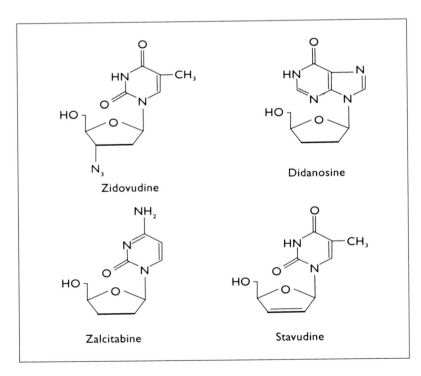

FIGURE 17-2 Inhibitors of reverse transcriptase are the most common drugs currently approved by the Food and Drug Administration (FDA) or under investigation for the treatment of HIV infection. The best known of these agents are dideoxynucleo- side analogs and include zidovudine (ZDV), didanosine (ddI), zal- citabine (ddC), and stavudine (d4T). (*Adapted from* Balzarini J, DeClercq E: Biochemical pharmacology of nucleoside analogs active against HIV. *In* Broder S, Merigan TC, Bolognesi D (eds): *Textbook of AIDS Medicine.* Baltimore: Williams & Wilkins; 1994:751–772.)

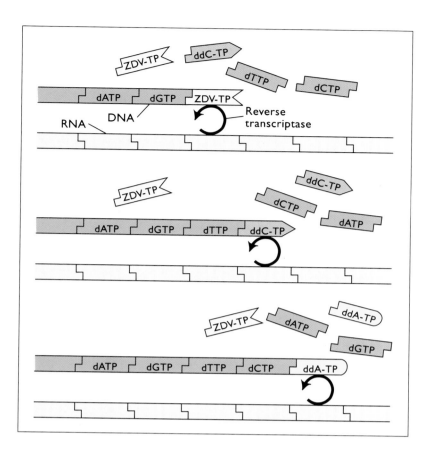

FIGURE 17-3 The dideoxynucleosides exert anti-HIV activity at the reverse transcriptase level. As triphosphates, they compete with cellular dideoxynucleoside-5'-triphosphates, and they act as chain terminators in the synthesis of proviral DNA, thereby interfering with elongation of the viral DNA chain. (dda-TP—the active triphosphate form of didanosine [ddI]). (*From* Fischl MA: Combination antiretroviral therapy for HIV infection. *Hosp Pract* 1994, 29:43–48; with permission.)

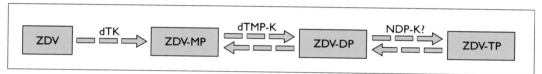

FIGURE 17-4 Zidovudine (ZDV) is a thymidine analog that is phosphorylated by cellular enzymes (2'-deoxy)thymidine kinase (dTK) to its monophosphate form (ZDV-MP), (2'-deoxy)thymidylate kinase (dTMP-K) to its diphosphate form (ZDV-DP), and nucleoside 5'-diphosphate kinase (NDP-K) to an active triphosphate form (ZDV-TP). Zidovudine triphosphate inhibits the replication of HIV by interfering with viral reverse transcriptase and elongation of the viral DNA chain. (*Adapted from* Balzarini J, DeClercq E: Biochemical pharmacology of nucleoside analogs active against HIV. *In* Broder S, Merigan TC, Bolognesi D (eds): *Textbook of AIDS Medicine.* Baltimore: Williams & Wilkins; 1994:751–772.)

ZIDOVUDINE EFFICACY

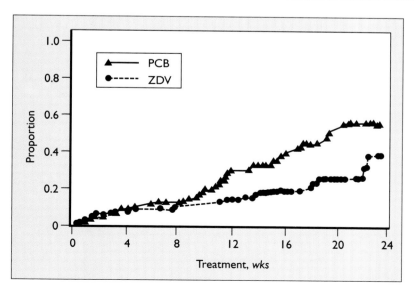

FIGURE 17-5 The first study on disease progression on zidovudine. The proportion of patients with opportunistic infections is shown for 85 AIDS patients assigned to receive 1500 mg/d of zidovudine (ZDV) and 75 to placebo (PCB). This subgroup of patients had AIDS prior to entry in the study. Because this was the first clinical trial to demonstrate the efficacy of zidovudine, no patient had any prior anti-HIV therapy. The probability of disease progression over 24 weeks was significantly lower, 0.23, for the zidovudine group than for the placebo group (0.43; $P<0.001$). (*From* Fischl MA, Richman DD, Grieco MH, *et al.*: The efficacy of azidothymidine [AZT] in the treatment of patients with AIDS and AIDS-related complex: A double-blind, placebo-controlled trial. *N Engl J Med* 1987, 317:185–191; with permission.)

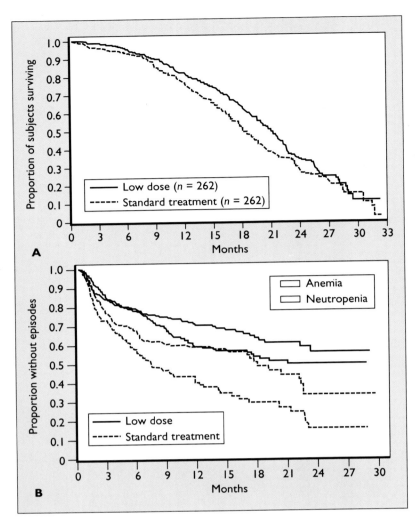

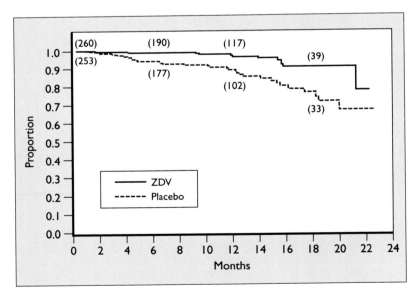

FIGURE 17-6 Low-dose vs high-dose zidovudine. Two hundred sixty-two patients were assigned to receive 600 mg/d of zidovudine (ZDV) and 262 patients to receive 1500 mg/d of ZDV (standard or high-dose treatment). Patients had a first episode of *Pneumocystis carinii* pneumonia with at least 2 weeks of enrollment in the study. **A**, Cumulative survival. Overall, 169 patients died in the 600-mg/d group and 188 in the 1500-mg/d group. A significantly better survival ($P=0.019$) was noted with low-dose zidovudine therapy (600 mg/d). However, a high fatality rate was noted over time for both groups. **B**, Overall, a significantly different delay in the time to a first episode of anemia (hemoglobin < 80 g/L) and neutropenia (< 750/mL) was noted for the low-dose zidovudine group (600 mg/d) compared with the high-dose group (1500 mg/d; $P=0.006$ and 0.009, respectively). The current recommended dose of zidovudine is 600 mg/d in patients with symptomatic HIV disease. (*From* Fischl MA, Parker CB, Pettinelli C, *et al.*: A randomized controlled trial of a reduced daily dose of zidovudine in patients with the acquired immunodeficiency syndrome. *N Engl J Med* 1990, 323:1009–1014; with permission.)

FIGURE 17-7 Cumulative disease-free survival, zidovudine vs placebo. Two hundred sixty patients were assigned to receive 1200 mg/d of zidovudine (*solid line*) and 260 to receive placebo (*dashed line*). Patients had minimally symptomatic HIV disease and 200–500 CD4 cells/mL. Overall, 12 patients in the zidovudine group had disease progression compared with 34 in the placebo group. Zidovudine therapy resulted in a more than threefold decrease in the risk of disease progression in this study compared with placebo by 18 months (3.23; 95% confidence interval [CI] = 1.67–6.24; $P=0.0002$). (*From* Fischl MA, Richman DD, Hansen N, *et al.*: The safety and efficacy of zidovudine [AZT] in the treatment of subjects with mildly symptomatic human immunodeficiency virus infection: A double-blind, placebo-controlled trial. *Ann Intern Med* 1990, 112:727–737; with permission.)

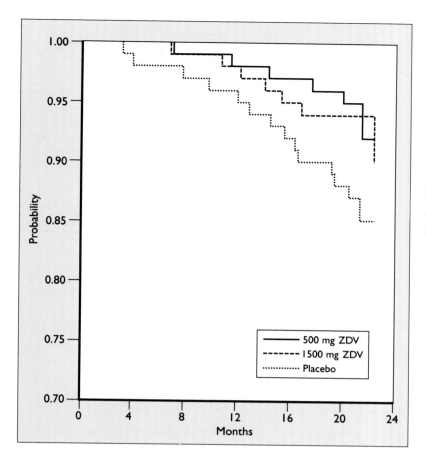

Figure 17-8 Cumulative AIDS-free survival, zidovudine vs placebo. Four hundred fifty-three patients were assigned to receive 500 mg/d of zidovudine (*solid line*), 457 to receive 1500 mg/d of zidovudine (*dashed line*), and 428 to receive placebo (*dotted line*). Patients had asymptomatic HIV disease and < 500 CD4 cells/mL. Overall, 11 patients in the 500-mg group, 14 in the 1500-mg group, and 33 in the placebo group developed AIDS. Zidovudine therapy resulted in a twofold decrease in the risk of AIDS for the 500-mg group (rate=2.3, *P*=0.002) and a threefold decrease for the 1500-mg group (rate=3.1; *P*=0.005) compared with placebo (rate=6.6) over 12 months. (*From* Volberding PA, Lagakos SW, Koch MA, *et al.*: Zidovudine in asymptomatic human immunodeficiency virus infection: A controlled trial in persons with fewer than 500 CD4-positive cells per cubic millimeter. *N Engl J Med* 1990, 322:941–949; with permission.)

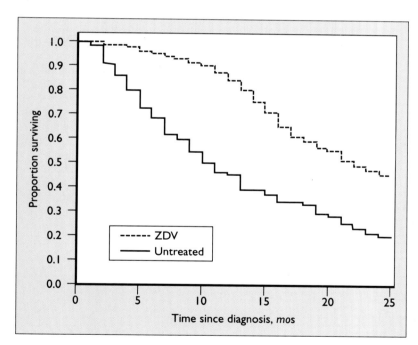

Figure 17-9 Cumulative survival, zidovudine vs no treatment. One hundred fifty-nine patients were treated with zidovudine (*dashed line*) and 112 were untreated (*solid line*) in a nonrandomized contemporary observational study. The median survival time for the zidovudine group was 22.1 months compared with 10.6 months in the untreated group. This study shows significant survival benefits for zidovudine over the 2-year follow-up period (*P*<0.001). (*From* Vella S, Giuliano M, Pezzotti P, *et al.*: Survival of zidovudine-treated patients with AIDS compared with that of contemporary untreated patients. *JAMA* 1992, 267:1232–1236; with permission.)

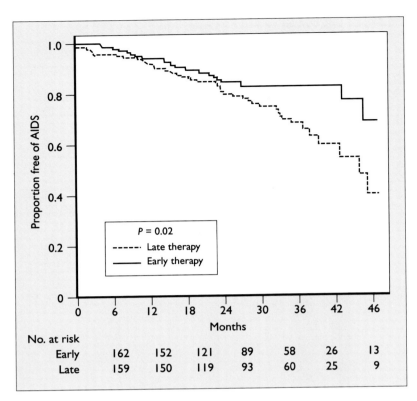

FIGURE 17-10 Cumulative AIDS-free survival, early vs late zidovudine. One hundred seventy patients with early zidovudine treatment (*solid line*) and 168 with late zidovudine treatment (*dashed line*) were compared. Patients had symptomatic HIV disease and 200–500 CD4 cells/mL. Delaying zidovudine therapy until the CD4 cell count fell to < 200 cells/mL or until the development of AIDS was associated with higher rates of disease progression, more rapid decline in CD4 cells, and greater risk for the development of p24 antigenemia. (*From* Hamilton JD, Hartigan PM, Simberkoff MS, *et al.*: A controlled trial of early versus late treatment with zidovudine in symptomatic human immunodeficiency virus infection: Results of the Veterans Affairs cooperative study. *N Engl J Med* 1992, 326:437–443; with permission.)

NUCLEOSIDE DRUG RESISTANCE

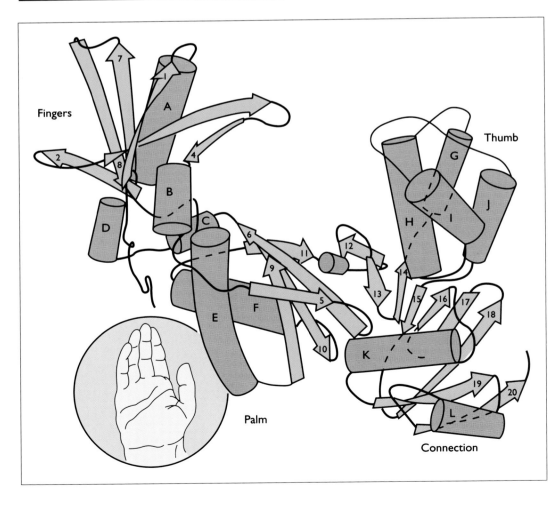

FIGURE 17-11 p66 subunit of HIV reverse transcriptase. The folding structure of the p66 subunit of the HIV reverse transcriptase has been compared to a right hand. Helical regions are presented by *letter tubes* and β-strands are presented by *number arrows*. This subunit is the target for reverse transcriptase inhibitors and identifies the binding sites for nucleoside and nonnucleoside reverse transcriptase inhibitors. Mutations in several amino acid residues will confer drug resistance to both nucleoside and nonnucleoside reverse transcriptase inhibitors. (*From* Richman DD: Viral resistance to antiretroviral therapy. *In* Broder S, Merigan TC, Bolognesi D (eds): *Textbook of AIDS Medicine.* Baltimore: Williams & Wilkins; 1994; with permission.)

HIV reverse transcriptase codon mutation site	Amino acid substitution	Associated resistance
41 Methionine	Leucine	ZDV
67 Aspartate	Asparagine	ZDV
69 Threonine 70 Lysine	Aspartate	ddC
74 Leucine	Arginine	ZDV
	Valine	ddl, ddC
215 Threonine	Tyrosine or phenylalanine	ZDV
219 Lysine	Glycine	ZDV

FIGURE 17-12 Specific mutation sites on the *pol* gene, which codes for the reverse transcriptase, have been noted to confer resistance to several nucleoside analogues. Zidovudine (ZDV) resistance is associated with a stepwise decrease in susceptibilities and associated with mutations at sites 41, 67, 70, 215, and 219, with sites 41, 70, and 215 being the most important sites of mutations. Didanosine (ddl) resistance has been associated with mutations at site 74 in patients with zidovudine resistance, and resistance to zalcitabine (ddC) has been associated with mutations at sites 69 and 74. (McLeod GX, Hammer SM: Nucleoside analogues: Combination therapy. *Hosp Prac (of Ed)* 1992, 27:14–25.)

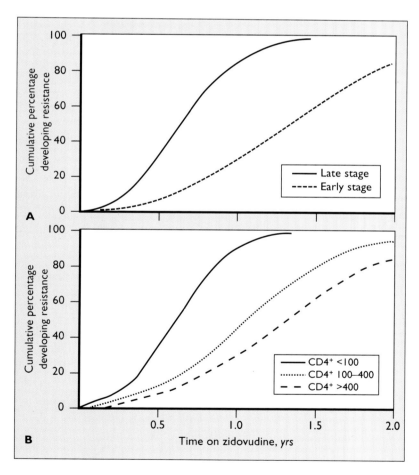

FIGURE 17-13 The rate of change in susceptibility of viral isolates to zidovudine is associated with the stage of disease. **A,** Patients with late-stage disease (AIDS or symptoms and < 200 CD4 cells/mL) are significantly more likely to develop resistance than those with early-stage disease (P=0.002). **B,** Similar findings have been noted when using pretreatment CD4 cell counts. Overall, patients with < 100 CD4 cells/mL are more likely to develop resistance earlier in the course of treatment than patients with > 100 CD4 cells/mL. (*From* Richman DD, Grimes JM, Lagakos SW: Effect of stage of disease and drug dose on zidovudine susceptibilities of isolates of human immunodeficiency virus. *J Acquir Immune Defic Syndr* 1990, 3:743–746; with permission.)

ZIDOVUDINE TOXICITY

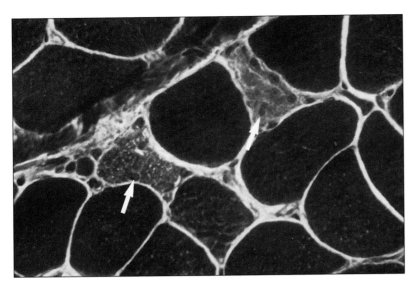

FIGURE 17-14 Zidovudine myopathy. A muscle biopsy specimen from a patient who had been treated with zidovudine for 24 months shows changes consistent with myopathy. Accumulation of fine reddish granules in the sarcoplasm, corresponding to mitochondria in atrophic fibers (trichrome; original magnification × 600), is noted. In addition, the fibers show marked myofilamentous abnormalities that include myofibrillar loss and cytoplasmic-body formation (*arrow*). Zidovudine myopathy is typically seen after prolonged therapy and is associated with muscle pain and tenderness, elevation in serum creatine kinase, and muscle wasting. (*From* Chariot P: Zidovudine myopathy. *N Engl J Med* 1993, 328:1675; with permission.)

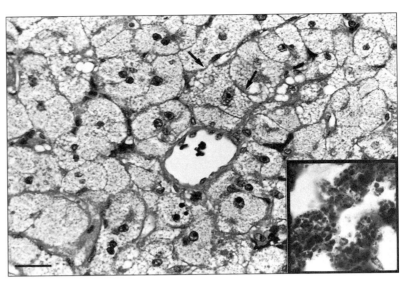

FIGURE 17-15 Liver toxicity. A liver biopsy specimen with microvesicular fatty changes following didanosine therapy. Hepatocytes surrounding a central vein show striking cytoplasmic clarity, resulting from microvesicular fatty changes (hematoxylin and eosin; original magnification × 600). Small droplet nature of these changes, shown on the inset, is confirmed by frozen-section fat stain (Oil Red; original magnification × 600). Steatosis associated with fulminant hepatic failure with or without lactic acidosis has been associated with nucleoside therapy, especially zidovudine and, to a lesser extent, didanosine. Elevation in serum transaminases with hepatosplenomegaly should alert the physician to this syndrome. (*From* Lai KK, Gang DL, Zawacki JK, Cooley TP: Fulminant hepatic failure associated with 2',3'-dideoxyinosine [ddI]. *Ann Intern Med* 1991, 115:283–284; with permission.)

DIDANOSINE

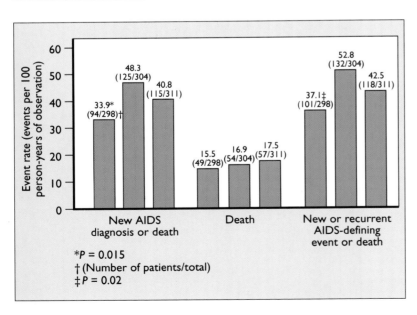

FIGURE 17-16 Disease progression, didanosine vs zidovudine. Event rates (per 100 person-years of observation) are shown for 298 patients assigned to 500 mg/d of didanosine (*solid bars*), 311 patients to 750 mg/d of didanosine (weight-adjusted, *crosshatched bars*), and 304 to 600 mg/d zidovudine (*open bars*). Patients had advanced HIV disease and < 300 CD4 cells/mL and had tolerated an average of 14 months of previous zidovudine therapy. Overall, the event rate (disease progression or death) was significantly lower for patients in the 500-mg/d didanosine group than the zidovudine group. (*From* Kahn JO, Lagakos SW, Richman DD, *et al.*: A controlled trial comparing continued zidovudine with didanosine in human immunodeficiency virus infection. *N Engl J Med* 1992, 327:581–587; with permission.)

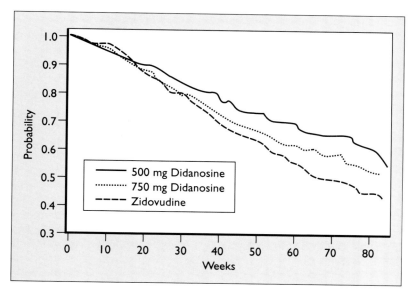

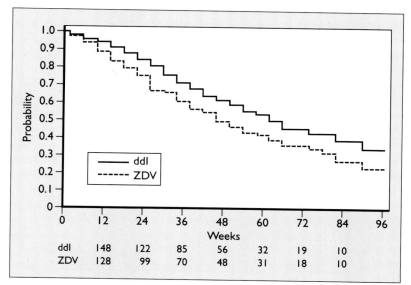

FIGURE 17-17 Probability of disease progression, didanosine vs zidovudine. Two hundred ninety-eight patients were assigned to receive 500 mg/d of didanosine (*solid line*), 311 to receive 750 mg/d of didanosine (*dotted line*), and 304 to receive 600 mg/d of zidovudine (*dashed line*). Patients had advanced HIV disease and < 300 CD4 cells/mL and had tolerated an average of 14 months of previous zidovudine therapy. 500 mg/d of didanosine was associated with a threefold decrease in disease progression compared with continuing zidovudine (relative risk [RR]=1.39; 95% CI=1.06–1.82; *P*=0.0015). Similar findings were not noted comparing 750 mg/d of didanosine with zidovudine (RR=1.10; 95% CI=0.86–142; *P*=0.45). (*From* Kahn JO, Lagakos SW, Richman DD, *et al.*: A controlled trial comparing continued zidovudine with didanosine in human immunodeficiency virus infection. *N Engl J Med* 1992, 327:581–587; with permission.)

FIGURE 17-18 Cumulative disease-free survival, didanosine vs zidovudine. One hundred sixty patients were assigned to receive didanosine (*solid line*) and 152 to receive 600 mg/d of zidovudine (*dashed line*). All patients had received and tolerated prior zidovudine therapy but had disease progression while on therapy. A total of 67 patients had disease progression or died in the didanosine group and 82 in the zidovudine group. Overall, didanosine was associated with a better outcome compared with continuing zidovudine in this group of patients (RR=1.5; 95% CI=1.1–2.0; *P*=0.02). (*From* Spotswood LS, Pavia AT, Peterson D, *et al.*: Didanosine compared with continuation of zidovudine in HIV-infected patients with signs of clinical deterioration while receiving zidovudine: A randomized, double-blind clinical trial. *Ann Intern Med* 1994, 120:360–368; with permission.)

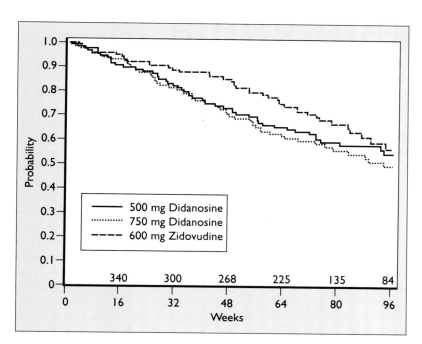

FIGURE 17-19 Cumulative disease-free survival, didanosine vs zidovudine. One hundred twenty-seven patients were assigned to receive 500 mg/d of didanosine (*solid line*), 122 to receive 750 mg/d of didanosine (*dotted line*), and 131 to receive 600 mg/d of zidovudine (*dashed line*). Patients had advanced HIV disease and < 300 CD4 cells/mL and had not received prior zidovudine therapy. Overall, 32% of patients had new disease progression or died in the 500-mg/d didanosine group, 37% in the 750-mg/d didanosine group, and 27% in the zidovudine group. Zidovudine was found to be superior to 750 mg/d of didanosine (RR=1.43, 90% CI=1.02–2.00) as initial therapy for the treatment of patients with advanced HIV disease. A similar trend was noted when comparing the zidovudine group with the 500-mg/d didanosine group (RR=1.21, 90% CI=0.86–1.71). (*From* Dolin R, Amato D, Fischl M, *et al.*: Efficacy of didanosine [ddl] versus zidovudine [ZDV] in patients with no or ≤ 16 weeks of prior ZDV therapy. Presented at the IX International Conference on AIDS, Berlin, June 1993, Abstract WS-B24-1.)

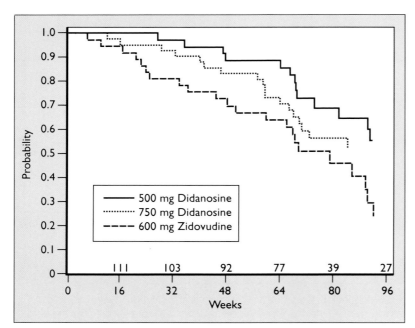

FIGURE 17-20 Cumulative disease-free survival, didanosine vs zidovudine. Thirty-six patients were assigned to receive 500 mg/d of didanosine (*solid line*), 42 to receive 750 mg/d of didanosine (*dotted line*), and 40 to receive 600 mg/d of zidovudine (*dashed line*). Patients had advanced HIV disease and < 300 CD4 cells/mL and had tolerated 8–16 weeks of prior zidovudine therapy. Overall, 25% of patients had new disease progression or died in the 500-mg/d didanosine group, 32% in the 750-mg/d didanosine group, and 53% in the zidovudine group. 500 mg/d of didanosine was associated with a twofold decrease in new disease progression compared with continuing zidovudine (RR=0.48, 90% CI=0.27–0.86). A similar trend was noted when comparing the 750 mg/d of didanosine to zidovudine (RR=0.61, 90% CI=0.36–1.03). (*From* Dolin R, Amato D, Fischl M, *et al.*: Efficacy of didanosine [ddI] versus zidovudine [ZDV] in patients with no or ≤ 16 weeks of prior ZDV therapy. Presented at the IX International Conference on AIDS, Berlin, June 1993, Abstract WS-B24-1.)

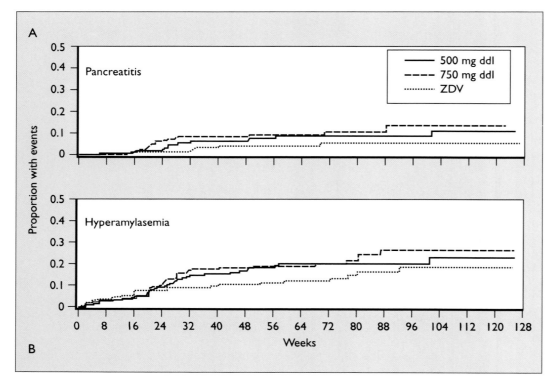

FIGURE 17-21 Toxicities of didanosine. One hundred ninety-seven patients were assigned to receive 500 mg/d of didanosine (*solid line*), 208 to receive 750 mg/d of didanosine (*dashed line*), and 212 to receive 600 mg/d of zidovudine (*dotted line*). All patients had advanced HIV disease and < 300 CD4 cells/mL, and had < 16 weeks of previous zidovudine therapy or no previous therapy. Toxicities in this study reflect use of a sachet formulation. **A,** Pancreatitis is the most common side effect to date associated with didanosine therapy. A slightly higher 1-year rate for pancreatitis is noted with the 750-mg/d didanosine group (9%) than the 500-mg/d didanosine group (7%). **B,** Annual rates for hyperamylasemia were 18% to 19%. Patients who had an elevation in serum amylase have a 2.5-fold increased risk for pancreatitis. (*From* Fischl MA, Dolin R, Cross A, *et al.*: Safety and tolerance of didanosine (ddI) in patients with advanced HIV disease. Presented at the IX International Conference on AIDS, Berlin, June 1993: PO-B26-2038.)

ZALCITABINE

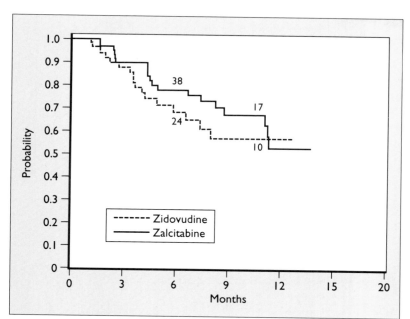

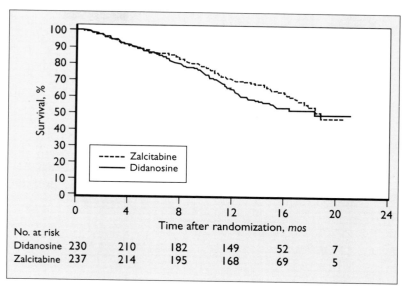

FIGURE 17-22 Disease progression, zidovudine vs zalcitabine. Estimated distributions of time to disease progression for 59 patients who received zidovudine (*dashed line*) and 52 patients who received zalcitabine (*solid line*). Patients had advanced HIV disease and had received and tolerated 48 weeks or more of prior zidovudine therapy. Due to poor accrual, the number of patients enrolled in the study was less than planned. In addition, a significantly larger number of patients self-withdrew from zidovudine compared with zalcitabine. Although these data potentially favor zalcitabine therapy, these results should be interpreted cautiously due to the accrual and self-withdrawal problems. (*From* Fischl MA, Olson RM, Follansbee SE, *et al.*: Zalcitabine compared with zidovudine in patients with advanced HIV-1 infection who received previous zidovudine therapy. *Ann Intern Med* 1993,118:762–769; with permission.)

FIGURE 17-23 Cumulative survival, zalcitabine vs didanosine. Two hundred thirty patients were assigned to receive 500 mg/d of didanosine (*solid line*) and 237 to receive 2.25 mg/d of zalcitabine (*dashed line*). Dosages were weight adjusted. All patients had received previous zidovudine therapy and had either disease progression or toxicity. A total of 100 patients died in the didanosine group and 88 in the zalcitabine group. After adjustments for CD4 cell count, Karnofsky score, and the presence of AIDS prior to treatment, there was a significant survival benefit associated with zalcitabine (RR=0.63; 95% CI=0.46–0.85; *P*=0.003). (*From* Abrams DI, Goldman AI, Launer C, *et al.*: A comparative trial of didanosine or zalcitabine after treatment with zidovudine in patients with human immunodeficiency virus infection. *N Engl J Med* 1994, 330:657–662; with permission.)

COMBINATION THERAPY

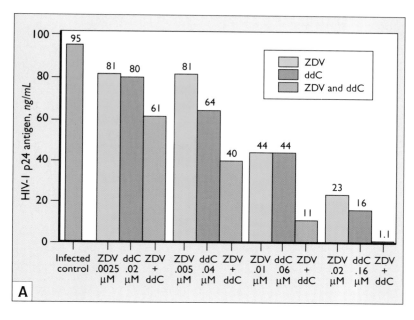

FIGURE 17-24 A and **B,** Inhibition of HIV-1 p24 antigen production by a zidovudine-sensitive isolate (*panel 24A*) and a zidovudine-resistant isolate (*panel 24B*) in acutely infected peripheral blood mononuclear cells treated with varying doses of zidovudine (ZDV), zalcitabine (ddC), or the combination of zidovudine and zalcitabine. These data show that the combination of zidovudine and zalcitabine synergistically inhibits HIV replication *in vitro* in both zidovudine-sensitive and -resistant isolates. These types of data resulted in several clinical trials to assess the utility of combination nucleoside analogue therapy. (*From* Eron JJ, Johnson VA, Merrill DP, *et al.*: Synergistic inhibition of replication of human immunodeficiency virus type 1, including that of zidovudine-resistant isolate, by zidovudine and 2',3'-dideoxycytidine *in vitro*. *Antimicrob Agents Chemother* 1992, 36:1559–1562; with permission.) *(continued)*

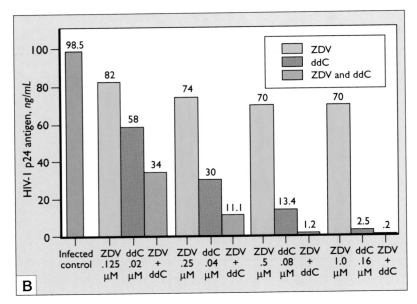

Figure 17-24 *(continued)*

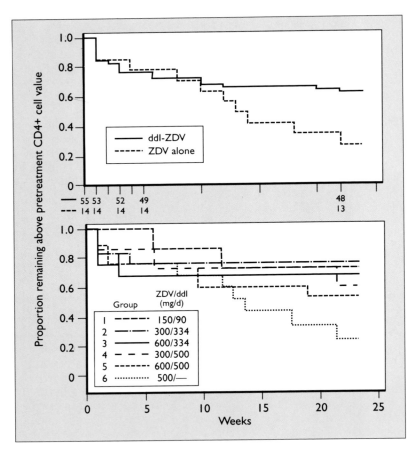

Figure 17-26 CD4 cell count changes, zidovudine and didanosine vs zidovudine. The proportion of patients with CD4 cell count values remaining above pretreatment values were compared for those treated with zidovudine (150, 300, or 600 mg/d) and didanosine (90, 334, or 500 mg/d) combination therapy vs zidovudine alone (600 g/d, *dashed line*). All patients had early HIV disease and had minimal or no prior antiretroviral therapy. Among patients receiving combination therapy, CD4 cell count changes were more persistent than with zidovudine alone. (*From* Collier AC, Coombs RW, Fischl MA, *et al.*: Combination therapy with zidovudine and didanosine compared to zidovudine alone in human immunodeficiency virus type one infection. *Ann Intern Med* 1993, 119:786–793; with permission.)

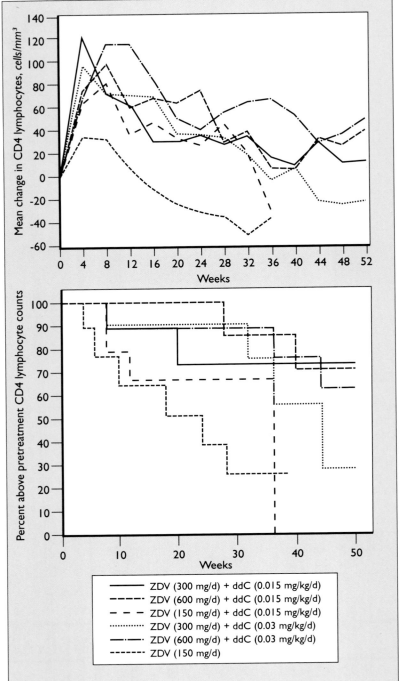

Figure 17-25 CD4 cell count changes, zidovudine and zalcitabine vs zidovudine. Patients with advanced HIV disease and no previous antiretroviral therapy received combination therapy with zidovudine (600, 300, or 150 mg/d) and zalcitabine (0.03 or 0.015 mg/kg/d) or zidovudine alone (150 mg/d). Among patients receiving combination therapy, CD4 cell count responses were both of a larger magnitude or more persistent than those with zidovudine alone. Similar findings were noted when comparing these responses with historical controls (600 mg/d of zidovudine monotherapy). (*From* Meng TC, Fischl MA, Boota AM, *et al.*: Combination therapy with zidovudine and dideoxycytidine in patients with advanced human immunodeficiency virus (HIV) infection. *Ann Intern Med* 1992, 116:13–20; with permission.)

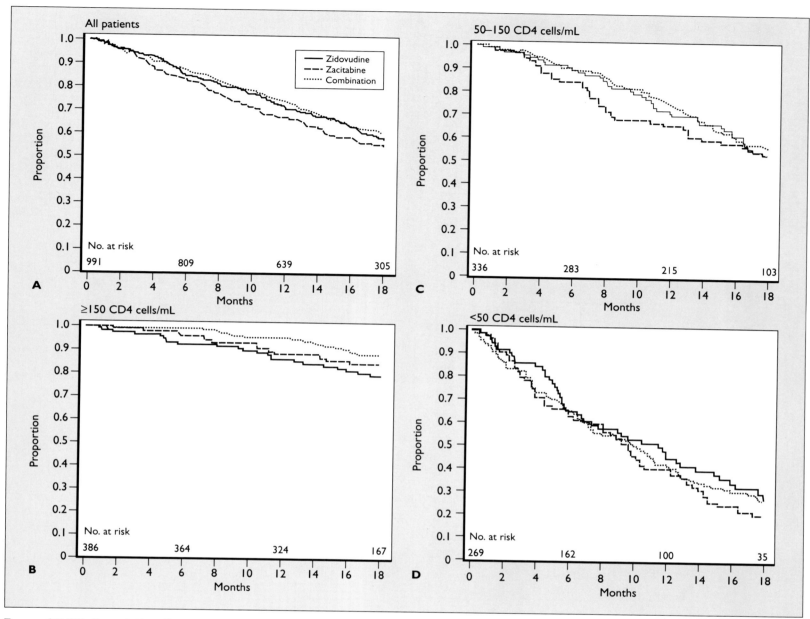

FIGURE 17-27 Cumulative disease-free survival, zidovudine vs zalcitabine vs combination of the two. Two hundred eighty-three patients were assigned to receive zidovudine (600 mg/d, *solid line*), 285 to receive zalcitabine (2.25 mg/d, *dashed line*), and 423 to receive the combination of zidovudine and zalcitabine (*dotted line*). Patients had advanced HIV disease and had received zidovudine therapy for an average of 18 months. No overall difference was noted among the three treatment groups. However, patients with pretreatment CD4 cell counts ≥ 150 cells/mL who received combination therapy had a better outcome than those who received zidovudine therapy. Similar findings were not noted for the other two CD4 cell subgroups (50–150 and < 50 cells/mL). (*From* Fischl MA, Collier AC, Stanley K, *et al.*: The safety and efficacy of zidovudine (ZDV) and zalcitabine (ddC) or ddC alone versus ZDV. Presented in part at the IX International Conference on AIDS, Berlin, June 1993: BS-B25-1.)

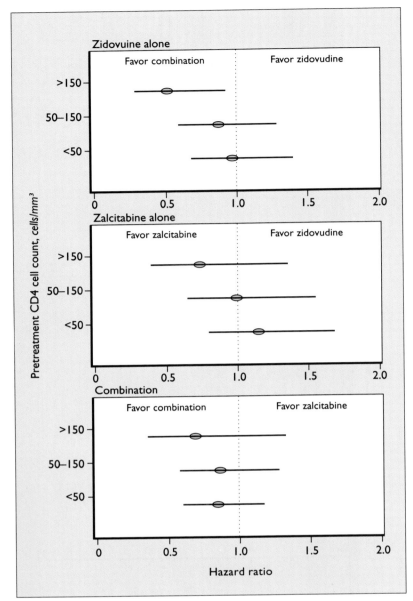

FIGURE 17-28 Time to disease progression, zidovudine vs zalcitabine vs combination. Hazard ratio comparisons for time to clinical disease progression or death, which ever occurred first, among patients who received zidovudine alone, zalcitabine alone, or the combination of zidovudine and zalcitabine by CD4 cell subgroups (< 50, 50–150, > 150 cells/mL). Patients had advanced HIV disease and had received zidovudine therapy for an average of 18 months. Although no difference was noted among the three treatment groups overall, a trend analysis showed a significantly lower progression rate for the combination therapy group relative to the zidovudine therapy group as the pretreatment CD4 cell count increased (P=0.027). (*From* Fischl MA, Collier AC, Stanley K, *et al.*: The safety and efficacy of zidovudine (ZDV) and zalcitabine (ddC) or ddC alone versus ZDV. Presented in part at the IX International Conference on AIDS, Berlin, June 1993: BS-B25-1.)

STUDY DESIGN STRATEGIES

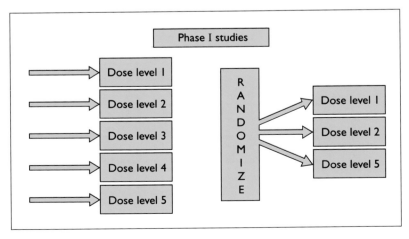

FIGURE 17-29 Phase I clinical trials are designed to evaluate single doses and multiple doses of new agents in order to assess pharmacokinetic parameters (peak concentration [C_{max}], time to peak concentration [T_{max}], and area under the concentration–time curve [AUC]). Parallel or dose escalation studies with 5–12 patients per dose level are typical. Small phase I studies can also be done to assess the initial anti-HIV activity of new agents in randomized trials of several doses of a new compound assessing surrogate markers (CD4 cell counts, viral burden as measured by p24 antigen levels, or plasma HIV RNA copy numbers or infectivity as measured by quantitative viral culture).

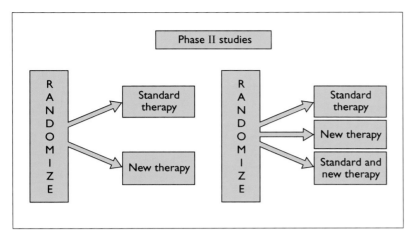

FIGURE 17-30 Phase II studies are designed to assess a particular dose of a new compound or to assess initial activity and safety of a new compound. Phase II studies typically include 60–400 patients in randomized, double-blind studies. These trials can be used to assess several dose levels of a new compound, a new compound compared with standard therapy, or the combination of a new compound with standard therapy.

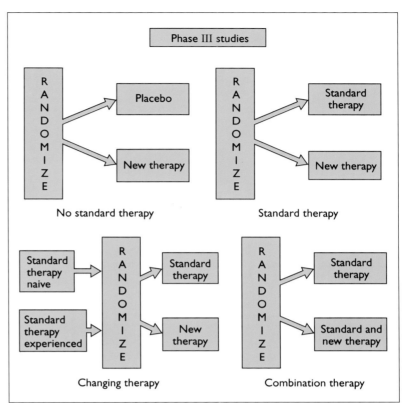

FIGURE 17-31 Phase II/III studies are designed to assess the safety and efficacy of new agents. Phase II/III studies are typically large studies of 400–1500 patients and randomized, double-blind controlled trials. These trials are used to assess the safety and efficacy of new regimens, and therefore these trials have clinical endpoints. These types of trial can be used to assess new regimens, including new agents, combination therapies, and new treatment strategies, such as switching therapies. (*From* Stanley K, Lagakos SW: Biostatistical considerations in the design and analysis of AIDS clinical trials. *In* Broder S, Merigan TC, Bolognesi D (eds): *Textbook of AIDS Medicine.* Baltimore: Williams & Wilkins; 1994:743–750; with permission.)

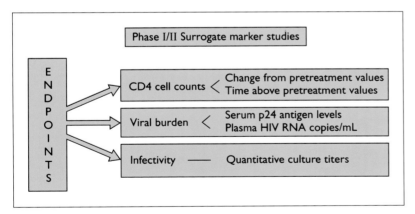

FIGURE 17-32 Surrogate markers for clinical disease progression in phase I/II HIV clinical trials. Due to the paucity of anti-HIV drugs, accelerated evaluation of potentially effective drugs through the use of surrogate markers for clinical disease progression has allowed a more rapid evaluation of new anti-HIV drugs and treatment strategies. Increases in CD4 cells, delays in CD4 cell count declines, and suppression of viral replication as measured by HIV p24 antigen levels, plasma HIV RNA copy numbers, and quantitative culture are associated with a better outcome and represent the current surrogate markers being used in the preliminary evaluation of new anti-HIV drugs and treatment strategies. None of these markers, however, completely predict clinical outcome in response to therapy.

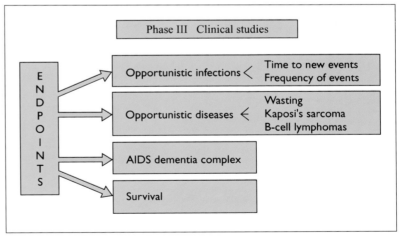

FIGURE 17-33 Clinical endpoints used in phase II/III HIV clinical trials. Because HIV infection results in a life-threatening disease, a logical endpoint for clinical trials is death. However, due to prolonged clinical latency and inadequacy of current anti-HIV drugs, death is not a feasible endpoint with the current sample sizes of studies. Survival has been used as a primary endpoint in only a few studies. Thus, serious or potentially life-threatening clinical disease progression, as noted, has been used as the primary clinical endpoints for most HIV clinical trials.

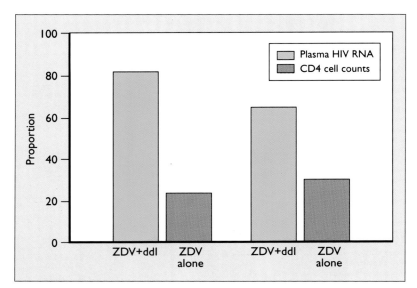

FIGURE 17-34 Surrogate marker responses, plasma HIV copies and CD4 counts. The proportion of patients with a one or more log reduction in plasma HIV RNA copies per milliliter and a 50-cell/mL or more increase in CD4 cell counts is noted for patients receiving combination therapy with varying doses of zidovudine (ZDV) and didanosine (ddI) compared with zidovudine alone. A significant reduction in plasma HIV RNA copies numbers and increase in CD4 cell counts were noted among patients receiving combination therapy versus monotherapy. The use of potential surrogate markers of HIV disease progression, as noted, are frequently used to rapidly evaluate new anti-HIV drugs and treatment strategies.

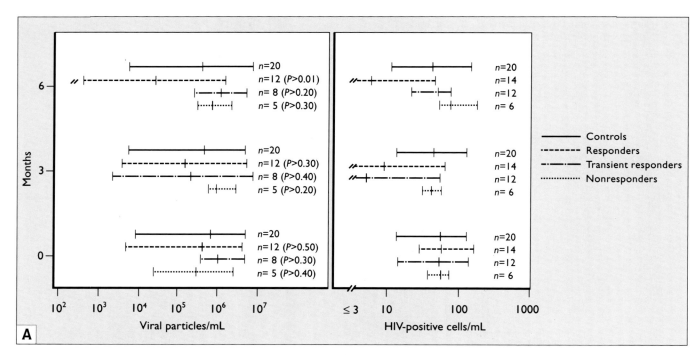

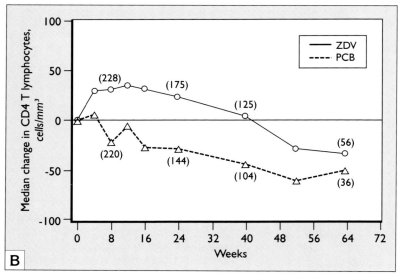

FIGURE 17-35 Methods of measuring antiviral activity for therapeutic agents. **A,** Antiviral activity of zidovudine therapy evaluated by measuring concentrations of infectious HIV-harboring cells in the blood (*left panel*) and RNA virus particles in serum (*right panel*). Data presented are for controls, responders, transient responders, and nonresponders. After 3 months of zidovudine therapy (500 mg/d) in patients with asymptomatic HIV infection, a significant reduction in cellular virus load was noted. (*From* Lu W, Andrieu JM: Early identification of human immunodeficiency virus-infected asymptomatic subjects susceptible to zidovudine by quantitative viral coculture and reverse transcription-linked polymerase chain reaction. *J Infect Dis* 1993, 167:1014–1020; with permission.) **B,** Antiviral activity of zidovudine therapy evaluated by measuring changes in median CD4 cell counts over time. After 40 weeks of follow-up, a significant increase in CD4 cell count is noted among patients with mildly symptomatic HIV disease and 200–500 CD4 cells/mL who received zidovudine therapy (1200 mg/d, *solid line*) vs placebo (*dashed line*). *(continued)*

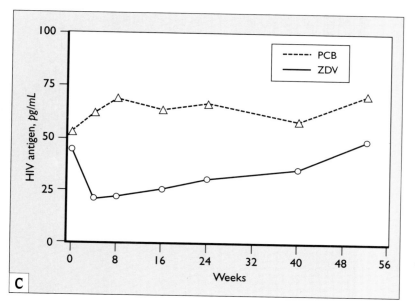

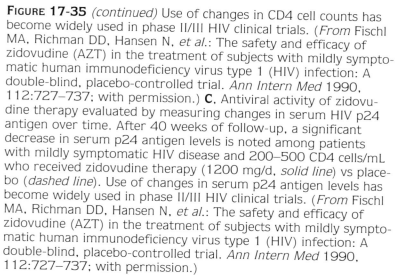

FIGURE **17-35** *(continued)* Use of changes in CD4 cell counts has become widely used in phase II/III HIV clinical trials. (*From* Fischl MA, Richman DD, Hansen N, *et al.*: The safety and efficacy of zidovudine (AZT) in the treatment of subjects with mildly symptomatic human immunodeficiency virus type 1 (HIV) infection: A double-blind, placebo-controlled trial. *Ann Intern Med* 1990, 112:727–737; with permission.) **C,** Antiviral activity of zidovudine therapy evaluated by measuring changes in serum HIV p24 antigen over time. After 40 weeks of follow-up, a significant decrease in serum p24 antigen levels is noted among patients with mildly symptomatic HIV disease and 200–500 CD4 cells/mL who received zidovudine therapy (1200 mg/d, *solid line*) vs placebo (*dashed line*). Use of changes in serum p24 antigen levels has become widely used in phase II/III HIV clinical trials. (*From* Fischl MA, Richman DD, Hansen N, *et al.*: The safety and efficacy of zidovudine (AZT) in the treatment of subjects with mildly symptomatic human immunodeficiency virus type 1 (HIV) infection: A double-blind, placebo-controlled trial. *Ann Intern Med* 1990, 112:727–737; with permission.)

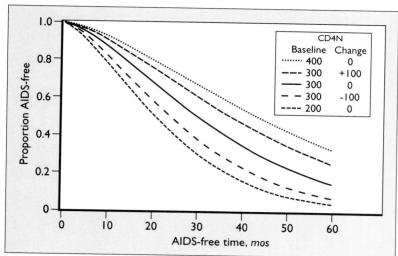

FIGURE **17-36** Estimating disease progression. Proportion of zidovudine-treated patients from the Multicenter AIDS Cohort Study (MACS) remaining without AIDS as estimated from pretreatment CD4 cell counts using a Wiebul model. These data suggest that improvements in AIDS-free time are associated with CD4 cell responses to zidovudine. Similar data were noted for survival time. This type of modeling, used to facilitate estimation of baseline risk of prediction of event probabilities over time, points out the importance of CD4 cell responses and number of CD4 cells at initiation of therapy in assessing anti-HIV therapies. (*From* Graham NM, Piantadosi S, Park LP, *et al.*: CD4+ lymphocyte response to zidovudine as a predictor of AIDS-free time and survival time. *J Acquir Immune Defic Syndr* 1993, 6:1258–1266; with permission.)

INITIATING ANTIRETROVIRAL THERAPY

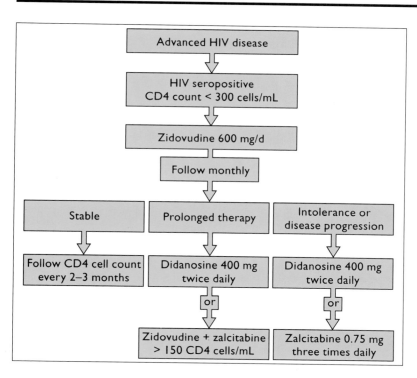

FIGURE **17-37** General guidelines for initiating antiretroviral therapy in patients with advanced HIV disease. Zidovudine has been shown to be superior to both didanosine and zalcitabine therapy as first-line therapy. However, due to the waning activity of zidovudine, switching antiretroviral therapy has been shown to be beneficial.

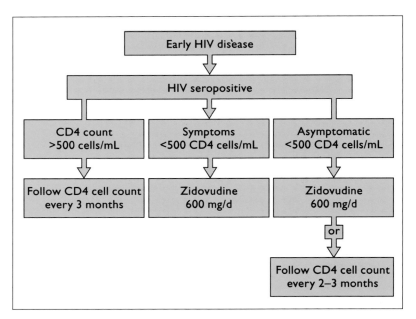

FIGURE 17-38 General guidelines for initiating antiretroviral therapy in patients with early HIV disease. Zidovudine is the only drug currently approved for first-line therapy of early HIV disease in patients with symptomatic or asymptomatic disease and 200–500 CD4 cells/mL. The role of early therapy vs delayed therapy has been raised with the Concorde study, and patients and physicians may wish to postpone early therapy with zidovudine alone in patients with higher CD4 cell counts and asymptomatic disease.

FIGURE 17-39 Toxicities experienced with the currently available nucleoside analogues. The common toxicities associated with zidovudine (ZDV) therapy include headache, malaise, anemia, and neutropenia. Anemia is less common with lower doses of the drug. The common toxicities seen with didanosine (ddI) include palatability of the current formulation, pancreatitis, hyperamylasemia, and peripheral neuropathy. Peripheral neuropathy appears less common with lower doses of the drug. The most common toxicities associated with zalcitabine (ddC) include initial problems with rash, fever, and stomatitis and longer-term problems with peripheral neuropathy. (*From* Saag MS: Nucleoside analogues: Adverse effects. *Hosp Pract* 1992, 27:26–36; with permission.)

	ZDV	ddI	ddC
Constitutional			
Fever	More common	Rare	Not reported
Malaise	More common	Less common	Not reported
Myalgias	More common	Rare	Rare
Headache	More common	Less common	Not reported
Altered taste	Rare	More common	Rare
Gastrointestinal			
Insomnia	Less common	Rare	Rare
Nausea	More common	More common	Rare
Vomiting	Rare	Rare	Rare
Diarrhea	Rare	Less common	Rare
Abdominal pain	Less common	More common	Rare
Pancreatitis	Less common	More common	Rare
Elevated transaminase	Less common	More common	Rare
Stomatitis	Not reported	Less common	More common
Hematologic			
Anemia	More common	Less common	Rare
Neuropenia	More common	Rare	Rare
Neuromuscular			
Myopathy	Less common	Rare	Rare
Peripheral neuropathy	Not reported	Less common	More common
Metabolic			
Hyperuricemia	Not reported	Not reported	Not reported
Hypertriglyceridemia	Not reported	Not reported	Not reported
Hyperamylasemia	Not reported	More common	Rare
Allergic			
Rash	Rare	Rare	Less common
Fever	Rare	Rare	Less common

○ More common   ● Rare   ▢ Less common   ▭ Not reported

Drugs whose toxicities may overlap with those of the nucleoside analogues

Gastrointestinal (nausea, vomiting)
Acyclovir
Azithromycin
Chemotherapeutic agents
Clarithromycin
Co-trimoxazole
Dapsone
Fluconazole
Flucytosine
Foscarnet
Ganciclovir
Interferon
Ketoconazole
Metronidazole

Hepatic
Acyclovir
Chemotherapeutic agents
Ethanol
Fluconazole

Ganciclovir
Intraconazole
Ketoconazole
Metronidazole
Trimetrexate

Renal
Acyclovir
Amphotericin B
Foscarnet
Ganciclovir
Sulfadiazine

Neuropathy
Dapsone
Ethionamide
Isoniazid
Metronidazole
Phenytoin
Pyridoxine

Vincristine

Hematologic (anemia, graulocytopenia)
Acyclovir
Amphotericin B
Chemotherapeutic agents
Co-trimoxazole
Dapsone
Flucytosine
Foscarnet
Ganciclovir
Interferon
Pentamidine
Pyrimethamine
Trimetrexate

Pancreatitis
Cimetidine
Ethanol

Pentamidine
Ranitidine
Sulfonamides

Neurologic (confusion, altered mental status)
Acyclovir
Compound Q
Ganciclovir
Interferon
Sulfadiazine
Trimetrexate

Dermatologic
Co-trimoxazole
Foscarnet
Fluconazole
Pentamidine
Pyrimethamine
Sulfadiazine

FIGURE 17-40 Drugs used in the treatment of HIV disease that have similar toxicity profiles and may increase toxicities of nucleoside analogues. Common concerns occur with overlapping hematologic toxicities with zidovudine, in which hematologic growth factors may be required to control concurrent additive toxicities. (*From* Saag MS: Nucleoside analogues: Adverse effects. *Hosp Pract* 1992, 27:26–36; with permission.)

NEW AND INVESTIGATIONAL AGENTS

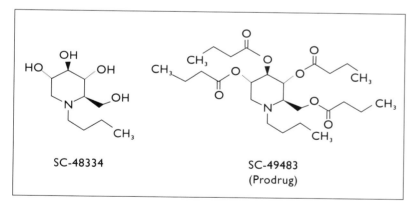

SC-48334

SC-49483
(Prodrug)

FIGURE 17-41 SC-48334, (*N*-butyl-deoxynojirmycin), an α-glucosidase I inhibitor, suppresses HIV-1 *in vitro* as measured by a reduction in HIV p24 core antigen and reverses transcriptase levels. The combination of SC-48334 and zidovudine has synergistic inhibitory activity against HIV *in vitro*. Phase I studies noted diarrhea as the major side effect. A prodrug that is converted to the active moiety in the intestinal wall is under evaluation and may cause substantially less diarrhea.

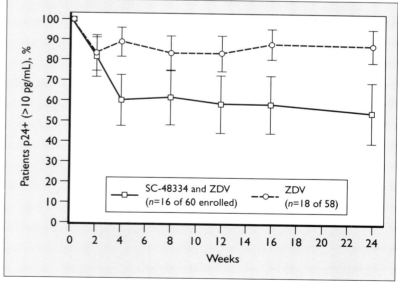

FIGURE 17-42 Changes in serum p24 antigen levels for 60 patients assigned to the combination of zidovudine (300 mg/d) and SC-48334 (3 g/d) (*solid line*), an α-glucosidase I inhibitor, and 58 to zidovudine (300 mg/d) alone (*dashed line*). These preliminary data suggest potential activity of this compound, and additional studies are under way. (*From* Fischl MA, Resnick L, Coombs R, *et al.*: The safety and efficacy of combination *N*-butyl-deoxynojirimycin (SC-48334) and zidovudine in patients with HIV-1 infection and 200–500 CD4 cells/mm³. *J Acquir Immune Defic Syndr* 1994, 7:139–147; with permission.)

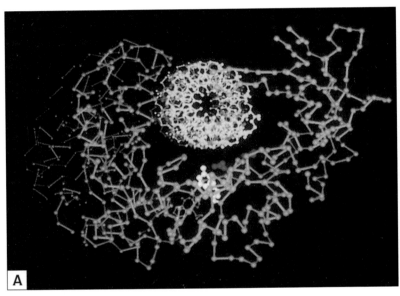

FIGURE 17-43 Inhibitors of reverse transcriptase by nonnucleoside analogues. These compounds directly bind to the functional reverse transcriptase enzyme and inhibit polymerization. This new class of anti-HIV agents showed initial promise in light of their marked inhibition of HIV *in vitro*, low toxicity profile, and synergy with nucleoside analogues. However, rapid emergence of resistance has been noted both *in vitro* and *in vivo*. (*From* Johnston MI, McGowan JJ: Strategies and progress in the development of antiretroviral agents. *In* DeVita VT, Hellman S, Rosenberg SA (eds): *AIDS: Etiology, Diagnosis, Treatment and Prevention*, 3rd ed. Philadelphia: J.B. Lippincott; 1992:357–371. Investigator Brochure for Delavirdine Mesylate (U-901525): A nonnucleoside reverse transcriptase inhibitor. Kalamazoo, MI: Upjohn Company; 1992.)

Delavirdine

Nevirapine

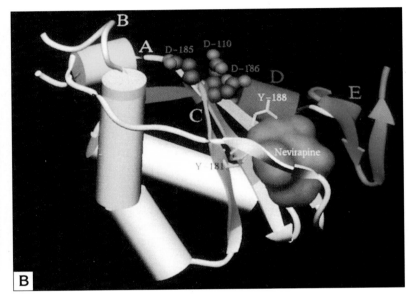

FIGURE 17-44 The position of nevirapine, a nonnucleoside reverse transcriptase inhibitor, bound to the p66 subunit of the reverse transcriptase is shown. The p66 subunit with model-built DNA (*blue* and *yellow*) showing the aspartic acid (*red*) at amino acid residues 185 and 186 at the presumed catalytic site nearby. Nevirapine (*green*) binds near the tyrosine (*white*) at residues 181 and 188. The aspartic acid at residue 110, 185, and 186 presumably participates in the catalytic site. Nevirapine fits into a pocket found by the β-strand comprised of residues 100–110 and 180–190. Mutations in these regions, including the tyrosine at 181 and 188 to which nevirapine binds, result in resistance to nevirapine and the other nonnucleoside reverse transcriptase inhibitors. (*From* Kohlstaedt LA, Wang J, Friedman JM, *et al.*: Crystal structure at 3.5 Å resolution of HIV-1 reverse transcriptase complexed with an inhibitor. *Science* 1992, 256:1783–1790; with permission.)

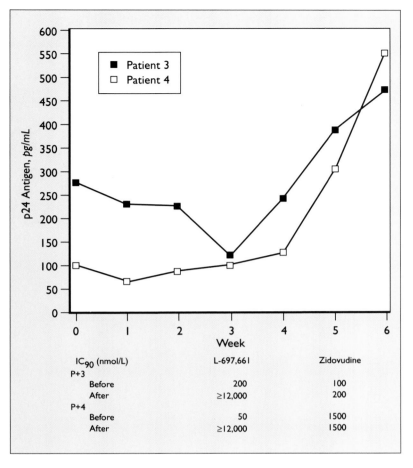

FIGURE 17-45 Plasma p24 antigen changes and 90% inhibitory concentration (IC_{90}) values for L-697,661 and zidovudine in HIV-1 isolates from representative patients treated with L-697,661. L-697,661 is a nonnucleoside inhibitor of HIV-1 reverse transcriptase. Nonnucleoside inhibitors directly inhibit HIV-1 reverse transcriptase and, unlike nucleoside analogues, are not incorporated into the elongating DNA strand. In this phase I study, a rapid dose-related decrease in plasma p24 antigen was noted, which disappeared after 6 weeks in some patients receiving L-697,661, which corresponded to emergence of resistant viruses. This was most prominent in patients receiving higher doses of the drug. (*From* Saag MS, Emini EA, Laskin OL, *et al.*: A short-term clinical evaluation of L-697,661, a non-nucleoside inhibitor of HIV-1 reverse transcriptase. *N Engl J Med* 1993, 329:1065–1072; with permission.)

FIGURE 17-46 The protease inhibitor Ro 31-8959 inhibits the processing of *gag* and *gag-pol* polyproteins, thereby blocking virion maturation and decreasing infectivity. Ro 31-8959 suppresses HIV-1 *in vitro* as measured by a reduction in HIV p24 antigen and syncytia formation. The combination of Ro 31-8959 with zidovudine, zalcitabine, or recombinant interferon-α has additive to synergistic inhibitory activity against HIV *in vitro*. Preliminary studies have noted increases in CD4 cell counts, and phase II/III trials to evaluate the safety and efficacy of this compound are under way. (Investigational Brochure: Ro 31-8959. Nutley, NJ: F. Hoffmann-LaRoche; 1992.)

SELECTED BIBLIOGRAPHY

Hirsch MS, D'Aquila RT: Therapy for human immunodeficiency virus. *N Engl J Med* 1993, 328:1686–1695.

Fischl MA, Parker CB, Pettinelli C, *et al.*: A randomized controlled trial of a reduced daily dose of zidovudine in patients with the acquired immunodeficiency syndrome. *N Engl J Med* 1990, 323:1009–1014.

Richman DD: Viral resistance to antiretroviral therapy. *In* Broder S, Merigan TC, Bolognesi D (eds): *Textbook of AIDS Medicine.* Baltimore: Williams & Wilkins; 1994:795–805.

Kahn JO, Lagakos SW, Richman DD, *et al.*: A controlled trial comparing continued zidovudine with didanosine in human immunodeficiency virus infection. *N Engl J Med* 1992, 327:581–587.

Abrams DI, Goldman AI, Launer C, *et al.*: A comparative trial of didanosine or zalcitabine after treatment with zidovudine in patients with human immunodeficiency virus infection. *N Engl J Med* 1994, 330:657–662.

CHAPTER 18

Pediatric HIV Infection

Ram Yogev

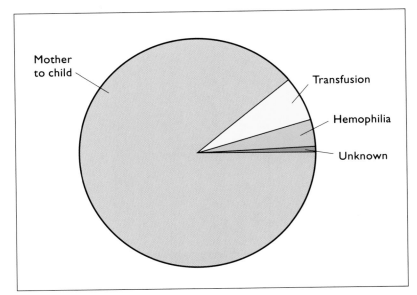

FIGURE 18-1 Mode of HIV transmission in children. The cumulative total of AIDS cases in children reported to the Centers for Disease Control and Prevention (CDC) through December 1993 is 5234. Vertical transmission from mother to child accounts for most new cases. The transmission rate from mother to child ranges from 15% to 30%. Multiple factors such as the mother's viral titers, disease status, or severity of the immune system deterioration affect the rate of transmission. Transmission through blood products is now very rare due to the initiation in the mid-1980s of regular screening of the blood supply and heat treatment of clotting factor. Few children have acquired the virus through sexual abuse. (Douglas GC, King BF: Maternal-fetal transmission of human immunodeficiency virus: A review of possible routes and cellular mechanisms of infection. *Clin Infect Dis* 1992, 15:678–691.)

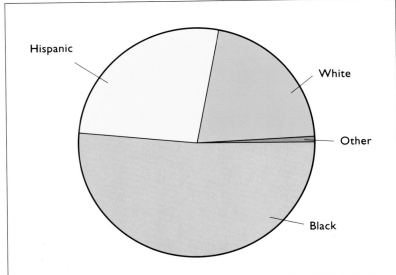

FIGURE 18-2 Percentage of pediatric AIDS cases by race and ethnicity. Most children with AIDS are African-American or Hispanic, with cumulative incidence rates of 17 and 7 times greater, respectively, than for white children. Maternal intravenous drug use and sexual contact with an intravenous drug user are the most common risk factors. Minorities will continue to make up the majority of infected women and children in coming years. (Centers for Disease Control: HIV prevalence estimates and AIDS cases projections for the United States: Report based upon a workshop. *MMWR* 1990, 39[RR16]:1–31.)

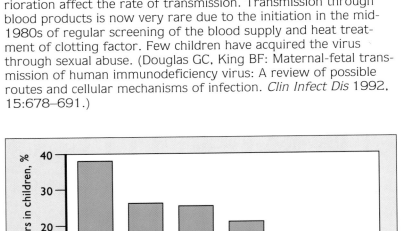
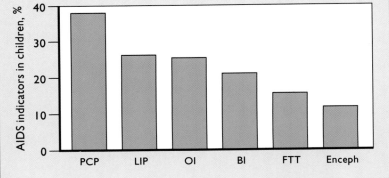

FIGURE 18-3 Percentage of AIDS-indicator diseases in children. The spectrum of HIV disease in children is very wide and creates a major difficulty in defining pediatric AIDS cases. In addition, some diseases common in healthy, uninfected children (*eg*, diarrhea, bacteremia, pneumonia) are also diseases frequently seen in HIV-infected children. Although *Pneumocystis carinii* pneumonia (PCP) is the leading AIDS-indicator disease in children (as in adults), lymphoid interstitial pneumonitis (LIP), opportunistic infections (OI), and recurrent bacterial infections (BI) are almost as common. It is important to note, however, that PCP is more common in the very young (< 1 year of age), whereas LIP is the leading AIDS-indicator disease in older children. Failure to thrive (FTT) and encephalopathy are the other common AIDS-indicator conditions.

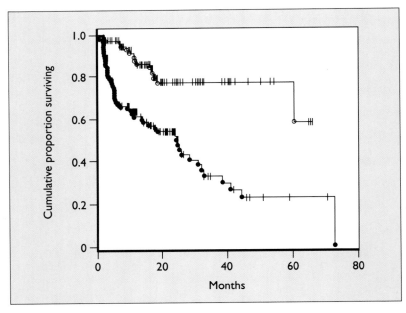

FIGURE 18-4 Survival in children with HIV-1 infection. Two patterns of HIV disease have been identified in children. About 20% present with a rapidly developing disease, with symptoms appearing early in life (around 6 months of age) (*bottom line*). The remaining 80% have a more indolent course with symptoms developing later in life (*top line*). (*From* Scott GB, Hutto C, Markuch RW, *et al.*: Survival in children with perinatally acquired human immunodeficiency virus type 1 infection. *N Engl J Med* 1989, 321:1971–1976; with permission.)

CLINICAL MANIFESTATIONS OF HIV INFECTION

Intermediate or Not Symptomatic

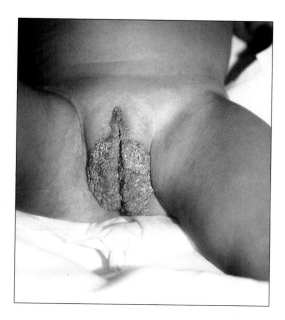

FIGURE 18-5 Large lesion of condyloma acuminata in the genital area occurring without severe depletion of CD4+ cells in the peripheral blood. (*Courtesy of* J. Oleske, MD.)

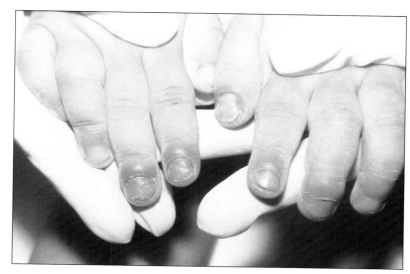

FIGURE 18-6 Candida paronychia with nail dystrophy. (*Courtesy of* N. Esterly, MD.)

Mildly Symptomatic Infection

Mildly symptomatic infection

Lymphadenopathy
Hepatomegaly
Splenomegaly
Dermatitis
Parotitis
Recurrent/persistent upper respiratory tract infection or sinusitis
Recurrent/persistent otitis media

FIGURE 18-7 Conditions reflective of mildly symptomatic HIV infection. This list includes examples of conditions appearing in HIV-infected children, which indicate a mild but increasing severity of HIV infection. (These conditions are proposed as category A in the upcoming CDC revised classification scheme [in preparation].)

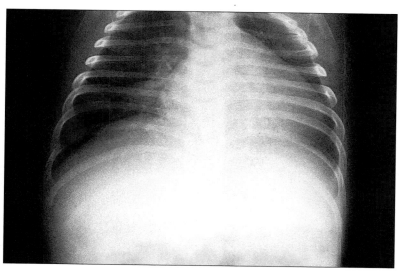

FIGURE 18-8 Hepatosplenomegaly. Although hepatosplenomegaly is one of the most common manifestations of HIV infection in children, hepatic dysfunction is rare. Mild elevation of transaminases is due to HIV infection and is found frequently, but it has no clinical importance. Marked elevation of transaminases may be the result of a toxic reaction to a therapeutic agent (*eg*, antiretroviral agents, sulfa drugs, fluconazole, dapsone) or viruses.

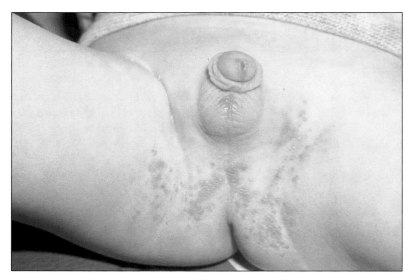

FIGURE 18-9 Candida diaper dermatitis. (*Courtesy of* Dr. N. Esterly.)

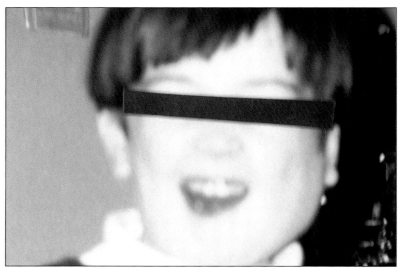

FIGURE 18-10 Parotid gland enlargement. The incidence rate is 10% to 15% in symptomatic HIV-infected children. Although the parotid gland is diffusely swollen, as seen here on the child's left side, there is no tenderness to touch or evidence of inflammation. Histologically, the gland is infiltrated with lymphocytes. The differential diagnosis includes acute suppurative parotitis, mumps, other viral infections (*eg*, parainfluenza, coxsackie, or influenza), tumors, and heavy metal or drug toxicity (*eg*, sulfisoxazole, iodides, etc.). Usually the HIV parotitis is chronic and painless. Treatment with zidovudine causes a rapid resolution in many patients, but the parotitis may recur when zidovudine is discontinued. (Rubinstein A: Pediatric AIDS. *Curr Probl Pediatr* 1986, 16:361–409.)

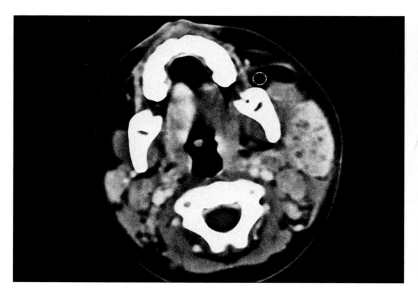

FIGURE 18-11 Computed tomographic (CT) scan of an enlarged parotid gland in an HIV infected child (seen in Fig. 18-10). The enlargement disappeared within 2 weeks of starting zidovudine therapy.

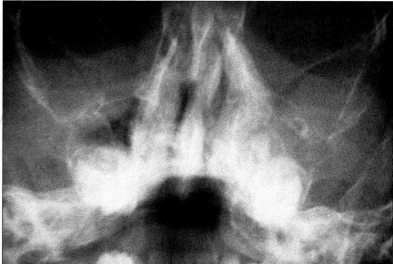

FIGURE 18-12 Sinusitis. This is a common condition in HIV-infected children. A sinus film shows opacification of the left maxillary sinus and mucosal thickening of the right maxillary sinus.

Moderately Symptomatic Infection

Moderately symptomatic infection

Anemia (< 8 g/mL) persisting ≥ 30 days
Neutropenia (< 1000 mm³) persisting ≥ 30 days
Thrombocytopenia (< 100,000 mm³) persisting ≥ 30 days
Bacterial meningitis, pneumonia, or sepsis (single episode)
Candidiasis, oropharyngeal (thrush), persistent (> 2 mo) in child
   > 6 mo of age
Cardiomyopathy
Cytomegalovirus infection (onset before 1 mo of age)
Diarrhea, recurrent or chronic
Hepatitis
Herpes stomatitis, recurrent (> 2 episodes in 1 yr)
Herpes simplex virus bronchitis, pneumonia, or esophagitis
   (onset before 1 mo of age)
Herpes zoster (shingles) (involving at least 2 distinct episodes or
   > 1 dermatome)
Leiomyosarcoma
Lymphoid interstitial pneumonitis (LIP) or pulmonary lymphoid
   hyperplasia complex (LPH)
Nephropathy
Nocardiosis
Persistent varicella zoster
Persistent fever > 1 mo
Toxoplasmosis (onset before 1 mo of age)
Varicella, disseminated (complicated chickenpox)

FIGURE 18-13 Conditions reflective of moderately symptomatic HIV infection. This list contains examples of conditions due to HIV infection and/or indicative of immunologic deficits attributable to HIV infection, which appear in HIV-infected children with a moderate severity of infection. It is not inclusive. Children with LIP are considered to have AIDS, although other conditions listed, appearing alone, are not considered indicative of full-blown AIDS. (These conditions are proposed as category B in the upcoming CDC revised classification scheme [in preparation].)

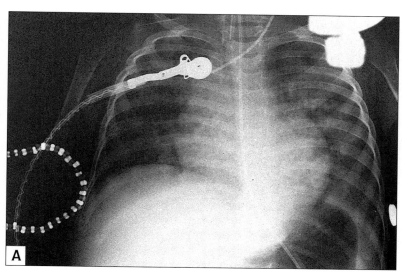
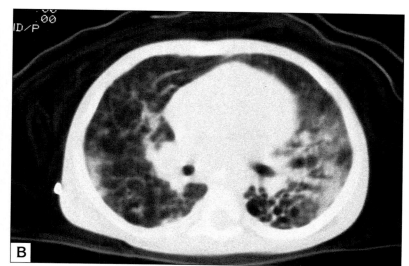

FIGURE 18-14 *Pseudomonas aeruginosa* pneumonia. Pseudomonas infections are an increasing problem in HIV-infected children. Most of these infections occur in patients with adequate neutrophil counts. Predisposing factors include central venous catheters and therapy with broad-spectrum antibiotics. With early diagnosis and therapy, the outcome is favorable. **A,** A chest radiograph shows diffuse bilateral alveolar infiltrates (*left side* worse). **B,** A CT scan of the same patient shows bilateral cavity lesions (*lower lobe*) with increased density of the lungs suggesting an infiltrative process. (Roilides E, Butler KM, Hussan RN: Pseudomonas infections in children with human immunodeficiency virus infection. *Pediatr Infect Dis J* 1992, 11:547–553.)

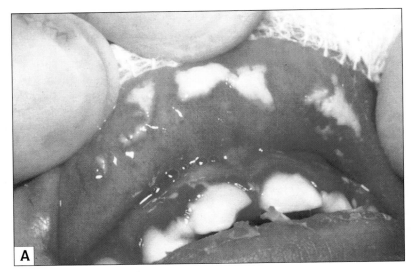
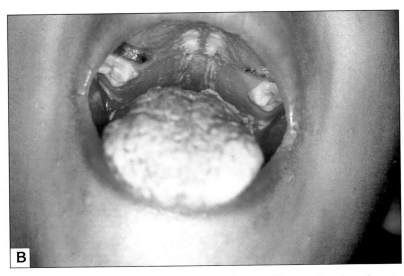

FIGURE 18-15 Oral candidiasis (persisting for 2 months or more). Oral candidiasis is common in HIV-infected children and > 25% of them may suffer from this disease. **A** and **B**. The clinical presentation varies from diffuse mucosal erythema with very few plaques (*panel 15A*) to angular cheilitis or extensive white pseudomembranous plaques on the tongue, buccal mucosa, hard palate, and gingivae (*panel 15B*). Oral hairy leukoplakia and chronic mucocutaneous candidiasis can present like oral candidiasis, but these diseases are very rare in HIV-infected children. Diagnosis of oral candidiasis is usually clinical, but scraping of lesions and culture provide the definitive diagnosis in atypical cases. Initial therapy should include nystatin suspension or clotrimazole troches for older children. For refractory infections, fluconazole (4–6 mg/kg/d orally) is the drug of choice. Recurrences are very common, and maintenance therapy with antifungal agents may be needed. (*Courtesy of* N. Toledo-de-Cabanellas, MD.)

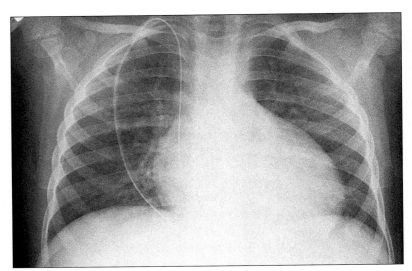
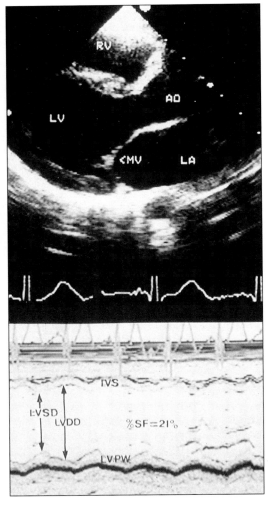

FIGURE 18-16 Cardiomyopathy, as evidenced by an enlarged cardiac silhouette on chest radiography. The incidence of this condition is unknown because the term cardiomyopathy is not well defined. Approximately 20% of children with symptomatic HIV infection develop some cardiac complications. It is speculated that either the HIV is cytopathic to the heart myocytes or that cardiomyopathy is an autoimmune disease. Some reports suggest that selenium deficiency contributes to the cardiomyopathy. (Lipshultz SE, Chanock S, Sanders SP: Cardiovascular manifestations of human immunodeficiency infection in infants and children. *Am J Cardiol* 1989, 63:1489–1497.)

FIGURE 18-17 Echocardiogram of a patient with HIV cardiomyopathy. The *top panel* shows a parasternal long axis view of the heart, demonstrating dilatation of the left ventricle (LV) and left atrium (LA). (AO—aorta; MV—mitral valve; RV—right ventricle.) The *bottom panel* is an M-mode tracing in the same patient from the same view, quantifying the dilated left ventricle and decreased contractility. Contractility is measured as the difference between the left ventricle diastolic dimension (LVDD) and left ventricular systolic dimension (LVSD), resulting in a shortening fraction (%SF) of 21% (normal is > 29%). (IVS—interventricular septum; LVPW—left ventricular posterior wall.)

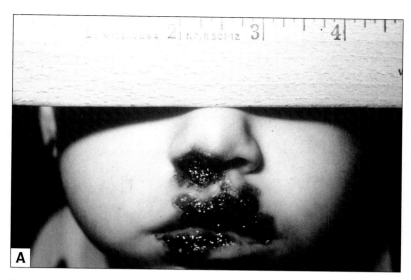

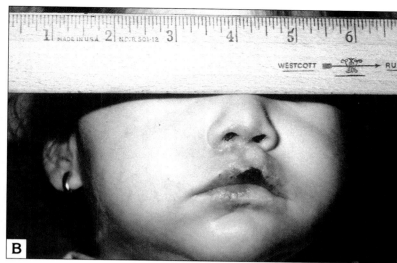

FIGURE 18-18 Herpes stomatitis (two or more episodes within a year). Oral lesions due to HSV occur commonly in HIV-infected children and have a tendency to recur. The frequency of the recurrences increases as the HIV disease progresses. Although in many patients, the lesions heal within 7–10 days, chronic infections that continue for weeks occur. Clinical diagnosis is usually easy, but atypical lesions should be scraped and examined for intranuclear inclusions and multinucleated giant cells (Tzank smear). Oral acy- clovir (750–1000 mg/m^2/d in divided doses every 6 or 8 hours) or foscarnet for acyclovir-resistant strains will reduce morbidity and potential serious complications. Intravenous therapy is required for more severe infections. In patients with frequent recurrences, chronic suppressive therapy with acyclovir is recommended. **A**, Extension of herpes simplex stomatitis to the nares. **B**, The same patient following therapy with foscarnet for an acyclovir-resistant strain. (*Courtesy of* C. Diaz, MD.)

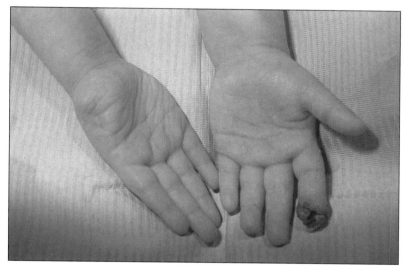

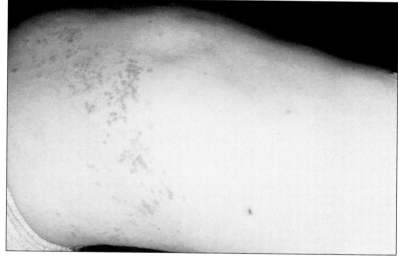

FIGURE 18-19 Herpetic whitlow. Herpes simplex infection on the finger was caused by the child's sucking on it during an episode of herpes gingivostomatitis. (*Courtesy of* N. Toledo-de-Cabanellas, MD.)

FIGURE 18-20 Multidermatomal herpes zoster infection. In HIV-infected children, cutaneous herpes zoster lesions can occur within a few months following chickenpox. As shown in this patient, the skin lesions can involve multiple dermatomes, sometimes imitating primary infection (*ie*, chickenpox) and can disseminate to visceral organs (*see* Fig. 18-22). (*Courtesy of* N. Esterly, MD.)

FIGURE 18-21 Recurrence and chronic herpes zoster are common in HIV-infected children. Therapy with high-dose acyclovir (1500–2000 mg/m^2/d every 8 hours for 7–10 days) is highly effective. For persistent lesions, chronic treatment with oral or intravenous acyclovir may be needed. In this patient, a chronic lesion of herpes zoster was reactivated anytime acyclovir was discontinued. The lesion is secondarily infected with *Listeria monocytogenes*. (*Courtesy of* N. Esterly, MD.)

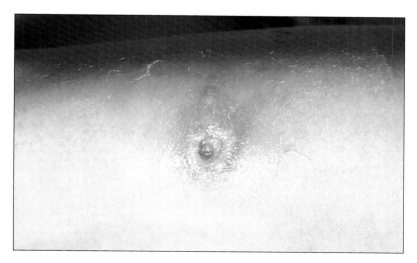

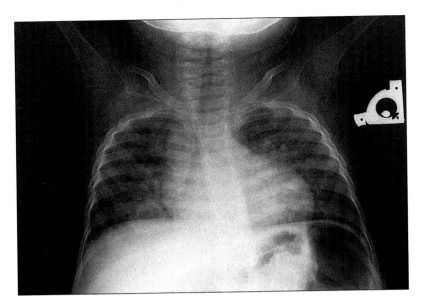

FIGURE 18-22 Disseminated herpes zoster. Varicella pneumonia appears as diffuse ill-defined opacities in both lungs on chest radiography.

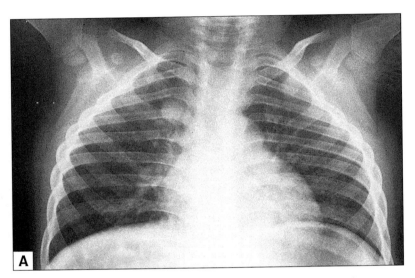

FIGURE 18-23 Leiomyomatoma. The origin of this tumor is smooth muscle. HIV itself or growth factors elaborated during HIV infection are suggested to contribute to its development. **A**, A chest radiograph reveals a masslike density (approximately 1.5 cm in diameter) in the right upper lobe. **B**, Histopathology of this tumor reveals well-defined and circumscribed round nodules composed of spindle cells organized in intersecting bundles. (Chadwick EG, Connor E, Hanson CG: Tumors of smooth muscle origin in HIV-infected children. *JAMA* 1990, 263:3182–3184.)

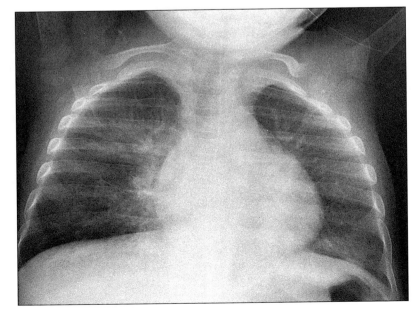

FIGURE 18-24 Lymphoid interstitial pneumonitis (LIP). A chest radiograph in an 8-month-old child shows prominent interstitial infiltrates, despite the lack of respiratory symptoms. The etiologic agent of LIP is not known. Some evidence suggests that Epstein-Barr virus may play a role in the pathogenesis, either by itself or by enhancing replication of HIV. The usual course of LIP is that of a slowly progressive, chronic pulmonary disease with intercurrent respiratory decompensation as the result of pulmonary infections. Serial cutaneous oxygen saturation determinations help in following the progression of LIP and development of hypoxemia. Children with LIP have a good prognosis compared with children with other AIDS-defining events (*eg*, PCP, encephalopathy). The use of steroids is associated with rapid improvement in respiratory symptoms and oxygenation. The usual dose is 2 mg/kg/d for 2–3 weeks followed by a tapering dose according to the O_2 saturation. (Scott GB, Hutto C, Markuch RW, *et al*. Survival in children with perinatally acquired human immunodeficiency virus type 1 infection. *N Engl J Med* 1989, 321:1971–1976.)

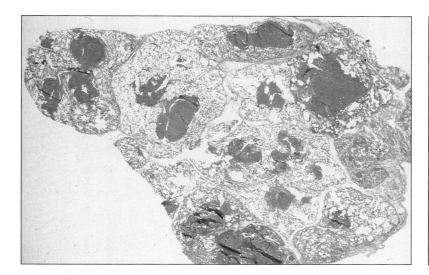

FIGURE 18-25 Histopathology of a lung biopsy specimen from a child with LIP (low magnification, hematoxylin-phyloxine-saffron stain). Definitive diagnosis of LIP can be done only by histologic examination of a lung biopsy specimen. Usually, the pathologic findings consist of peribronchial lymphoid nodules, without involvement of blood vessels or destruction of the lung architecture. (*Courtesy of* Dr. J. Oleske, MD.)

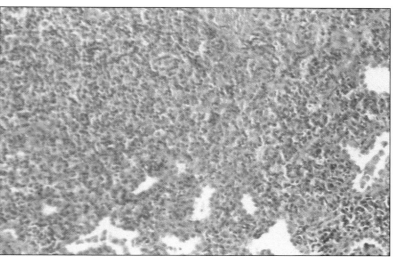

FIGURE 18-26 Hematoxylin-eosin staining of a lung biopsy specimen demonstrating LIP. Diffuse infiltration of alveolar space by lymphocytes and plasma cells. The infiltrated lymphocytes are both B cells and T cells with predominance of T-suppressor cells. (*Courtesy of* J. Oleske, MD.)

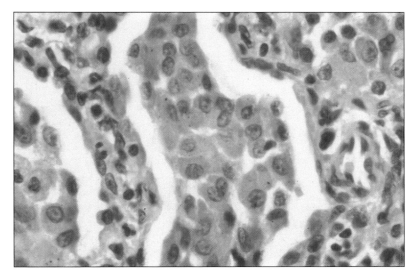

FIGURE 18-27 Desquamative interstitial pneumonitis (DIP), a manifestation of lung injury in children with LIP, is typified by the intra-alveolar collection of mononuclear cells and metaplasia of the alveolar epithelium. DIP is not specific to LIP but represents a nonspecific process of lung injury. Thus, DIP can be found also in patients with PCP or *Cytomegalovirus* pneumonitis. (*Courtesy of* J. Oleske, MD.)

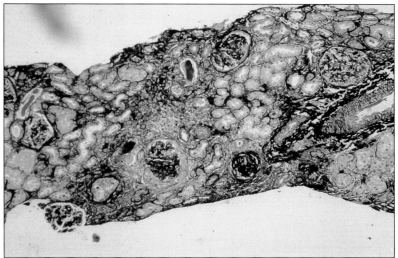

FIGURE 18-28 Nephropathy. The incidence of nephropathy is estimated to be 5% to10%. Most patients demonstrate tubular dysfunction, whereas fewer develop glomerulopathy. The pathologic findings include glomerulosclerosis (focal changes are illustrated in this figure), nephrocalcinosis, interstitial nephritis, acute tubular necrosis, or minimal changes. The role of the HIV infection in the evolution of nephropathy is unclear. (Strauss AC, Zilleruelo G: Renal disease in children with the acquired immunodeficiency syndrome. *N Engl J Med* 1989, 321:625–630.) (*Slide courtesy of* J. Oleske, MD.)

Severely Symptomatic Infection (AIDS)

Severely symptomatic infection (AIDS-indicator conditions)

Serious bacterial infections, multiple or recurrent
Candidiasis, esophageal or pulmonary
Coccidioidomycosis, disseminated
Cryptococcosis, extrapulmonary
Cryptosporidiosis or isosporiasis (diarrhea persisting > 1 mo)
Cytomegalovirus disease (onset of symptoms after 1 mo of age)
   (other than liver, spleen, or lymph nodes)
Encephalopathy (persisting for > 2 mo)
Herpes simplex virus infection causing mucocutaneous ulcers
   (persisting > 1 mo) or bronchitis, pneumonitis, or esophagitis
   (onset after 1 mo of age)
Histoplasmosis, disseminated
Kaposi's sarcoma
Lymphoma, primary, brain
Lymphoma, small noncleaved cell (Burkitt's) or immunoblastic
   or large cell lymphoma of B-cell or unknown immunologic
   phenotype
Mycobacterium tuberculosis, disseminated or extrapulmonary
Mycobacterium, other or unidentified species
Mycobacterium avium complex or *M. kansasii*, disseminated
Pneumocystis carinii pneumonia
Progressive multifocal leukoencephalopathy
Salmonella (nontyphoid) septicemia, recurrent
Toxoplasmosis of brain (onset after 1 mo of age)
Wasting syndrome

FIGURE 18-29 Conditions reflective of severely symptomatic HIV infection (AIDS). Children who are HIV-infected and who have any condition listed (also including LIP, which is a symptom of "moderate severity") are considered to have AIDS. These children are reportable to state and local health departments as having AIDS. This list includes examples of AIDS-indicator conditions from the 1987 CDC classification as well as other conditions recognized to be reflective of the severe immunosuppression due to HIV infection. (These conditions are proposed as category C in the upcoming CDC revised classification scheme [in preparation].)

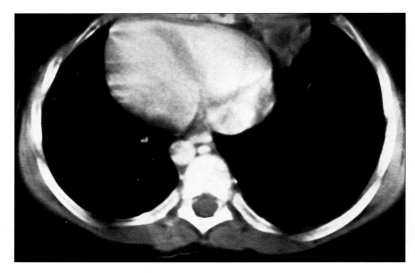

FIGURE 18-30 Lung abscess. Lung abscess rarely occurs in HIV-infected children. The clinical manifestations, which include low-grade fever, dyspnea, and anorexia, may resemble the clinical features of the primary disorder (HIV infection), making the diagnosis very difficult. Although chest radiography will usually show the abscess, a CT scan is more helpful in localizing the abscess. The patient here presented with right upper quadrant abdominal pain. A chest radiograph was negative. CT scan shows involvement of the medial segment of the right middle lobe with central low attenuation.

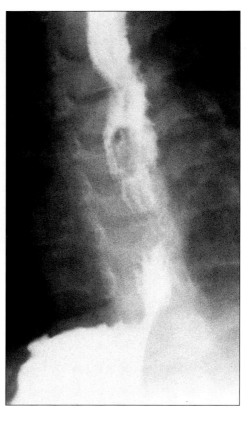

FIGURE 18-31 Esophageal candidiasis. Diffuse marked mucosal irregularity and ulceration are seen radiographically. Although oral candidiasis occurs in > 25% of children with HIV infection, esophageal candidiasis is much less common and can occur with or without the oropharyngeal presentation. Common symptoms include dysphagia and substernal pain, but asymptomatic cases also occur. Thus, a high index of suspicion is important in high-risk patients. Fluconazole (4–6 mg/kg/d) is very effective with rapid resolution of symptoms. Only in severe cases that do not respond to fluconazole, amphotericin B (0.5–1 mg/kg/d) should be given.

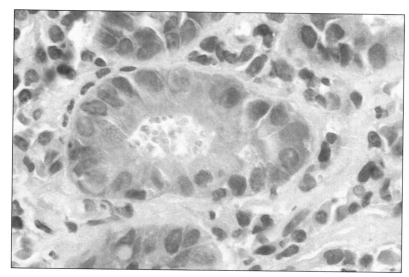

FIGURE 18-32 Chronic cryptosporidiosis (persisting > 1 mo). Duodenal mucosa with *Cryptosporidium* organisms seen along the glandular lumina filling the glandular lumen. Transmission from person to person occurs through fecally contaminated food and water. Because *Cryptosporidium* is resistant to chlorine, water filtration must be a part of the public water supply. The parasite may cause profuse watery diarrhea with severe weight loss by disrupting the absorptive surfaces of the small intestine. There is no good specific therapy against *Cryptosporidium*. Trials with spiramycin and paromomycin may be helpful in some patients. Hyperimmune bovine colostrum is being evaluated for its efficacy.

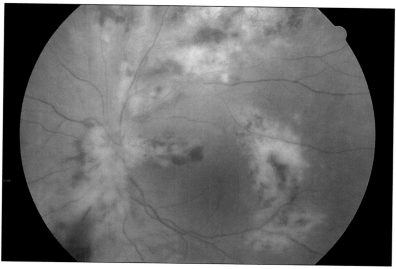

FIGURE 18-33 Cytomegalovirus (CMV) retinitis. Large white perivascular exudates (resembling cottage cheese) and hemorrhages are seen. Early in the disease, the lesions involve only the periphery of the retina, but later the macula and optic disc are also involved, causing blindness. CMV is common in pediatric AIDS patients. Almost half of them will either have an asymptomatic shedding or an infection such as pneumonitis, hepatitis, chorioretinitis, encephalitis, or gastrointestinal involvement. (*Courtesy of* D. Weinberg, MD.)

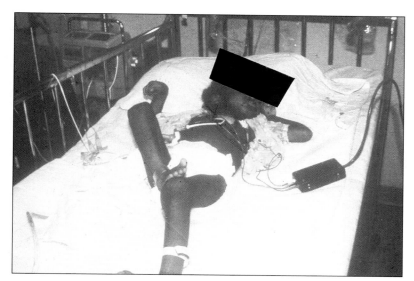

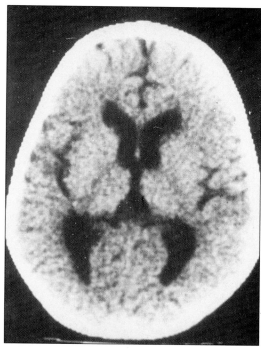

FIGURE 18-35 CT scan of a child with progressive encephalopathy secondary to HIV infection, showing diffuse atrophy. (*Courtesy of* J. Oleske, MD.)

FIGURE 18-34 Central nervous system (CNS) dysfunction occurs in 20% to 30% of HIV-infected children. In symptomatic children, the incidence is even higher (> 40%). Some infants develop encephalopathy as their first AIDS-defining illness, whereas most children have deterioration of CNS function as part of the systemic progression of the disease. Severely affected infants present with progressive deterioration in their motor, language, and cognitive abilities. Loss of acquired developmental milestones is common. With more advanced disease, paresis, hypertonicity, and spasticity (as seen in this patient) appear with or without extrapyramidal dysfunction signs (*ie*, rigidity and dystonia). Cerebral atrophy with enlargement of the ventricles (*see* Fig. 8-35) and bilateral calcifications, especially in the basal ganglia (*see* Fig. 8-36), are some of the manifestations of impaired brain growth. (*Courtesy of* J. Oleske, MD.)

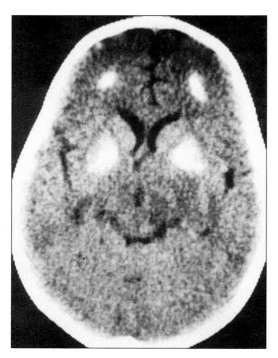

FIGURE 18-36 CT scan showing bilateral symmetrical calcification of the basal ganglia. (*Courtesy of* J. Oleske, MD.)

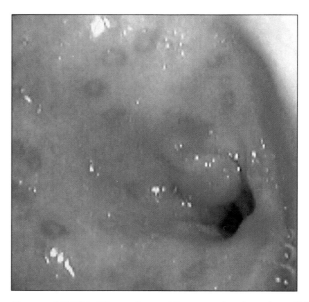

FIGURE 18-37 Disseminated herpes simplex virus (HSV) infection (with onset after 1 month of age). Esophageal involvement in a 12-year-old child. The incidence of HSV esophagitis in children is unknown, although this disease is relatively common in adult AIDS patients. The clinical symptoms include dysphagia, anorexia, and retrosternal pain. The symptoms are indistinguishable from esophagitis caused by candida, other bacteria, or drug toxicity. Therefore, esophagoscopy and biopsy of lesions for histology and culture are necessary for diagnosis. Acyclovir (750 mg/m²/d in divided doses every 8 hours) is the drug of choice. For acyclovir-resistant strains, foscarnet or vidarabine is a successful alternative.

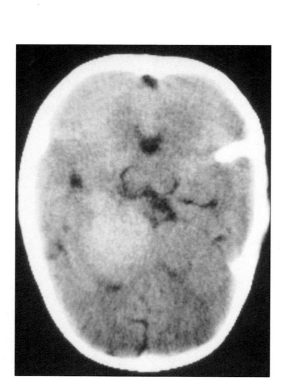

FIGURE 18-38 Primary lymphoma of the brain. Malignancy is an uncommon AIDS-defining illness in pediatric patients (only 2%). Non-Hodgkin's lymphoma (NHL), predominantly high-grade B-cell tumors, heads the list of malignancies. Among pediatric AIDS patients with malignancy, primary lymphoma of the brain is relatively common. As seen in this figure, CT scan of the brain usually demonstrates a hypodense or isodense single lesion, which enhances with contrast. The prognosis is poor, with a median survival of < 6 months. (Beral V, Peterman T, Berkelman R, Jaffe H: AIDS-associated non-Hodgkin's lymphoma. *JAMA* 1991, 337:805–809.) (*Slide courtesy* of J. Oleske, MD.)

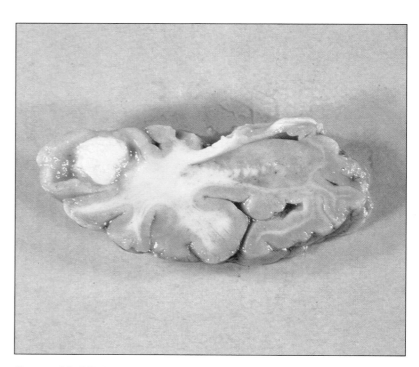

FIGURE 18-39 Non-B-cell lymphoma of the brain (gross pathology). (*Courtesy of* J. Oleske, MD.)

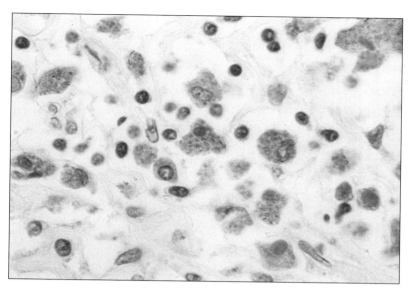

FIGURE 18-40 Disseminated *Mycobacterium avium-intracellulare* (MAI) infection. Histopathology of a pericolonic lymph node. Reports of disseminated MAI in pediatric AIDS patients are increasing. It is estimated that about 10% of HIV-infected children will develop such an infection. In addition, up to 25% of patients with < 100 CD4+ cells will suffer this disease. The clinical symptoms are nonspecific and include fever, weight loss, malaise, anorexia, and profuse diarrhea. Severe anemia and neutropenia are reported to be relatively common in these patients. Blood cultures (at least three sets at different times) are helpful in diagnosis of MAI bacteremia. Positive acid-fast smear of a nonconcentrated stool is a good predictor of disseminated MAI infection, but examination of a biopsy specimen from an abdominal lymph node or the intestinal tract is necessary in patients without detectable bacteremia. Combination therapy with clarithromycin, ethambutol, and rifabutin has shown some promise in slowing the progression of the disease. (Hoyt L, Oleske J, Holland B, Connor E: Non-tuberculous mycobacteria in children with acquired immunodeficiency syndrome. *Pediatr Infect Dis J* 1992, 11:354–360.)

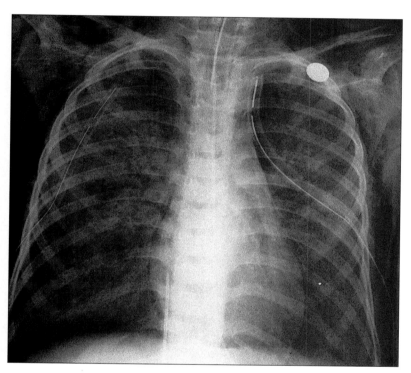

FIGURE 18-41 *Pneumocystis carinii* pneumonia (PCP). PCP is the most common opportunistic infection in children, especially in infants younger than 6 months of age. In almost all pediatric cases it is confined to the lungs, where it typically appears on chest radiographs as a diffuse bilateral infiltrate, as shown in this figure. The CD4+ lymphocyte count is not an accurate predictor of risk for PCP in infants younger than 1 year of age. Therefore, HIV-infected infants < 1 year of age should receive prophylaxis regardless of their CD4+ counts. The prophylaxis of choice is with trimethoprim/sulfamethoxazole (150 mg/m2/d in divided doses given twice daily 3 days a week). In most cases, respiratory symptoms progress rapidly, but a more insidious course of 2–3 weeks of progressive cough and tachypnea has been reported. Thus, any infant at risk for HIV infection who develops progressive respiratory symptoms should be considered for bronchopulmonary lavage, the diagnostic method of choice. The collected specimen should be stained with methenamine-silver nitrate, which will help identify both the *P. carinii* cyst and trophozoite. Trimethoprim/sulfamethoxazole is the drug of choice. Patients with intolerance to this drug should be treated with intravenous pentamidine (4 mg/kg/d). Corticosteroids (prednisone, 2 mg/kg/d) should be added to the treatment because they increase the efficacy of therapy. (Connor E, Bagarazei M, McSherry G: Clinical and laboratory correlates of *Pneumocystis carinii* pneumonia in children infected with HIV. *JAMA* 1991, 265:1693–1697.)

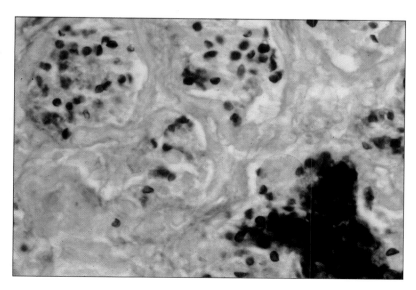

FIGURE 18-42 Histopathology of lung with PCP. Many *P. carinii* organisms are found in the alveoli with invasion of the interstitial area. As the disease progresses, an extensive desquamative alveolitis occurs. (*Courtesy of* J. Oleske, MD.)

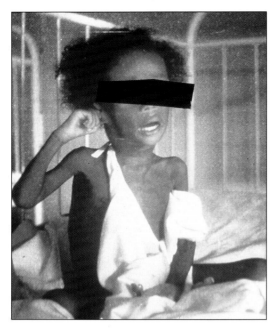

FIGURE 18-43 Severe failure to thrive. The incidence of this condition ranges from 25% to 75% in symptomatic HIV-infected children. The hypermetabolic state during fever and infections, gastrointestinal malabsorption and accelerated losses (*eg*, diarrhea), limited caloric intake, central nervous system impairment (which affects appetite or swallowing), and abnormalities of the endocrine system are some of the multiple factors that contribute to failure to thrive. Treatment should include optimization of nutritional status through the use of high caloric supplements and appetite stimulants (*eg*, megestrol acetate). If oral feeding is insufficient, enteral tube feeding (nasogastric or gastrostomy) should be done, and as a last resort, total parenteral nutrition should be considered. Severe failure to thrive is part of the HIV wasting syndrome. (*Courtesty of* J. Oleske, MD.)

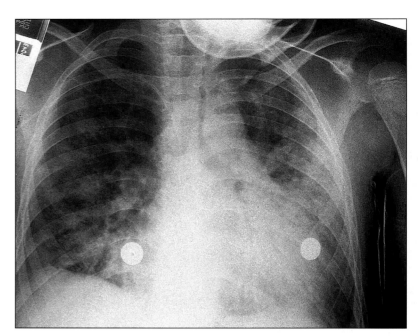

FIGURE 18-44 Disseminated *Aspergillus fumigatus* infection. Aspergillosis develops late in the course of AIDS. Neutropenia, corticosteroid therapy, and treatment with broad-spectrum antibiotics are among the most common predisposing factors. Clinical symptoms are not specific and include insidious cough and fever. Pleuritic pain and hemoptysis may occur. A chest radiograph, as presented here, shows bilateral mixed interstitial and alveolar infiltrates, although it may fail to detect the infiltrate caused by the invasive aspergillosis. If the patient produces large intrabronchial plugs, the aspergillus hyphae may be seen; otherwise an open lung biopsy is needed for diagnosis. The prognosis is poor and treatment with amphotericin B generally has a poor outcome. (Denning DW, Fallansbee SE, Scolard M: Pulmonary aspergillosis in the acquired immunodeficiency syndrome. *N Engl J Med* 1991, 324:654–662.)

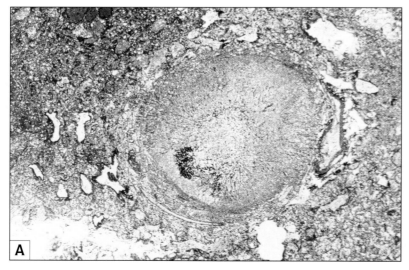

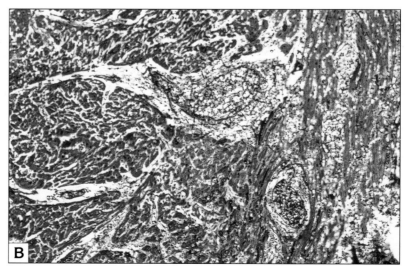

FIGURE 18-45 Histopathology of angioinvasive *A. fumigatus* infection. Most cases of disseminated aspergillosis in adult AIDS patients are in the central nervous system. Involvement of the heart, thyroid, kidney, lymph nodes, and sinuses have also been described. Because the fungus is angioinvasive, it can spread to any organ in the body. **A,** Involvement of the pulmonary vessels. **B,** Involvement of the cardiac vessels.

OTHER CONDITIONS COMMONLY SEEN IN HIV-INFECTED CHILDREN

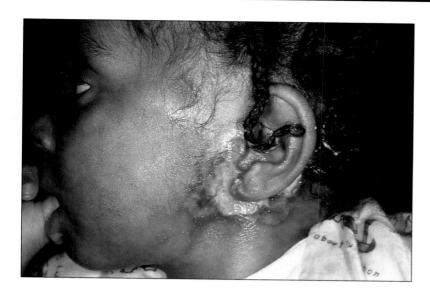

FIGURE 18-46 Pyoderma gangrenosum. An expanding cutaneous ulcer with undermined borders typifies this lesion. The base of the ulcer reveals subcutaneous fat with granulation tissue and necrosis.

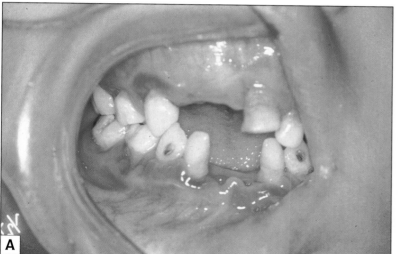

A

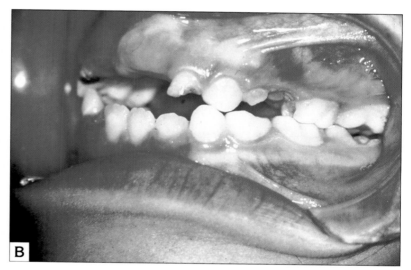

B

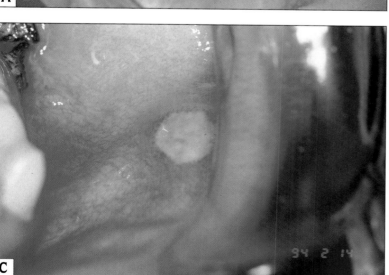

C

FIGURE 18-47 Oral manifestations. Although oral manifestations are commonly seen in HIV-infected children, their appearance may not be due to the HIV infection but rather may relate to the use of various medications in these children. **A**, Severe periodontitis. **B**, Rampant caries. **C**, Aphthous stomatitis. (*Courtesy of* N. Toledo-de-Cabanellas, MD.)

1987 CDC classification system for HIV in children

P-0 Indeterminate infection
P-1 Asymptomatic infection
  P-1A Normal immune function
  P-1B Abnormal immune function
  P-1C Immune function not tested
P-2 Symptomatic infection
  P-2A Nonspecific findings
  P-2B Progressive neurologic disease
  P-2C Lymphoid interstitial pneumonitis
  P-2D Secondary infectious disease
  P-2E Secondary cancers
  P-2F Other diseases (possibly due to HIV)

FIGURE 18-48 1987 CDC classification system for HIV infection in children. In 1987, the CDC published a classification system for use in children under 13 years of age, which listed conditions as reflective of the severity of underlying HIV infection. The CDC continues to work on a revised system to replace this one, and it should appear in the near future. (Centers for Disease Control: Classification system for human immunodeficiency virus (HIV) infection in children under 13 years of age. *MMWR* 1987, 36:225–230, 235.)

SELECTED BIBLIOGRAPHY

Yogev R, Conner E: *HIV infection in infants and children*. St. Louis: Mosby Year Book, Inc; 1992.

Pizzo PA, Wilfert CM: *Pediatric AIDS: the challenge of HIV infection in infants, children and adolescents*: 2nd ed., Baltimore: Williams and Wilkins, 1993.

Fauci AS: Multifactorial nature of immunodeficiency virus disease: Implications for therapy. *Science* 1992, 262:1011–1018.

Guidelines for the care of children and adolescents with HIV infection: Report of the NY state department of health AIDS institute criteria committee for the care of HIV-infected children. *J Pediatr 1991*, 119 (July suppl): S1–S68.

Levy JA: Pathogenesis of human immunodeficiency virus infection. *Microbiol Rev* 1993, 57:183–289.

American Academy of Pediatrics: Report of the committee on infectious diseases. Elk Grove Village, IL: American Academy of Pediatrics; 1991.

CHAPTER 19

HIV Infection in Women

Mary Ann Chiasson
Thomas C. Wright, Jr.

EPIDEMIOLOGY

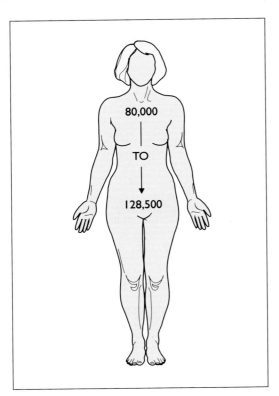

FIGURE 19-1 Estimates of the number of HIV-infected women in the United States vary from 80,000 to 128,500. The lower estimate was extrapolated from the number of infected childbearing women (Gwinn M, Pappaioanou M, George JR, *et al.*: Prevalence of HIV infection in childbearing women in the United States: Surveillance using newborn blood samples. *JAMA* 1991, 265:1704–1708), whereas the higher estimate was developed from a mathematical model of all infected women (Mann J, Tarantola D, Netter T, eds: *AIDS in the World*. Boston: Harvard University Press, 1992:30).

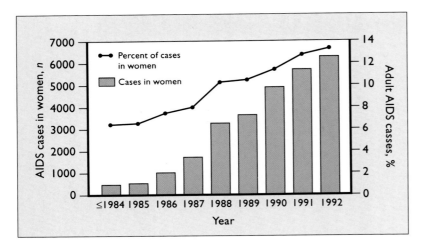

FIGURE 19-2 Incidence and percentage of female adult and adolescent AIDS cases by year in the United States, 1981–1992. Nationally, women (> 12 years of age) represent an increasing number and percentage of adults with AIDS. The *bars* represent the number of women reported with AIDS before 1985 and each year since. The *line* represents the percentage of all adult AIDS cases that occurred among women. In 1985, 541 cases, about 7% of adult cases, were reported among women. Through 1992, more than 27,000 AIDS cases among women in the United States had been reported to CDC. (*Courtesy of* the Centers for Disease Control and Prevention [CDC].)

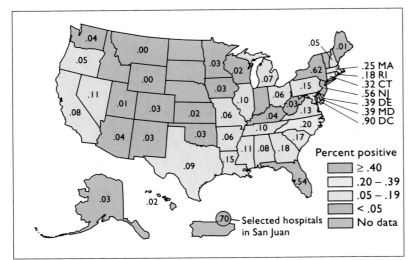

FIGURE 19-3 HIV seroprevalence among childbearing women in the United States, 1991. To estimate the HIV seroprevalence among women who deliver live births, blood specimens that are routinely collected from newborn infants for metabolic screening are also tested for HIV, after removal of personal identifiers. Antibody status of the neonate represents infection status of the mother, because the infant, whether infected or not, passively acquires HIV antibody from the mother during pregnancy. Among 44 states reporting data in 1991, the states with the highest rates were New York, New Jersey, and Florida—the three states with the highest incidence of AIDS in women and perinatally acquired AIDS in children. Seroprevalence rates in childbearing women varied markedly within, as well as among, the states. In general, HIV infection was more prevalent among women residing in metropolitan counties than in other areas. Also, seroprevalence rates in black women were 5–15 times higher than in white women in the same states, whereas rates in Hispanic women were intermediate between those in black and white women in most states. (*Courtesy of* the CDC.)

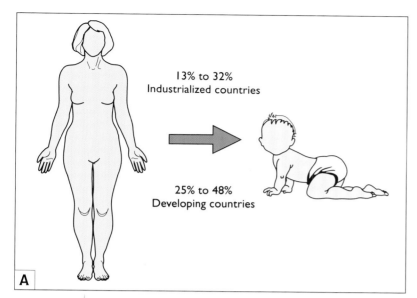

B. Possible factors related to maternal transmission of HIV

Impaired clinical status of mother
Impaired immunologic status of mother
HIV seroconversion during pregnancy
Shortened duration of pregnancy
Chorioaminionitis
Vaginal delivery
Prolonged complicated delivery
Breast feeding

FIGURE 19-4 A, Frequency of maternal–infant transmission of HIV. Numerous studies in both developing and industrialized countries are examining the frequency of transmission from HIV-infected mother to infant. The Ghent Workshop developed standardized criteria for determining the rate of transmission and published rates of 13% to 32% for industrialized countries and 25% to 40% in developing countries. (Dabis F, Msellati P, Dunn D, *et al.*: Estimating the rate of mother-to-child transmission of HIV: Report of a workshop on methological issues, Ghent [Belgium]. *AIDS* 1993, 7:1139–1148.) **B,** Possible factors related to maternal–infant transmission. Factors that increase the exposure of the baby *in utero* or intrapartum to maternal blood or other HIV-infected body fluids increase transmission. Breast feeding provides an additional risk of infection. The passive transfer of maternal antibodies to all newborns makes it difficult to accurately determine which infants are truly infected until maternal antibodies wane at about 15–18 months. (Dabis F, Msellati P, Dunn D, *et al.*: Estimating the rate of mother-to-child transmission of HIV: Report of a workshop on methological issues, Ghent [Belgium]. *AIDS* 1993, 7:1139–1148.)

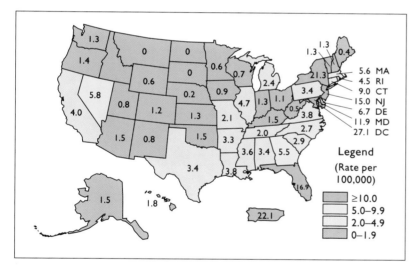

FIGURE 19-5 Women with AIDS by state of residence in the United States, 1992. All but three states reported AIDS cases in women in 1992; however, the incidence rates for the various states differed markedly. Four states—New York, Florida, New Jersey, and Maryland—along with the District of Columbia and Puerto Rico, all of which are *orange* on this map, had incidence rates greater than 10 cases/100,000 women. Twenty states, colored *green*, *yellow*, or *red* had rates between 2 and 10 cases/100,000; the remaining 26 states, in *blue*, had rates < 2. Except for Nevada, all areas that reported rates of five or more AIDS cases/100,000 women were located on the east coast or in Puerto Rico. (*Courtesy of* the CDC.)

Women with AIDS: Number and incidence by race/ethnic group

Race/ethnic group	Patients, *n* (%)	Incidence/100,000 women
Black	3394 (54)	27
White	1458 (23)	2
Hispanic	1337 (21)	13
Other	52 (1)	3
Total*	6255 (100)	6

*Includes 14 women of unknown race/ethnicity.

FIGURE 19-6 Women with AIDS by race/ethnicity. In 1992, 54% of women reported with AIDS in the United States were black, 23% were white, and 21% were Hispanic. These percentages have not changed markedly since 1988. The incidence of AIDS cases per 100,000 women in 1992 was 27 in blacks, compared with 13 in Hispanics and 2 in whites. Accordingly, black and Hispanic women had incidence rates approximately 13 and 6 times, respectively, the rate for white women. (*Courtesy of* the CDC.)

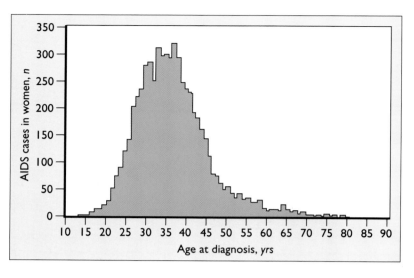

FIGURE 19-7 Age at diagnosis. Most women with AIDS are young. About one quarter of the women reported with AIDS in 1992 were between 20–29 years of age at diagnosis. This age distribution suggests that many of these women were infected as teenagers, because the median period from HIV infection to AIDS is about 10 years. In addition, almost half of the women with AIDS were in their 30s when diagnosed. About 85% of the women with AIDS were of reproductive age (15–44 years) at the time of diagnosis. (*Courtesy of* the CDC.)

Women with AIDS: 10 most common AIDS-indicator diseases in the US

Rank	Disease	Patients, %*
1	*Pneumocystis carnii* pneumonia	43
2	HIV wasting syndrome	21
3	Candidiasis, esophageal	21
4	HIV encephalopathy	6
5	Herpes simplex	6
6	Toxoplasmosis (brain)	6
7	Mycobacterium avium complex	6
8	Cryptococcus (extrapulmonary)	4
9	Cytomegalovirus disease	3
10	Cytomegalovirus retinitis	3

*Some women were reported with multiple diagnoses.

FIGURE 19-8 Common AIDS-indicator diseases in women. In 1992, the most common AIDS-indicator disease in US women was *Pneumocystis carinii* pneumonia, which was diagnosed in about 40% of women reported with AIDS. Both HIV wasting syndrome and esophageal candidiasis were diagnosed in about 20% of women reported with AIDS, whereas each of the other diseases was diagnosed in < 7% of the women with AIDS. The percentages of conditions listed are based primarily on information from women recently diagnosed with AIDS, and some women with AIDS were reported with multiple diagnoses. Accordingly, this list probably underestimates AIDS-indicator diseases that occur later in the course of AIDS. (*Courtesy of* the CDC.)

ETIOLOGIC FACTORS

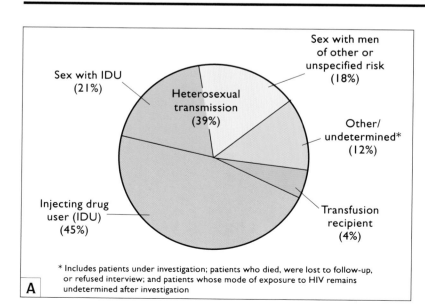

* Includes patients under investigation; patients who died, were lost to follow-up, or refused interview; and patients whose mode of exposure to HIV remains undetermined after investigation

A

FIGURE 19-9 A, Mode of transmission for women with AIDS in the United States. In 1992, heterosexual transmission, which has increased significantly in the past several years, was associated with 39% of reported AIDS cases in women. About half of these women had a history of sex with an injecting drug user, whereas the other half had sex with men with other or unspecified risks. Injection drug use was associated with 45% of reported AIDS cases in women. In addition, 4% of the women with AIDS reported receipt of blood or blood components, and 12% had other or undetermined risks. Most persons with undetermined risk are reclassified as more information becomes available. Since 1987, the percentage of women with AIDS associated with transfusions has decreased from 12% to 4%, whereas the percentage of women with AIDS attributed to heterosexual contact has increased from 30% to 39%. (*Courtesy of* the CDC.) (*continued*)

B. Women with AIDS: Transmission category of race/ethnic group reported in the US

Transmission category	White, n (%)	Black, n (%)	Hispanic, n (%)	Total, n (%)*
Intravenous drug use	617(42)	1600(47)	581(43)	2815(45)
Heterosexual contact	535(37)	1328(39)	549(41)	2437(39)
Transfusion	143(10)	78(2)	49(4)	279(4)
Other/undetermined	163(11)	388(11)	158(12)	724(12)
	1458(100)	3394(100)	1337(100)	6255(100)

*Includes 66 women of unknown or other race/ethnic groups.

FIGURE 19-9 (*continued*) **B**, Mode of transmission by race/ethnicity. In 1992, the overall percentages of women with AIDS who were white, black, or Hispanic tended to be similar for each transmission category. Injection drug use was the most common means of transmission for all three groups, followed by heterosexual contact, undetermined route, and finally transfusion. (*Courtesy of* the CDC.)

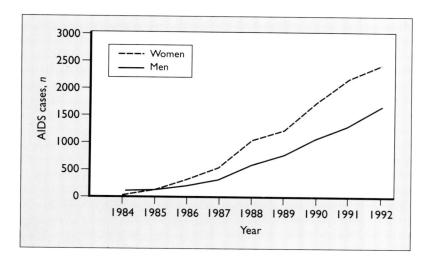

FIGURE 19-10 Reported AIDS cases associated with heterosexual transmission of HIV have been increasing steadily since 1984, with cases occurring more frequently among women than men. "Heterosexual contact" is considered to be the mode of transmission for persons whose only reported risk is heterosexual contact with a person who is either (1) HIV-infected or at increased risk for HIV infection, or (2) born in a country where heterosexual transmission predominates. (*Courtesy of* the CDC.)

Factors that may influence heterosexual transmission of HIV

Infectivity factors
Advanced HIV infection
Early HIV infection
Genital ulcer disease
Other sexually transmitted disease
Antiretroviral therapy (may decrease infectivity)

Susceptibility factors
Genital ulcer disease
Other sexually transmitted diseases
Lack of circumcision (men)
Traumatic sex
Defloration
Cervical ectopy
Oral contraceptive
Anal intercourse (women)
Age (women)

FIGURE 19-11 Factors that may influence heterosexual transmission of HIV. **A**, Infectivity factors. A number of biologic factors increase infectivity of HIV-positive individuals. The increased viremia found in early and late stages of HIV infection may explain the higher frequency of heterosexual transmission during these periods. Similarly, the occurrence of open lesions and disrupted genital epithelium, which are associated with sexually transmitted diseases, appear to enhance sexual transmission of HIV. A few studies have suggested that infected individuals may be less likely to transmit HIV when taking antiretroviral therapy. (Holmberg SD, Horsburgh CR Jr, Ward JW, Jaffe HW: Biologic factors in the sexual transmission of human immunodeficiency virus. *J Infect Dis* 1989, 160:116–125.) **B**, Susceptibility factors. Numerous studies have shown that the occurrence of open lesions and disrupted genital epithelium, in individuals with sexually transmitted diseases, provide HIV with ready access to target cells. Similarly, lack of circumcision in men, traumatic sex, defloration, cervical ectopy (ectropion), and anal intercourse may all result in disrupted genital epithelium, destroying the mechanical barrier to viral entry. The association between oral contraceptive use and increased HIV infection has been observed in African prostitutes but may be mediated by an increased area of ectopy (ectropion), which results in a more friable cervix. Young women also have larger areas of ectopy, whereas postmenopausal women may be at increased risk because of senile atrophic vaginitis. (Holmberg SD, Horsburgh CR Jr, Ward JW, Jaffe HW: Biologic factors in the sexual transmission of human immunodeficiency virus. *J Infect Dis* 1989, 160:116–125.)

Genital Ulcers

Most common etiologic agents of genital ulcers in the US
Treponema pallidum *Herpes simplex virus type 2* *Haemophilus ducreyi*

FIGURE 19-12 Common etiologic agents of genital ulcer disease in the United States. Although the association between genital ulcers and sexual transmission of HIV in developing countries is well recognized, genital ulcers are also common in the United States. In 1992, 33,973 cases of primary syphilis, 200,000–500,000 first patient visits for genital herpes, and 1886 cases of chancroid were reported. (Division of STD/HIV Prevention: *Sexually Transmitted Disease Surveillance, 1992.* Atlanta, CDC, 1993.)

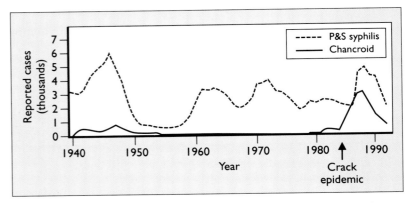

FIGURE 19-13 Incidence of syphilis and chancroid in New York City, 1940–1992. In New York, like many other areas along the eastern seaboard, an epidemic of genital ulcer disease occurred coincident with the crack cocaine epidemic in the late 1980s and early 1990s. The effects of these twin epidemics on the heterosexual transmission of HIV will not be fully evaluable until the late 1990s.

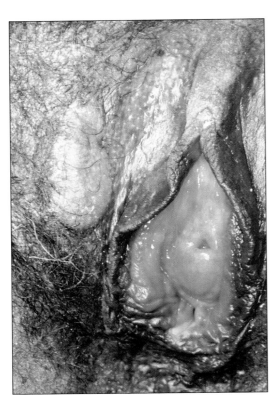

FIGURE 19-14 Secondary syphilis in HIV infection. A 34-year-old HIV-infected woman had a 3 × 2-cm swollen, indurated, and grayish area of leathery consistency on the right labia majora. Her VDRL test was positive with a titer of 1:32, and a Papanicolaou smear showed trichomoniasis. (*Courtesy of* K. LaGuardia, MD.)

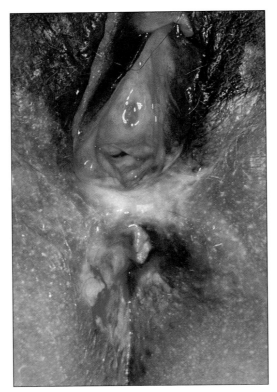

FIGURE 19-15 Herpetic lesion, acyclovir resistant. A 31-year-old HIV-infected woman with a 4-year history of recurrent genital herpes infection presented with a chronic (7-month-old) perianal ulcer, which was resistant to treatment with acyclovir. Her herpes culture showed acyclovir resistance. Her ulcer healed within 4 weeks after initiating therapy with intravenous gancyclovir. (*Courtesy of* K. LaGuardia, MD.)

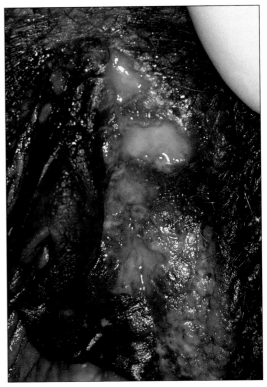

FIGURE 19-16 Recurrent genital herpes. Multiple recurrent ulcers in an HIV-infected women. Herpetic lesions can become quite large, become secondarily infected, and assume an unusual appearance in HIV-infected patients.

Stages of Cervical Ectopy

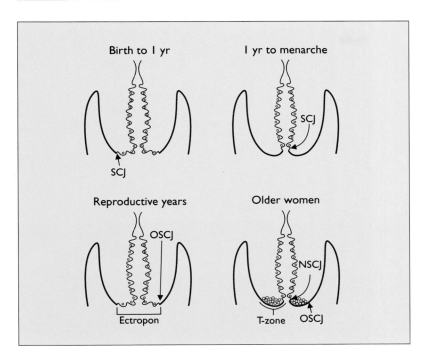

FIGURE 19-17 At birth, mucin-secreting columnar endocervical epithelium is present on the outer surface (portio) of the cervix. This columnar epithelium is frequently referred to as *cervical ectopy* (or ectropion). Hormonal and other physical factors influence the amount and distribution of this endocervical columnar epithelium on the portio surface of the cervix (*ie*, ectopy). At about 1 year after birth, the cervix begins to elongate, which alters the shape and size of the cervical portio. As a result of this elongation, the endocervical mucin-secreting columnar epithelium becomes displaced inward, reducing the amount of columnar epithelium on the outer surface of the cervix (*ie*, reducing the size of the ectopy). At puberty, both the uterus and cervix begin to enlarge, and endocervical columnar epithelium becomes displaced onto the portio surface of the cervix. Subsequently, over a period of years, the squamous epithelium grows inward toward the endocervical canal, a process termed *squamous metaplasia*, and replaces the mucin-producing columnar epithelium with a stratified squamous epithelium. The end result of this ingrowth is the total loss of cervical ectopy (ectropion). (SCJ—squamocolumnar junction; T-zone—transformation zone; OSCJ and NSCJ—original and native squamocolumnar junction.)

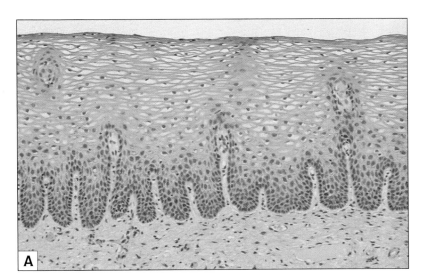

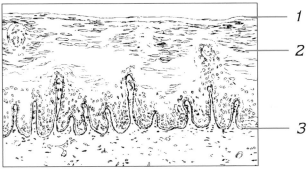

FIGURE 19-18 A, Normal squamous epithelium. The exposed, or vaginal, portion of the cervix is generally lined by a nonkeratinizing, stratified squamous epithelium, referred to as the *native portio epithelium*. Histologically, the mature squamous epithelium of the native portio is divided into three zones: (*1*) the superficial zone, containing the most mature cell population; (*2*) the midzone or stratum spinosum, which comprises the majority of the epithelium; and (*3*) the basal or germinal cell layer, which is responsible for continuous epithelial renewal. The mature squamous epithelium of the portio is considered to be quite resistant to physical trauma and many infectious agents. **B,** Mucin-producing columnar epithelium. The mucosa of the cervical canal (endocervix) is composed of a single layer of tall columnar mucin-secreting epithelium, which lines both the surface and the underlying glandular structures. These cells are considered to be more susceptible to trauma than the stratified squamous epithelium of the portio and are more susceptible to various microbial pathogens, such as *Neisseria gonorrhoeae* and *Chlamydia trachomatis.* (*continued*)

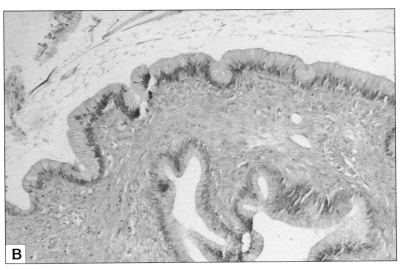

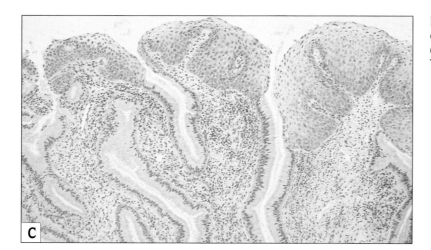

FIGURE 19-18 (*continued*) **C,** Squamous metaplasia. Small islands of stratified squamous epithelium can be seen replacing the columnar, endocervical-type, mucosa of the cervical epithelium. This is a normal physiologic process occurring after puberty.

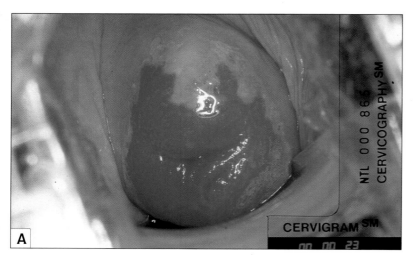

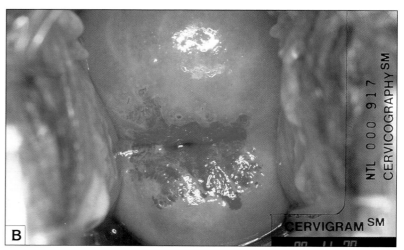

FIGURE 19-19 A, Cervical ectopy (ectropion). When viewed with the naked eye, the endocervical mucosa of the cervical ectopy appears as a red, velvety zone, sharply contrasting with the neighboring pink and shiny squamous portio epithelium. This is a large cervical ectopy in a young female. **B,** With time, the cervical ectopy becomes reduced, as a pink, metaplastic squamous epithelium replaces the red columnar epithelium. Tongues of metaplastic epithelium are seen growing into the cervical ectopy. **C,** Mature cervix. In older women, the process of squamous metaplasia totally replaces the cervical ectopy, and the external surface of the portio cervix becomes covered by a stratified squamous epithelium.

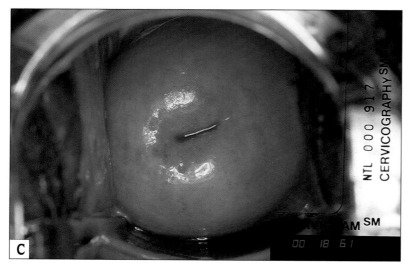

Determinants of cervical ectopy
Age
Time since last pregnancy
Progestin administration
Cervical infections
Cervical pH

FIGURE 19-20 Determinants of cervical ectopy. Although there has been no definitive study of factors influencing cervical ectopy, its presence has been inversely related to age and directly associated with pregnancy and oral contraceptive usage in some studies. The process of squamous metaplasia is primarily dependent on local (vaginal) environmental factors. (Coppleson M, Reid B: *Preclinical Carcinoma of the Cervix Uteri*. Oxford: Pergamon Press, 1967. Linhartova A: Extent of columnar epithelium on the ectocervix between the ages of 1 and 13 years. *Obstet Gynecol* 1978, 52:451–455). The initial stimulus for squamous metaplasia is thought to be the low (acid) pH of the vagina after puberty. Under the influence of estrogen, the vaginal mucosal cells become rich in glycogen, and this may allow the number of acid-secreting Döderlein's bacteria to increase, thus resulting in a lower vaginal pH. Trauma, chronic irritation, or cervical infection may also play a role in the development and maturation of the cervix by stimulating repair and remodeling. In some studies, cervical ectopy has been associated with *Chlamydia trachomatis* infection. (McCormack W, Rosner B: Infection with *Chlamydia trachomatis* in female college students. *Am J Epidemiol* 1985, 121:107–115).

GYNECOLOGIC CONDITIONS IN HIV-INFECTED WOMEN

Important gynecologic conditions in HIV-infected women

Cervical cancer
Cervical intraepithelial neoplasia
Vulvovaginal intraepithelial neoplasia
Condyloma acuminatum
Candidiasis
Trichomoniasis
Pelvic inflammatory disease

FIGURE 19-21 HIV infection is thought either to increase the prevalence or exacerbate the clinical course of four gynecologic conditions: invasive cervical cancer and its precursor lesion (cervical intraepithelial neoplasia), vulvovaginal human papillomavirus (HPV)-associated clinical lesions (*ie*, condyloma accuminata and intraepithelial neoplasia), vulvovaginal infections including chronic candidiasis, and pelvic inflammatory disease.

Cervical Cancer

Cervical cancer risk factors

Number of sexual partners
Sex at an early age
Early first pregnancy
Parity
Pap smear interval
Oral contraceptive use
Low socioeconomic class
Human papillomavirus
Herpes simplex virus
Cigarette smoking
Immunosuppression
Vitamin deficiencies

FIGURE 19-22 Risk factors for the development of cervical cancer in women (with or without HIV infection). Infection with either herpes simplex virus type 2 or specific HPV types (*ie*,16 or 18) are key risk factors, as is a history of abnormal Papanicolaou smears. (Brinton LA: Oral contraceptives and cervical neoplasia. *Contraception* 1991, 43:581–595.)

HIV and cervical disease: Reasons for concern

Both HIV infection and HPV infection can be sexually transmitted
Well-recognized increase in anogenital cancers in immunosuppressed women

FIGURE 19-23 There are reasons to be concerned that women with HIV infection may be at special risk for cervical cancer. It is well established that most anogenital squamous cell carcinomas are associated with specific types of HPV, which are sexually transmitted agents. (Schiffman MH, Bauer HM, Hoover RN, *et al.*: Epidemiological evidence that human papillomavirus infection causes most cervical intraepithelial neoplasia. *J Natl Cancer Inst* 1993, 85:958–964. zur Hausen H: Human papillomaviruses in the pathogenesis of anogenital cancer. *Virology* 1991, 184:9–13.) Many HIV-infected women become infected through heterosexual contact and would be presumed to be at risk for the acquisition of a second sexually transmitted disease, *eg*, HPV. In addition, women who are immunosuppressed for reasons other than HIV infection are at increased risk for developing invasive squamous cell carcinomas and intraepithelial squamous neoplasia of the anogenital tract. (Penn I: Cancers of the anogenital region in renal transplant recipients. *Cancer* 1986, 58:611–616.)

Transplant recipients—Cincinnati transplant tumor registry

777 tumors in women, 6% anogenital (includes carcinoma *in situ*)
Tumors often multiple, extensive, refractive to therapy

FIGURE 19-24 Anogenital cancers and neoplasia in transplant recipients. One of the largest studies of anogenital tumors in transplant recipients is by Penn, who maintained a registry of tumors in transplant recipients. This registry included 777 "tumors" in female transplant recipients. Six percent of these "tumors" were of the anogenital tract and included 20 cases of intraepithelial neoplasia and 29 cases of invasive squamous cell carcinoma of the vulva, vagina, or cervix. Of note, vulvar lesions were more than twice as common as cervical lesions in the cases referred to this registry. Lesions in immunosuppressed women were frequently multicentric, and recurrent/persistent disease was common after standard therapy. (Penn I. Cancers of the anogenital region in renal transplant recipients. *Cancer* 1986, 58:611–616.)

Aggressive anogenital cancers

Author	Site	Unusual aspects
Rellihan	Cervix	Clitoral metastasis, dead in 5 months
Schwartz	Cervix	Iliopsoas metastasis, dead in 5 months
Giorda	Vulva	Recurrence in 2 months

FIGURE 19-25 Aggressive anogenital cancers in HIV-infected women. Two case reports of rapidly progressive invasive cervical cancers that metastasized to unusual sites have been described in HIV-infected women. One case was a 32-year-old HIV-seropositive patient with a FIGO stage IIB carcinoma who developed disseminated carcinomatosis, relapsed at a periclitoral site 2 months after radiation therapy, and died < 5 months after diagnosis. (Rellihan MA, Dooley DP, Burke TW, *et al.*: Rapidly progressive cervical cancer in a patient with human immunodeficiency virus infection. *Gynecol Oncol* 1990, 36:435–438.) Another case report described a 25-year-old woman with a FIGO stage IIIB cervical cancer who developed a metastases to the iliopsoas muscle and also died within 5 months of diagnosis. (Schwartz LB, Carcangiu ML, Bradham L, Schwarz PE: Rapidly progressive squamous cell carcinoma of the cervix coexisting with human immunodeficiency virus infection: Clinical opinion. *Gynecol Oncol* 1991, 41:255–258.) In addition, there has been a single case report of an invasive vulvar carcinoma developing in an HIV-infected patient. (Giorda G, Vaccher E, Volpe R, *et al.*: Case report: An unusual presentation of vulvar carcinoma in a HIV patient. *Gynecol Oncol* 1992, 44:191–194.)

Cervical cancers in HIV-infected women

Author	Country	HIV+	Cervical cancer
Provencher	US	213	–
Carpenter	US	100	–
Vermund	US	47	–
Schafer	Germany	111	5
Kreiss	Kenya	42	–
Wright	US	430	–
Laga	Zaire	41	–
Maggwa	Kenya	205	–

FIGURE 19-26 A. Cervical cancers in HIV-infected women. Many studies have used either cytology or a combination of cytology and colposcopy to screen HIV-infected women for cervical cancer. For the most part, these studies have failed to detect invasive cervical cancers in the women screened. The only exception is a study of Schafer from Berlin. However, this study enrolled women from the inpatient gynecologic service of a Berlin teaching hospital, which might explain the large number of invasive cancers detected. (Provencher D, *et al.*: *Gynecol Oncol* 1988, 31:184–188. Carpenter CCJ, *et al.*: *Medicine* 1991, 70:307–325. Vermund SH, *et al.*: *Am J Obstet Gynecol* 1991, 165:392–400. Schafer A, *et al.*: *Am J Obstet Gynecol* 1991, 164:593–599. Kreiss JK, *et al.*: *Sex Trans Dis* 1992, 19:54–59. Wright T, *et al.*: First National Conference on Human Retroviruses and Related Infections, Washington, DC, 1993:61. Laga M, *et al.*: *Int J Cancer* 1992, 50:45–48. Maggwa B, *et al.*: *AIDS* 1993, 7:733–738.)

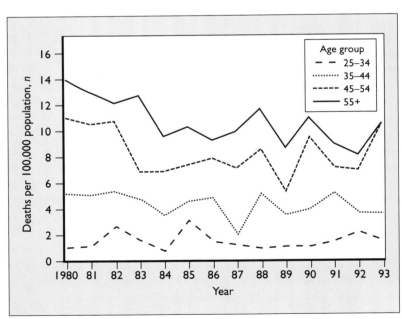

FIGURE 19-27 Cervical cancer mortality in New York City, 1980–1993. No overall increase in deaths or death rates (per 100,000 population) due to cervical cancer have been observed in New York City women in the decade since HIV infection emerged. As the epicenter of the AIDS epidemic in women in the United States, New York would be expected to show an increase in mortality if an epidemic of cervical cancer were occurring in these women. Thus far, only 42 of 11,006 women with AIDS from New York City have been reported to have invasive cervical cancer. (New York City Department of Health: *AIDS Case Surveillance Report*, January 1994.)

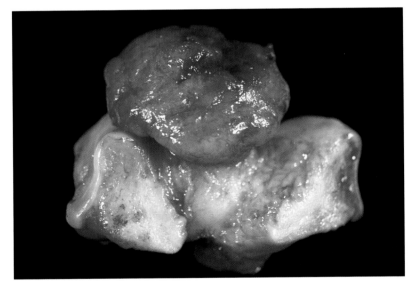

FIGURE 19-28 Gross appearance of a typical, exophytic invasive cervical cancer. Although this tumor is from an HIV-seronegative patient, there are no reported differences in the gross appearances of invasive cancers between HIV-infected and uninfected women.

Cervical Intraepithelial Neoplasia

Cervical disease in HIV-infected women

Author	Patients, *n*	Method	CIN, *n* (%)
Bradbeer	9	Colposcopy	5 (56%)
Spurrett	6	Colposcopy	1 (17%)
Crocchiolo	24	Colposcopy	6 (25%)
Byrne	15	Cytology	4 (27%)

FIGURE 19-29 The first report linking cervical intraepithelial neoplasia (CIN), a cervical cancer precursor, to HIV infection appeared in 1987. Eight (73%) of the 11 HIV-infected women who were enrolled from a London HIV clinic had an abnormal Papanicolaou smear, and 56% of those who underwent colposcopy had biopsy-proven CIN. Subsequently, other small series confirmed a high rate of cervical disease in HIV-infected women. (Bradbeer C: Is infection with HIV a risk factor for cervical intraepithelial neoplasia? *Lancet* 1987, ii:1277–1278. Spurrett B, Jones DS, Stewart G: Cervical dysplasia and HIV infection. *Lancet* 1988, i:238–239. Crocchiolo P, Lizioli A, Goisis F, *et al.*: Cervical dysplasia and HIV infection [letter]. *Lancet* 1988, i:238–239. Byrne M, Taylor-Robinson D, Harris JRW: Cervical dysplasia and HIV infection. *Lancet* 1988, i:238–239.)

Pap smears in HIV-infected women

Author	Seropositive patients, *n* (% abnormal)	Seronegative source (% abnormal)
Provencher	201 (63%)	Serotesting (5%)
Marte	135 (26%)	Amb. care (6%)
Schafer	111 (41%)	IVDUs (9%)
Vermund	51 (33%)	Methadone (13%)
Laga*	41 (27%)	Prostitutes (3%)
Maggwa*	205 (5%)	Gyn. clinic (2%)
ter Meulen*	41 (2%)	Gyn. clinic (3%)
Kreiss*	42 (26%)	Prostitutes (24%)

*African studies.

FIGURE 19-30 Papanicolaou smears in HIV-infected women. The early cytologic studies found an increased prevalence of cytologic abnormalities among HIV-infected women. Although these studies lacked control groups and involved relatively small numbers of women, their conclusions have now been confirmed by larger studies comparing HIV-infected and uninfected women. Even though evidence appears to be convincing for an association between CIN and HIV infection, two recent African studies have failed to detect significantly higher rates of cytologic abnormalities in HIV-infected women compared with controls. The reasons for the findings of these two studies are unknown but may relate to the fact that few of the HIV-infected women enrolled in the study were symptomatic from their HIV infections. (Provencher D, *et al.*: *Gynecol Oncol* 1988, 31:184–188. Marte C, *et al.*: *Am J Obstet Gynecol* 1992, 166:1232–1237. Schafer A, *et al.*: *Am J Obstet Gynecol* 1991, 164:593–599. Vermund SH, *et al. Am J Obstet Gynecol* 1991, 165:392–400. Laga M, *et al.*: *Int J Cancer* 1992, 50:45–48. Maggwa B, *et al.*: *AIDS* 1993, 7:733–738. ter Meulen J, *et al.*: *Int J Cancer* 1992, 51:515–521. Kreiss JK, *et al.*: *Sex Trans Dis* 1992, 19:54–59.)

Effects of immunosuppression

Author	Patients, *n*	Immune status	Abnormal pap, %
Schafer	111	CD4+ >250	39%
		CD4+ <250	53%
Vermund	51	Asymptomatic	17%
		Symptomatic	42%
Marte	135	CD4+ >400	26%
		CD4+ <400	45%
Smith	43	Asymptomatic	22%
		Symptomatic	100%

FIGURE 19-31 Effects of immunosuppression. The degree of HIV-related immunosuppression has been associated with the presence of cervical disease in a number of studies. These studies have used CD4+ T-lymphocyte counts or the presence of HIV-associated symptoms to estimate the degree of immunosuppression. (Schafer A, *et al.*: The increased frequency of cervical dysplasia-neoplasia in women infected with the human immunodeficiency virus is related to the degree of immunosuppression. *Am J Obstet Gynecol* 1991, 164:593–599. Vermund SH, *et al.*: High risk of human papillomavirus infection and cervical squamous intraepithelial lesions among women with symptomatic human immunodeficiency virus infection. *Am J Obstet Gynecol* 1991, 165:392–400. Marte C, *et al.*: Papanicolaou smear abnormalities in ambulatory care sites for women infected with human immunodeficiency virus. *Am J Obstet Gynecol* 1992, 166:1232–1237. Smith JR, *et al.*: Is HIV infection associated with an increase in the prevalence of cervical neoplasia? *Br J Obstet Gynaecol* 1993, 100:149–153.)

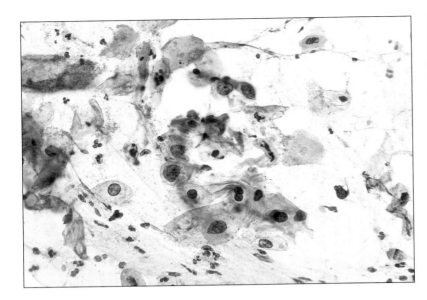

FIGURE 19-32 Low-grade squamous intraepithelial lesion. A Papanicolaou smear from an HIV-infected woman diagnosed with a low-grade squamous intraepithelial lesion (LoSIL). There are prominent koilocytes and multinucleated cells present. Koilocytes are the cells with prominent perinuclear halos and dense, atypical nuclei. They are typically found in HPV-infected squamous epithelium.

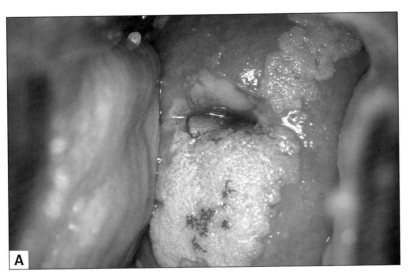

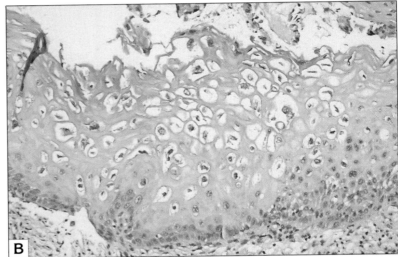

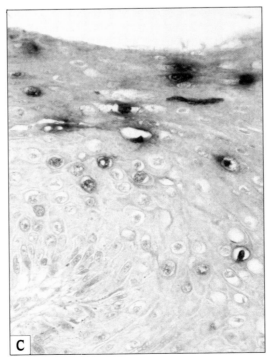

FIGURE 19-33 Low-grade cervical intraepithelial neoplasia. **A,** A colpophotograph from an HIV-infected woman shows a low-grade CIN. The lesional tissue is dense white after the application of 5% acetic acid (vinegar) and is slightly raised. Abnormal vessels are not present, and the appearance of the lesion is quite bland. Because of its exophytic appearance, some clinicians might call this a cervical condyloma acuminata. However, because pathologists have difficulty in distinguishing between a low-grade CIN lesion and condyloma acuminata, biopsy specimens from these lesions are usually diagnosed as low-grade CIN. **B,** A photomicrograph from a cervical biopsy specimen of the lesion in *panel 33A*. The epithelium is thickened and has squamous epithelial cells with nuclear atypia, prominent perinuclear halos, and multinucleation. These cells are identical to the koilocytes observed in the Papanicolaou smear in Figure 19-32 and are diagnostic of an HPV-associated lesion. **C,** *In-situ* hybridization for HPV-DNA. A cervical biopsy specimen from a low-grade CIN lesion processed for *in-situ* hybridization using probes for HPV-16 or 18 DNA. The nuclei of those superficial squamous epithelial cells that had nuclear atypia and perinuclear halos are stained dark blue, indicating the presence of HPV-DNA.

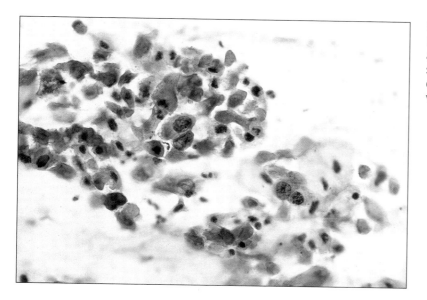

FIGURE 19-34 High-grade squamous intraepithelial lesion. A Papanicolaou smear from an HIV-infected woman was diagnosed as a high-grade squamous intraepithelial lesion (HiSIL). The superficial squamous cells and the parabasal and basal cells all have nuclear and cytoplasmic changes. The nuclei are enlarged and hyperchromatic, with an increase in the nuclear-to-cytoplasmic ratio.

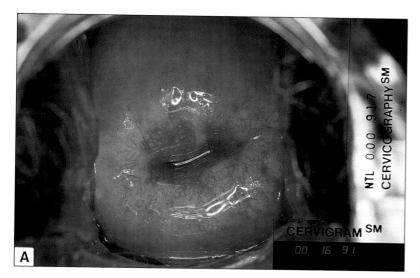

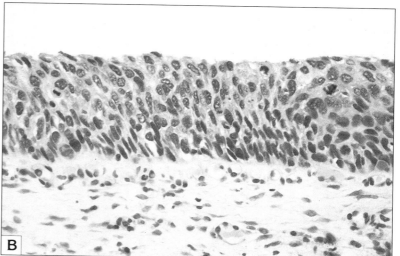

FIGURE 19-35 High-grade cervical intraepithelial neoplasia. **A**, A colpophotograph from an HIV-infected woman with high-grade CIN shows a flat, dense, acetowhite lesion with sharp margins. There are prominent blood vessels forming a mosaic pattern in the lesional tissue. These are the features of high-grade CIN lesions and (in our experience) are similar in HIV-infected and uninfected women. **B**, A photomicrograph of a cervical biopsy specimen of the lesion in *panel*

35A. The maturation of the squamous epithelium is markedly altered and the epithelium has been replaced by small, hyperchromatic cells with an increase in the nuclear-to-cytoplasmic ratio. Mitotic figures are present in the upper two thirds of the epithelium. Although lesions with this histologic appearance are almost universally associated with HPV, the typical HPV cytopathic effects of multinucleation and perinuclear halos are usually minimal.

Treatment of CIN in HIV-infected women

Method	Study	Patients, *n*	Failure
Conization	Spinillo	6	17%
	Maimen	8	13%
Cautery	Spinillo	16	0
Cryosurgery	McGuiness	18	78%
	Maimen	27	48%
Laser	Maiman	9	33%
LEEP	Wright	34	56%

FIGURE 19-36 Treatment of cervical intraepithelial neoplasia. A number of studies have looked at the responses of CIN lesions in HIV-infected women to standard therapies. In the first study, conducted in Italy, excellent success rates after treatment using either electrocautery or cone biopsy were reported. More recent studies from the United States have reported poor outcomes after treatment with either cryosurgery or laser ablation. (Spinillo A, *et al.*: Prevalence, diagnosis and treatment of lower genital neoplasia in women with human immunodeficiency virus infection. *Eur J Obstet Gynecol* 1992, 43:235–241. Maiman M, *et al.*: Recurrent cervical intraepithelial neoplasia in human immunodeficiency virus-seropositive women. *Obstet Gynecol* 1993, 81:170–174. McGuinness K, LaGuardia K: Cryotherapy in the management of cervical dysplasia in HIV infected women. Presented at the IX International Conference on AIDS, Berlin, 1993:409. Wright T, *et al.*: Treatment of cervical intraepithelial neoplasia in HIV-infected women with loop electrosurgical excision. Presented at the 1st National Conference on Human Retroviruses and Related Infections, Washington, DC, 1993:61.)

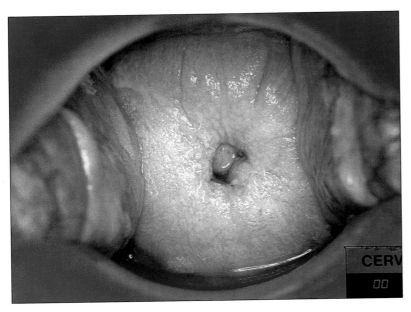

FIGURE 19-37 Failure of loop electrosurgical excision for CIN. An HIV-infected patient was treated for low-grade CIN using loop electrosurgical excision. Four months after treatment, she returned with extensive recurrent/persistent low-grade CIN involving the entire cervix and extending to the vagina. This pattern is observed in up to one third of HIV-infected women who develop recurrent/persistent CIN after loop excision. (Wright T, *et al.*: Treatment of cervical intraepithelial neoplasia in HIV-infected women with loop electrosurgical excision. Presented at the 1st National Conference on Human Retroviruses and Related Infections, Washington, DC, 1993:61.)

Vulvovaginal Human Papillomavirus-Associated Lesions

Vulvovaginal HPV lesions

Author	HIV+, *n*	Lesion	Patients, *n (%)*
Carpenter	200	Condyloma	32 (16%)
Byrne	19	VIN	3 (16%)
Smith	50	VIN & VAIN	4 (9%)
Chiasson	398	Condyloma	22 (6%)
		VIN	2 (<1%)

FIGURE 19-38 Although there are fewer data on the prevalence of vulvovaginal HPV-associated lesions in HIV-infected women than there are for cervical disease, several studies suggest an increased prevalence of condyloma accuminata as well as vulvar and vaginal intraepithelial neoplasia (VIN and VAIN) in this population (Carpenter CCJ, *et al.*: Human immunodeficiency virus infection in North American women: Experience with 200 cases and a review of the literature. *Medicine* 1991, 70:307–325. Bryne M, *et al.*: Cervical dysplasia and HIV infection. *Lancet* 1988, i:238–239. Chiasson MA, *et al.*: Vulvovaginal condyloma and intraepithelia neoplasia in HIV-infected and uninfected women. Presented at the 1st National Conference on Human Retroviruses and Related Infections, Washington, DC, 1993.)

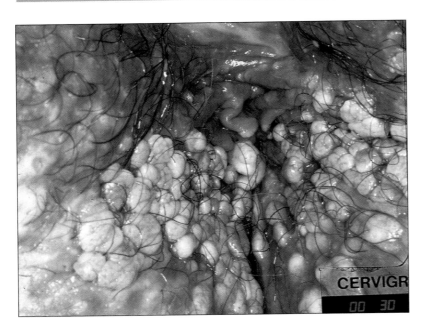

FIGURE 19-39 Anogenital condyloma. In our experience, condylomas have an identical appearance in HIV-infected and uninfected women. They typically present as raised, white growths involving the vulva, perianal area, urethra, and vagina. In HIV-infected women, they can become large and can be difficult to treat with standard therapies such as trichloroacetic acid or electrocautery. Pigmented or ulcerated lesions should always undergo biopsy, as should lesions that are refractory to therapy, to rule out an intraepithelial neoplasia or squamous cell carcinoma.

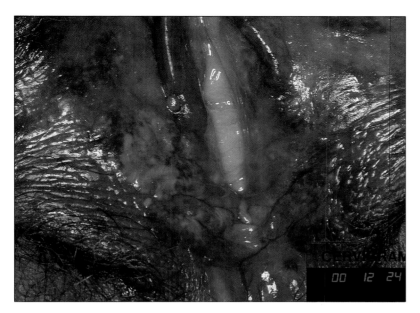

FIGURE 19-40 Vulvar intraepithelial neoplasia (VIN). In the HIV-infected patient, VIN is frequently multifocal and presents as discrete, pigmented, slightly raised lesions. These lesions are frequently asymptomatic and can easily be overlooked (especially in dark-skinned patients). VIN can sometimes be symptomatic and associated with severe pruritus. VIN is considered to be a precursor to invasive vulvar carcinoma, and all pigmented lesions of the anogenital region should undergo biopsy.

Vulvovaginal Infections

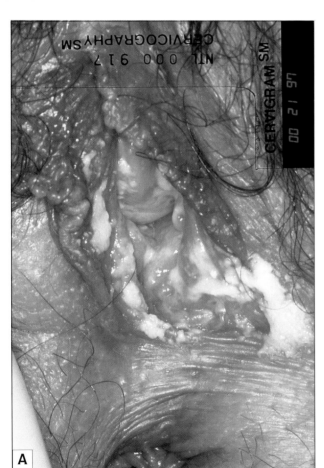

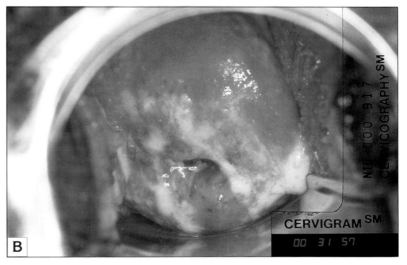

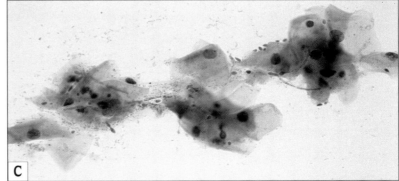

FIGURE 19-41 Candidiasis. **A,** Chronic vulvovaginal candidiasis is a common gynecologic complaint in HIV-infected women. Patients frequently present with pruritis (which can be severe), an irritating discharge, and sometimes vulvar pain and dyspareunia. Vulvar erythema and edema are frequently present and usually most prominent between the labia minora. However, a discharge is not always present, and in those cases in which it is present, the characteristics of the discharge can be highly variable. **B,** Typically, the discharge of candidiasis is described as containing thick, white, cottage cheese–like material. In other patients, the discharge can be thin and watery. The easiest way to confirm the diagnosis is to perform a microscopic examination of the discharge after suspending it in 10% potassium hydroxide. **C,** Large numbers of yeastlike organisms are observed in a Papanicolaou smear from an HIV-infected patient with candidiasis. Yeast forms (blastocyts) as well as long, nonbranching pseudohyphae are present.

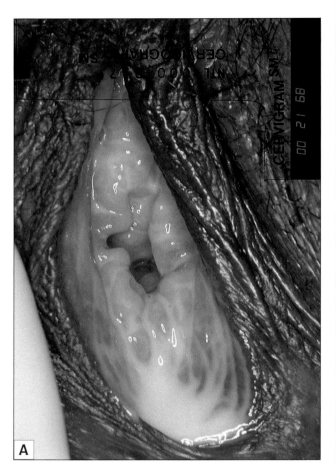
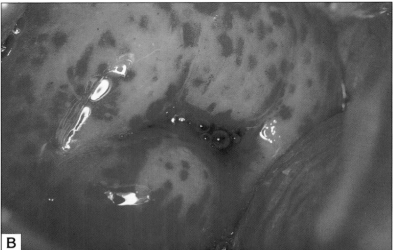
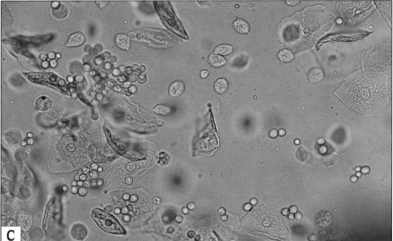

FIGURE 19-42 Trichomoniasis. **A**, Trichomoniasis is a common, sexually transmitted vulvovaginal infection in HIV-infected women. It is caused by *Trichomonas vaginalis.* Patients with documented trichomoniasis frequently complain of a profuse, frothy discharge which is associated with vulvovaginal pruritus, tenderness, and burning. The vulva and vagina are frequently erythematous and sometimes edematous. **B**, The cervix and vagina frequently develop small, red, punctated lesions in severe cases of trichomoniasis. These produce a classic "strawberry" appearance. **C**, Diagnosis of trichomoniasis is most easily made through microscopic examination of the discharge (ie, wet mount). Because of their motility, the small, pear-shaped organisms can easily be detected on a wet mount. Cultures can also be useful to document the presence of *T. vaginalis* in women with clinical manifestations of trichomoniasis but with repeatedly negative wet mounts.

Pelvic Inflammatory Disease

Pelvic inflammatory disease in HIV-infected women
1 million cases of salpingitis yearly
10% to 15% of US women have had an episode of salpingitis
PID may be more common and difficult to treat in HIV+ women

FIGURE 19-43 Pelvic inflammatory disease (PID) is common in the United States, and there is growing evidence that it may occur more frequently in HIV-infected women and may be more difficult to treat in them.

HIV infection and pelvic inflammatory disease

Author	Site	Patients, *n*	HIV+, %
Sarfrin	San Francisco	333	6.7
Hoegsberg	Brooklyn	110	13.6
Sperling	New York	30	16.7

FIGURE 19-44 Investigators from three sites have reported an increased prevalence of HIV infection in women with PID. (Safrin S, et al.: Seroprevalence and epidemiologic correlates of human immunodeficiency virus infection in women with acute pelvic inflammatory disease. *Obstet Gynecol* 1990, 75:666–670. Hoegsberg B, et al.: Sexually transmitted diseases and HIV infection among women with PID. *Am J Obstet Gynecol* 1990, 163:1135–1139. Sperling R, et al.: Seroprevalence of human immunodeficiency virus–women admitted to the hospital with pelvic inflammatory disease. *J Reprod Med* 1991, 2:122–124.)

PID in hospitalized women: Clinical signs

Factor	HIV+ (*n* = 23)	HIV– (*n* = 108)
Tenderness score	1.5	2.0*
Admission WBC	9.0	13.0*
Admission ESR	44	33
Abscess formation	4%	13%
Surgical intervention	17%	4%*

Korn *et al*, Obstet Gynecol 82:765 (1993).
*$P < 0.05$.

FIGURE 19-45 Clinical symptoms of PID. From a series of hospitalized women, Korn *et al.* reported that although HIV-seropositive women reported less tenderness and had a lower leukocyte count on admission, they were more likely to undergo surgical intervention. (Korn AP, Landers DV, Green JR, Sweet RL: Pelvic inflammatory disease in human immunodeficiency virus-infected women. *Obstet Gynecol* 1993, 82:765–768.)

SURVIVAL

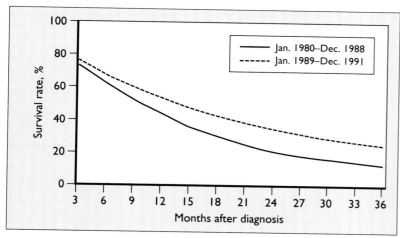

FIGURE 19-46 Survival trends for 2327 women diagnosed with AIDS in New York City from the beginning of the epidemic through December 1988 and 3833 women diagnosed from January 1988 through December 1991 are compared. Both median survival and the proportion of women surviving > 3 years after a diagnosis of AIDS have increased over time. The 1987 AIDS case definition expansion may have had a small effect on the increase in survival. Among women diagnosed more recently, about 35% of those surviving at least 1 month after diagnosis are expected to survive at least 3 years.

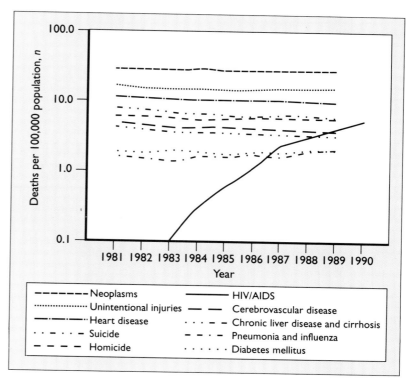

FIGURE 19-47 Death rates for HIV/AIDS and other leading causes in women in the United States, 1981–1990. HIV infection has emerged as an important cause of mortality in young women (aged 25–44 years) in the United States. The *solid line* represents the death rate due to HIV infection in women, which has increased rapidly since 1983, whereas the rates for other leading causes of mortality have remained relatively stable. In 1989, HIV infection was the sixth leading cause of death among women 25–44 years of age. By 1992, HIV/AIDS rose to the fourth leading cause of death for this age group. (*Courtesy of* the CDC.)

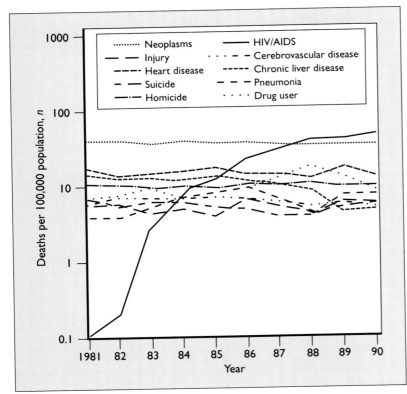

FIGURE 19-48 Age-specific death rates for young women for leading causes in New York City, 1981–1990. Although HIV/AIDS was
only the seventh leading cause of death nationally among women
aged 25–44 years in 1988, it has had a much more dramatic
effect on mortality in cities such as New York, which have a dis-
proportionate share of AIDS cases. As evidenced by the rapidly rising *solid line* in this graph, HIV/AIDS became the leading cause of
death among women aged 25–44 in New York City in 1988. It is
likely to remain so into the next century.

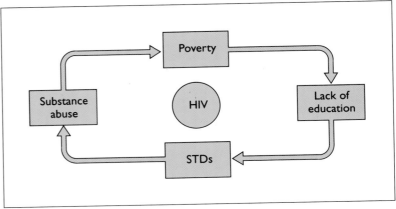

FIGURE 19-49 HIV in the social context of women's lives. When
caring for HIV-infected women or those at high risk, it is essential
to consider the links between poverty, lack of education, sub-
stance abuse, and prevalence of other sexually transmitted diseases that make successful treatment and prevention so difficult.

SELECTED BIBLIOGRAPHY

Carpenter CCJ, Mayer KH, Stein MD, *et al.*: Human immunodeficiency virus infection in North American women: Experience with 200 cases and a review of
the literature. *Medicine* 1991, 70:307–325.

Ellerbrock TV, Bush TJ, Chamberland ME, Oxtoby MJ: Epidemiology of women
with AIDS in the United States, 1981 through 1990: A comparison with
heterosexual men with AIDS. *JAMA* 1991, 265:2971–2975.

Farizo KM, Buehler JW, Chamberland ME, *et al.*: Spectrum of disease in persons
with human immunodeficiency virus infection in the United States. *JAMA*
1992, 267:1798–1805.

Holmberg SD, Horsburgh CR, Ward JW, Jaffe HW: Biologic factors in the sexual
transmission of human immunodeficiency virus. *J Infect Dis* 1989,
160:116–125.

Wright TC, Ellerbrock TV, Chiasson MA, *et al.*: Cervical intraepithelial neoplasia in
women infected with human immunodeficiency virus: Prevalence, risk factors, and validity of Pap smears. *Obstet Gynecol*, in press.

INDEX

Cytokines
  CD4⁺ T-cell production of, 3.7
  in HIV infection, 3.12–3.14
Cytomegalovirus
  encephalitis due to, 10.6–10.7
  gastrointestinal manifestations of, 9.2–9.3, 9.9, 14.2
  microbiology of, 13.14–13.15
  neuropathy due to, 10.7
  pneumonitis due to, 8.6
  retinitis due to, 6.6–6.8, 14.2
    pediatric, 18.11
    treatment of, 15.18–15.19
  skin lesions due to, 14.3
Cytopenias, 12.2–12.3

Dapsone/pyrimethamine, aerosolized pentamidine vs, in toxoplasmosis
    prophylaxis, 15.11–15.12
Death *see also* Mortality
  causes of, in United States, 1.7
  rate attributable to HIV infection, in United States, 1.7
  rates for women, 19.17–19.18
Delayed-type hypersensitivity, in anergic state, 3.12
Dementia, 10.3 *see also* Neurologic manifestations
Demyelination, in progressive multifocal leukoencephalopathy, 10.9
Dendritic herpes simplex virus infection, corneal, 6.4
De novo lipogenesis, 11.3
Dermatitis *see also* Skin rash
  diaper, candidal, 18.4
  occupational exposures and, 1.17
  photoallergic, 5.14
  seborrheic, 5.4
Dermatophytes, tinea infections with, 5.3
Dermatoses, papular, pruritic, 5.6
Desquamative interstitial pneumonitis, pediatric, 18.9
Diagnosis of HIV infection, 2.9–2.15
  age at, in women, 19.4
  differential, 4.5
Diaper dermatitis, candidal, 18.4
Diarrhea
  cryptosporidial, 9.5–9.6
  HIV enteropathy and, 9.4
  Kaposi's sarcoma and, 9.8
  microsporidial, 9.6–9.7
  proctitis and, 9.9
Didanosine, 17.8–17.10 *see also* Therapies, anti-HIV
  in combination therapy, 17.12
  disease progression with
    zalcitabine vs, 17.11
    zidovudine vs, 17.8–17.10
  for Kaposi's sarcoma, 16.9
  toxicities of, 17.10
Dideoxynucleosides, 17.3 *see also* Reverse transcriptase inhibitors; *specific dideoxynucleoside*
Differential diagnosis, 4.5
DIP *see* Desquamative interstitial pneumonitis
Distal sensory polyneuropathy, 10.5
DNA amplification, branched-chain, 2.13

Drugs *see also* Adverse drug reactions; *specific drug or type of drug*
  anti-HIV, development of, 17.2–17.3
Duodenal ulcer, CMV and, 9.3

EBV *see* Epstein-Barr virus
Ectopy, cervical, 19.7–19.9
ELISA antibody test, 2.10, 2.12
Encephalitis
  CMV, 10.6–10.7
  HIV, 10.4
  toxoplasmic, 14.12, 15.10–15.13
Encephalopathy, pediatric, 10.4–10.5, 18.11
Endogenous bacterial retinitis, 6.11–6.12
Endophthalmitis
  exogenous, 6.13
  fungal, 6.9
Endothelial cells, 12.9
Enhancing antibodies, 3.4
Enterocytozoon bineusi, 9.6–9.7
Enteropathy, 9.3–9.4
env, V-loop regions in, and antigenic variations, 2.8
Envelope glycoprotein complex of HIV-1, 2.8
Envelope subunit products, vaccines using, 1.15
Enzyme-linked immunosorbent assay (ELISA), 2.10, 2.12
Eosinophilic pustular folliculitis, 5.7
Epidemiology
  of U.S. epidemic, 1.4–1.8
  in women, 19.2–19.4
  of world pandemic, 1.2–1.3
Epithelioid angiomatosis, 5.13, 14.5
Epotin alfa, 12.10, 12.11
Epstein-Barr virus, CNS lymphoma and, 10.11
Epstein-Barr virus mononucleosis, primary HIV-1 infection vs, 4.5
Esophageal candidiasis, 4.6, 14.9, 18.10
Esophagitis, CMV, 9.2
Ethnic minorities *see* Minorities
Exogenous endophthalmitis, 6.13
Exudative lesions, occupational exposures and, 1.17
Eye, 6.2–6.13 *see also specific disorders*

Failure to thrive, 18.14
Fat loss, in wasting syndrome, 11.2
Fatty acids, synthesis of, 11.3
Feet, tinea pedis of, 5.3
Filgrastim, 12.11
Fluconazole
  for cryptococcal meningitis, 15.16
    amphotericin B vs, 15.15
  resistance to, 15.14
Flucytosine, for cryptococcal meningitis, 15.15
Folate metabolism, intracellular, PCP treatment and, 15.2
Folliculitis, pustular, eosinophilic, 5.7
Foscarnet
  ganciclovir vs, for CMV retinitis, 15.18–15.19
  vidarabine vs, for acyclovir-resistant herpes infections, 15.18